Step into the world of anatomy and

G-W PUBLISHER

PREPARING FOR
A&P

BASIC SCIENCE AND BIOLOGY

Michael Crandell

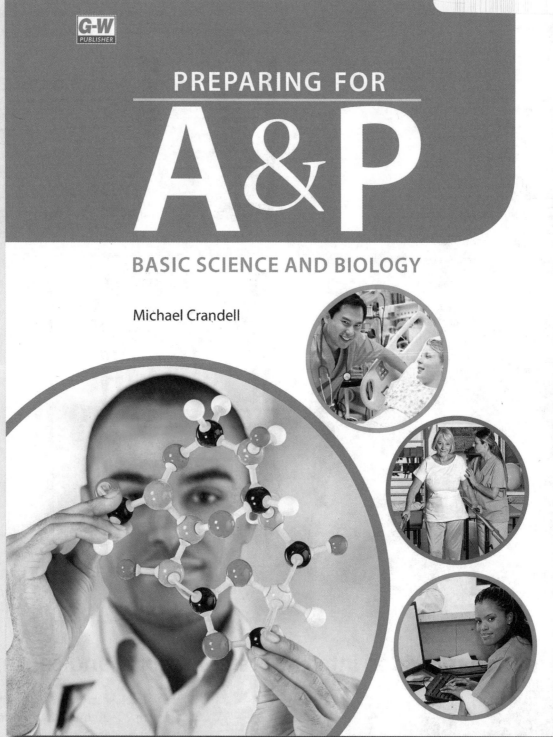

and build a solid foundation in

science	math	body tissues
study skills	chemistry	anatomical terms
scientific terminology	cell biology	human body systems

A step-by-step approach builds your science knowledge

Concepts build on each other, progressing from simple to more complex

Sections dig progressively deeper, gaining complexity as your science knowledge grows

Concept 1: Cubic Centimeters and Milliliters

Liquid volume is the amount of liquid in a three-dimensional object, usually a cylinder. Whereas dry volume is measured in cubic centimeters, liquid volume is measured using *milliliters* (mL) or *liters* (L). There are 1000 cubic centimeters in 1 liter, and there are 1000 milliliters in 1 liter (L). Therefore, the volume contained in 1 cubic centimeter (cc or cm³) is equal to the volume contained in 1 milliliter (mL).

Concept 2: Reading a Meniscus

Liquid volume can be measured using a *graduated cylinder*, a narrow cylinder with milliliter increments. When liquid fills and climbs up the side of the graduated cylinder, a meniscus will form. The *meniscus* is the semicircular surface of liquid in a cylinder. To determine the volume of liquid, read the cylinder at the *bottom* of the meniscus (Figure 4.21).

10 —— Meniscus

Read the level here, at the bottom of the meniscus

Figure 4.21 To measure liquid volume, read the measurement at the bottom of the meniscus.

Chapter 5
Chemistry

Section 5.1: Atoms
Section 5.2: The Periodic Table of Elements
Section 5.3: Atomic Diagrams
Section 5.4: Ionic Bonding
Section 5.5: Covalent Bonding
Section 5.6: Hydrogen Bonding
Section 5.7: Carbohydrates
Section 5.8: Lipids
Section 5.9: Proteins
Section 5.10: Enzymes
Section 5.11: Nucleic Acids
Section 5.12: pH

Section 5.1 Atoms

Atoms, also known as *elements*, are extremely small particles that make up the universe. You might be familiar with some atoms. Some examples of atoms are hydrogen, carbon, and helium. Atoms contain subatomic particles and can be classified by symbol, number, and mass. In this section, you will learn about atoms and their properties.

The terms below are some of those that will be introduced in Section 5.1. To become familiar with these terms, reproduce each term as you write it. Pronounce each term as you write it. You will learn the definitions of these words as you complete this section.

Section 5.2 The Periodic Table of Elements

Atoms are organized on the periodic table of elements. As you have learned, an *element* is another word used to describe an *atom*. In this section, you will learn about the periodic table of elements and the atoms it contains.

The terms below are some of those that will be introduced in Section 5.2. To become familiar with these terms, reproduce each word on the line beside it. Pronounce each term as you write it. You will learn the definitions of these words as you complete this section.

Chapters culminate in an introduction to the human body systems

Chapter 10
Human Body Systems

Section 10.1: The Integumentary System
Section 10.2: The Skeletal System
Section 10.3: The Muscular System
Section 10.4: The Nervous System
Section 10.5: The Endocrine System
Section 10.6: The Respiratory System
Section 10.7: The Cardiovascular System
Section 10.8: The Lymphatic System
Section 10.9: The Digestive System
Section 10.10: The Urinary System
Section 10.11: The Reproductive Systems

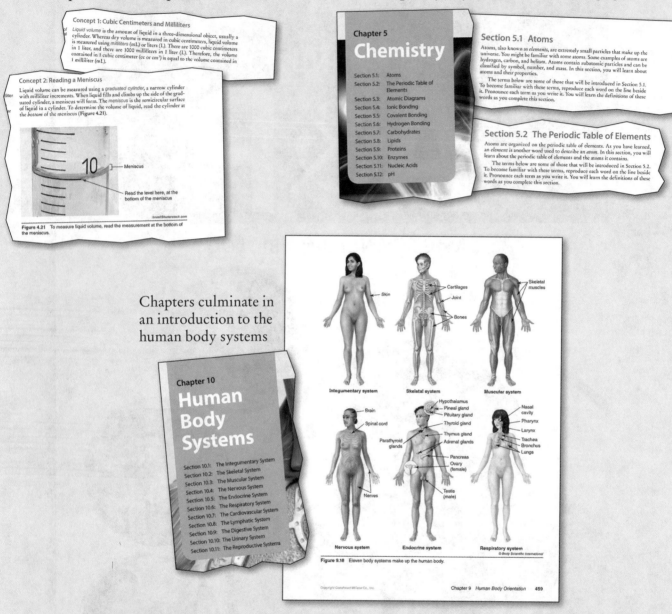

Integumentary system   Skeletal system   Muscular system

Skin   Cartilages   Joint   Bones   Skeletal muscles

Nervous system   Endocrine system   Respiratory system

Brain   Spinal cord   Nerves

Hypothalamus   Pineal gland   Pituitary gland   Thyroid gland   Parathyroid glands   Thymus gland   Adrenal glands   Pancreas   Ovary (female)   Testis (male)

Nasal cavity   Pharynx   Larynx   Trachea   Bronchus   Lungs

Figure 9.18 Eleven body systems make up the human body.
© Body Scientific International

Information is divided into chapters, sections, and concepts

Chapter 6
Cell Morphology

Section 6.1: Overview of the Cell
Section 6.2: Plasma Membrane
Section 6.3: Nucleus
Section 6.4: Endoplasmic Reticulum and Golgi
Section 6.5: Cytoplasm
Section 6.6: Outside the Cell

Concept 2: Chromosomes and Chromatin

chromosome a structure inside the nucleus that contains packaged DNA during cell division

chromatin a structure inside the nucleus that contains packaged DNA most of the time

A cell's operating instructions, encoded in DNA, are located on chromosomes (Figure 6.7). A *chromosome* is a structure inside the nucleus that contains packaged DNA. However, DNA is only packaged in chromosomes during cell division. When a cell is *not* dividing—which is most of the time—DNA is packaged as *chromatin*.

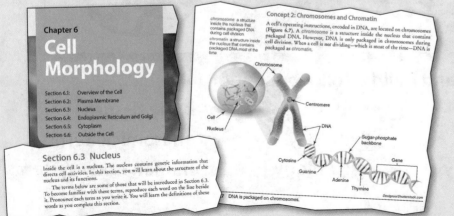

Chromosome   Cell   Nucleus   Centromere   DNA   Sugar-phosphate backbone   Cytosine   Guanine   Adenine   Thymine   Gene

DNA is packaged on chromosomes.
Designua/Shutterstock.com

Section 6.3 Nucleus

Inside the cell is a nucleus. The nucleus contains genetic information that directs cell activities. In this section, you will learn about the structure of the nucleus and its functions.

The terms below are some of those that will be introduced in Section 6.3. To become familiar with these terms, reproduce each word on the line beside it. Pronounce each term as you write it. You will learn the definitions of these words as you complete this section.

Each section can be completed in 20–30 minutes, making it perfect for a quick but thorough review

Sections are divided into concepts to break down the material to be learned

Repetition and reinforcement help you remember material

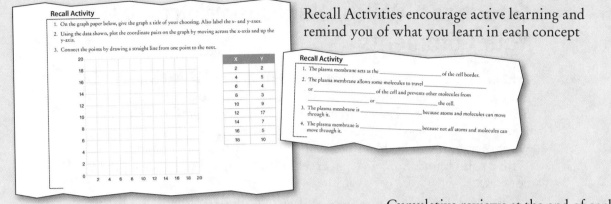

Recall Activities encourage active learning and remind you of what you learn in each concept

Cumulative reviews at the end of each section and chapter make connections to content learned in previous chapters

Section reinforcements provide consistent checkpoints to map your progress

You can practice your test-taking skills by completing chapter reviews

Clear, colorful illustrations help you envision concepts

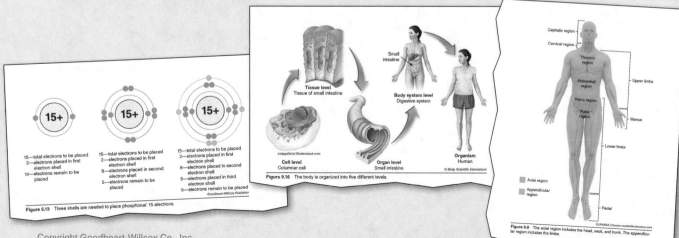

Goodheart-Willcox Publisher Welcomes Your Comments

A leader in educational publishing since 1921, Goodheart-Willcox Publisher is continuously developing print and digital products for Health and Health Sciences courses and needs. *Preparing for A&P: Basic Science and Biology* is written with you—the student—in mind. By reading and completing this work text, you will build a solid foundation in science and biology basics. With a solid foundation, you can excel in A&P and other advanced science courses.

With each new product, our goal at Goodheart-Willcox Publisher is to deliver superior educational materials that effectively meet the ever-changing, increasingly diverse needs of students and teachers. To that end, we welcome your comments and suggestions regarding *Preparing for A&P: Basic Science and Biology*. Please send any comments and suggestions to the managing editor of our Health Sciences Editorial Department. You can send an e-mail to editorial@g-w.com, or write to:

Managing Editor—Health Sciences
Goodheart-Willcox Publisher
18604 West Creek Drive
Tinley Park, IL 60477-6243

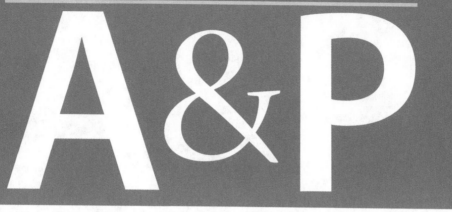

PREPARING FOR
A&P

BASIC SCIENCE AND BIOLOGY

by

Michael Crandell
Professor of Biology
Carl Sandburg College
Galesburg, Illinois

Publisher
The Goodheart-Willcox Company, Inc.
Tinley Park, IL
www.g-w.com

About the Author

Michael Crandell teaches face-to-face, blended, and online classes in General Biology and Fundamentals of A&P as a Professor of Biology at Carl Sandburg College in Galesburg, Illinois. He strives to make the classroom a welcoming environment, where each student is valued and encouraged. In 1999 and in 2015, he was awarded Carl Sandburg ICCTA Faculty of the Year. Crandell's other experiences include being an autobody repair instructor at Carl Sandburg College (for 19 years), a part-time biology instructor at Illinois Central College (for 25 years), and the vector control sanitarian at Peoria City/County Health Department (for 20 summers). Crandell has written several books and related manuals, including *Auto Collision Repair and Refinishing*. He has an associate's degree in Biology from Illinois Central College, a bachelor's degree in Biology from Illinois State University, and a master's degree in Environmental Biology from Eastern Illinois University.

Reviewers

Goodheart-Willcox Publisher would like to thank the following instructors who reviewed select manuscript chapters and provided valuable input into the development of this book.

Charles Beaman
Adjunct Professor
Austin Community College
Austin, TX

Samuel Clifford
Adjunct Faculty Biology
Austin Community College
Austin, TX

Mary Colon
Professor of Biology
Seminole State College of Florida
Sanford, FL

Sheree Daniel
Biology Professor
Trinity Valley Community College
Terrell, TX

Carol Garrett
Adjunct Faculty Biology
Hagerstown Community College
Hagerstown, MD

David Gonzales
Associate Professor of Biology
Montgomery County Community College
Pottstown, PA

Kathryn Gubista
Adjunct Faculty Biology
Asheville-Buncombe Technical Community
  College
Asheville, NC

Dale Horeth
Associate Professor of Biology
Tidewater Community College
Virginia Beach, VA

Jacki Houghton, DC
Adjunct Professor
Moorpark College and Los Angeles Valley College
Moorpark and Valley Glen, CA

Karen Huffman
Assistant Professor of Biology
Genesee Community College
Batavia, NY

Carol Keating
Associate Professor of Biology
Union County College
Cranford, NJ

Alrena Lightbourn
Adjunct Faculty Biological Sciences
Tallahassee Community College
Tallahassee, FL

Maxine Medaglia
Adjunct Faculty Biology
Hagerstown Community College
Hagerstown, MD

Rita Pagano
Biology Laboratory Technician
Camden County College
Blackwood, NJ

Laura Ritt
Assistant Professor of Biology
Rowan College at Burlington County
Mt. Laurel, NJ

Samuel Schwarzlose
Associate Professor of Biology
Amarillo College
Amarillo, TX

Acknowledgments

The author would like to thank the following individuals: Janine Crandell, for her help with computers and education strategies; Carl Sandburg instructors Susan Buck, David Burns, Kelli Mayes-Denker, Gail Hannam, David Kellogg, Gary Miracle, Carla Murray, Kylie Price, Marjorie Smolensky, and Keith Williams for their advice and encouragement; and Cindy Arthur at the Carl Sandburg College Faculty Teaching and Learning Center for video creation and guidance with computers.

Contents in Brief

Contents

To the Student

Too many students who enter an A&P course are not prepared. In fact, nationwide, only about one-quarter of high school graduates are ready for college-level science. Maybe you struggled with science in high school; maybe you have been out of school for years. Regardless, enrolling in a science class that will lead to a healthcare program will strengthen your chance of finding a good job and improving your life. I celebrate your courage, diving into the challenging world of science. Don't let the challenge make you give up your dream and quit.

This book is written to guide you toward success as you step up to college-level science. As you work through this book, you will learn how to study as you understand and master the basics of college chemistry, biology, and A&P. This book is written with you, the student, in mind. Chapters progress from simple to more complicated, with each science topic building on previous knowledge. Chapters are divided into sections, which can be completed in 20–30 minutes, and sections are divided into concepts that teach information clearly and concisely. Regular recall and reinforcement activities will help you remember what you learn and build upon knowledge gained in previous sections. By the end of this book, you will have a solid foundation in the science basics you need to excel in A&P. With a solid foundation in science basics, there is no limit to where you can go.

Chapter 1
Learning About Science

Introduction

If you are studying this book, it is because you are stepping into the world of science. The field of science can be challenging, full of terminology and technical concepts that are sometimes difficult to comprehend. Students approach these challenges in different ways and with varying results. However, success in science is possible with the right attitude, practice, and knowledge. This book is designed to help you step up to science. Through the exercises in this book, you will study an array of skills and science concepts. When you master the information in this book, you will be well prepared for a class in anatomy and physiology, general biology, or general chemistry.

Objectives

After completing this chapter, you will be able to
- understand how this book is organized
- explain how this book promotes active learning
- know how to use the features of this book
- define *science*
- understand the difference between natural and supernatural explanations
- know that, in science, a statement is tested with facts
- understand that science cannot be 100% certain that an explanation is correct
- describe the areas of biology
- explain the importance of having a good attitude about learning science
- use mnemonics to remember words and concepts
- demonstrate study skills

Key Terms

The following terms and phrases will be introduced and explained in Chapter 1. Read through the list to become familiar with the words.

active learning	mnemonic
anatomy	natural
attitude	phenomenon
biology	physiology
cytology	reinforce
fact	science
genetics	studying
histology	supernatural
key term	terminology

Section 1.1 Using This Book

As you get ready to read this book, you are embarking on a journey to construct your foundation in science and biology concepts. Building yourself a solid foundation will prepare you for more advanced science courses, such as anatomy and physiology. This book is interactive and will help you understand and apply what you learn. In this section, you will learn about how to use this book and reach your full potential for succeeding in science.

The terms below are some of those that will be introduced in Section 1.1. To become familiar with these terms, reproduce each word on the line beside it. Pronounce each term as you write it. You will learn the definitions of these words as you complete this section.

1. key term _____

2. active learning _____

3. reinforce _____

Concept 1: Building Your Knowledge

This book is designed to help you build your science knowledge using a series of steps. Science builds upon itself. Basic science concepts enable you to understand science concepts that are more complicated. That is why, with each concept, section, and chapter, this book progresses from simple to more complex. The first concept in each section is the most basic, and successive concepts add information to build an understanding of the topic. The sections in each chapter also provide a step-by-step path through the chapter topic.

Concept 2: Becoming Familiar with Terminology

The sections in this book teach many new words, and this book's organization will help you comprehend and recall vocabulary terms. Each chapter in this book begins with an alphabetical list of the key terms that will be introduced. Before you start reading through a chapter, read this list of terms to establish links for the information you will encounter later. Each section also begins with a list of words that will be introduced, except this list presents the words in order of appearance within the section. Before you start reading the first concept, write each key term on the line beside it and say the word as you write it. This exercise in reading, speaking, hearing, and writing the terms will reinforce your knowledge.

Concept 3: Learning in Brief Sessions

A person can only stay focused on a task for about 20–30 minutes. For that reason, each concept in this book presents only a small amount of information. Most concepts are not more than 10 sentences in length. As you study, devote your full attention to learning each section. Read the sentences aloud if it will help you understand the topic. Work for 20–30 minutes, and then reward yourself for completing a section by doing some type of physical activity (for example, walking) while reviewing the section in your mind (**Figure 1.1**).

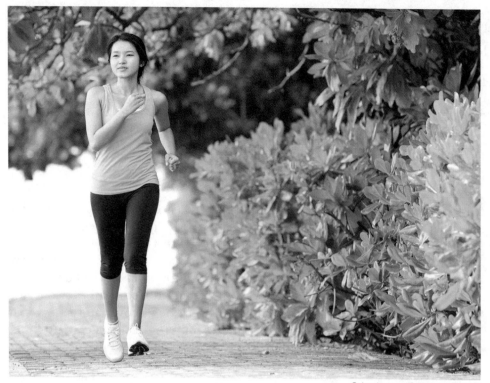

Figure 1.1 You can engage in physical activity while reviewing a section in your mind.

Concept 4: Recognizing Terminology

As you read each concept, you will recognize the terms introduced. *Key terms* are shown in red and are italicized throughout this book. Definitions in the margins also define key terms where they are introduced and make it easy to review new terminology. You can reinforce your knowledge of new words by reviewing the marginal definitions in the book. You can look at a word and say its definition or look at a definition and say the word. Do this at least five times each day over several days. Repeatedly writing, reading, hearing, and speaking the words will help you remember them.

key term a word essential to understanding a concept

Concept 5: Active Learning

This book encourages you to use a practice known as active learning. *Active learning* is using your hands or feet—by writing, typing, or walking, for example—while studying material. For most students, learning through a variety of activities (for example, reading, speaking, listening, and writing) reinforces knowledge. After each concept in this book, you will have the opportunity to take a turn at applying what you just learned. In Recall Activity sections, write answers to questions and draw diagrams using the knowledge you've gained. These exercises help create short-term memories and reinforce long-term memory. Walking or engaging in other physical activity while reviewing a section in your mind is also active learning and will help you remember.

active learning the practice of using your hands or feet while studying material

Recall Activity

1. Using your hands or feet while studying material is _____.

2. Exercises at the end of each concept help create _____ memories and reinforce _____ memory.

Concept 6: Reinforcing Knowledge

reinforce to strengthen one's knowledge of material

As you read this book, stop regularly to *reinforce* (strengthen your knowledge of) what you have learned. Recall Activity exercises give you regular opportunities to stop and reinforce each concept. Each section ends with a section reinforcement that covers all the concepts in a section. A comprehensive review follows to help you retrieve information from sections you worked on days or weeks before. Chapter reviews give you the chance to recall all the concepts in a chapter, and end-of-chapter comprehensive reviews cover all the material up until that point in the book. Opportunities for reinforcement contain a mix of questions (fill-in-the-blank, multiple choice, matching, and true/false, for example) to help you understand the material from different perspectives.

Recall Activity

1. During reinforcement, you _____ your knowledge of what you have learned.

2. What reinforcement opportunities are available at the end of each section? _____

_____

Concept 7: Checking Your Work

As you complete the exercises in this book, check your understanding by referring to the answer key in the back of the book. In the answer key, you will find answers for Recall Activity, section reinforcement, comprehensive review, and chapter review sections. If your answers to the reinforcement questions are correct, move on to the next concept, section, or chapter. If your answers are not correct, reread the material you do not understand and study the correct answers. Science builds upon itself. For example, knowledge about the molecular structure of water allows you to understand why some substances dissolve in water and why other substances do not. Because of this, it is important that you check your work and understanding before moving on to the next concept, section, or chapter.

Recall Activity

1. If your answers to reinforcement questions are not correct, you should _____ the material you do not understand.

2. Why should you check your work and understanding before moving on to the next section?

   _____

   _____

Concept 8: Testing Yourself

Once you have completed a chapter, test yourself on the sum of what you have learned. Each chapter in this book has a chapter review that contains questions similar to those you might encounter on an exam. The purpose of these questions is twofold: to help you retrieve information and to help you practice for an exam. Retrieval over a period of time—minutes, hours, or days—creates additional memory links and reinforces learning. Testing yourself at the end of each chapter will help you retrieve information you've learned and will hone your skills in test taking so you can excel in an anatomy and physiology course (**Figure 1.2**).

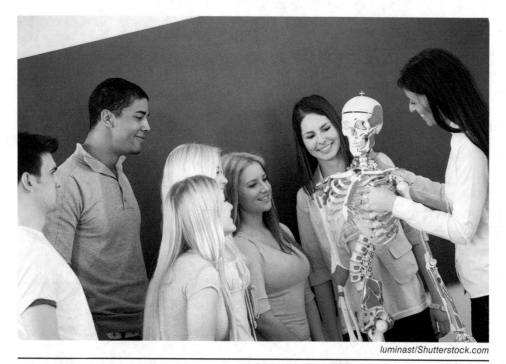

luminast/Shutterstock.com

Figure 1.2 Skills in test taking are vital to success in an anatomy and physiology course.

Recall Activity

1. What is the purpose of testing yourself on what you have learned?_____

_____

2. Retrieval over a period of time creates additional _____ links and

_____ learning.

Section 1.1 Reinforcement

Answer the following questions using what you learned in this section.

1. A person can only stay focused on a task for about _____ minute(s).

2. *True or False.* You should not complete the Recall Activity exercises in the book until you've

completely read a section. _____

3. What reinforcement opportunities are available at the end of each section?_____

_____

4. Write the letters backward: ecrofnier. Define the word that is formed. _____

_____

5. _____ science concepts enable you to understand science concepts that are

more _____.

6. Which of the following words is misspelled?

   A. reinforce   C. learning

   B. anwser   D. section

7. What is active learning? _____

8. *True or False.* Each concept, section, and chapter in this book progresses from complex to more

simple. _____

9. Key terms are shown in _____ and are _____
throughout this book.

10. Where do marginal definitions for key terms appear in this book? _____

_____

11. Explain why you should check your answers to the questions in this book before moving on to the

next section. _____

_____

12. When reading this book, it is recommended that you work for 20–30 minutes, and then reward

yourself for completing a section by doing some type of _____.

13. What reinforcement opportunities are available at the end of each chapter? _____

_____

14. *True or False.* Most concepts are not more than five sentences in length. _____

15. If your answers to the questions in this book are not correct, you should _____ the material you do not understand and study the _____ answers.

16. Repeatedly _____, _____, _____, and _____ words will help you remember them.

17. How many times a day should you review the marginal definitions in this book? _____

18. Science builds upon _____.

19. Which of the following exercises does *not* appear at the end of each section?
    A. section reinforcement   C. chapter review
    B. comprehensive review

20. Why should you test yourself using the chapter reviews for this book? _____
    _____

Comprehensive Review (Chapter 1)

Answer the following question using what you have learned so far in this book.

21. How long can a person stay focused on a task? _____

Section 1.2 What Is Science?

The study of biology and anatomy and physiology is a science. Science enables you to understand your world, including your human body. The concepts of science build on one another and open the door to greater and more detailed understanding. This section will introduce you to the world of science and explain what science is and what science seeks. By the end of this section, you will understand what it means that biology and anatomy and physiology are sciences.

The terms below are some of those that will be introduced in Section 1.2. To become familiar with these terms, reproduce each word on the line beside it. Pronounce each term as you write it. You will learn the definitions of these words as you complete this section.

1. science _____

2. phenomenon _____

3. fact _____

4. natural _____

5. supernatural _____

6. biology _____

7. genetics _____

8. cytology _____

9. histology _____

10. anatomy _____

11. physiology _____

Concept 1: Defining Science

science the body of
knowledge and techniques
that enables mankind to
explain the natural world

To learn about science, you must first understand what science is. *Science* is the body of knowledge and techniques that enables mankind to explain the natural world. This body of knowledge is made up of facts that scientists have accumulated and recorded about the natural world. Scientific techniques are the scientific methods used to obtain facts. The natural world is based on the properties of subatomic particles, atoms, molecules, cells, and organisms—all of which you will learn about in this book.

Recall Activity

1. Science's body of knowledge includes _____ that scientists have accumulated about the natural world.

2. _____ is the body of knowledge and techniques that enables mankind to explain the natural world.

3. The natural world is based on the properties of _____ particles,

_____, _____, _____, and

_____.

Concept 2: What Science Seeks

phenomenon a physically
observable fact or event

Science has a purpose: to seek natural explanations to phenomena. A *phenomenon* is a physically observable fact or event. For example, a phenomenon might be a flash of lightning or the spread of a disease. The word *phenomena* is the plural form of phenomenon.

Recall Activity

1. A(n) _____ is a physically observable fact or event.

2. Science seeks _____ explanations to phenomena.

3. The plural form of phenomenon is _____.

Concept 3: Facts

Science is concerned with facts. A *fact* is a confirmed observation. You are surrounded by facts. For example, a microscopic examination of a cross-section of a frog intestine will show that the tissue layers of the intestine are composed of cells. The cell composition of the intestine is a fact. Facts are not opinions. Whereas an opinion is what someone believes about a subject, facts are independent of people and opinions. You cannot argue against a fact.

fact a confirmed observation

Science is based on facts, not opinions. Science connects facts to explain the natural world, and facts are used as evidence to support scientific explanations.

Recall Activity

1. A(n) _____ is a confirmed observation.

2. Whereas a(n) _____ is what someone believes about a subject, facts are independent of _____ and _____.

3. Science _____ facts to explain the natural world.

Concept 4: Natural Explanations

Science seeks natural explanations. An explanation is *natural* if it is observable and testable. A natural explanation could involve the masses of objects, magnetism, opposite charges, or concentration. If an explanation is natural, it can be measured or tested and proven to be false.

natural observable and testable

Recall Activity

1. Science seeks _____ explanations.

2. A natural explanation can be _____ or _____ and proven to be false.

Concept 5: Supernatural Explanations

supernatural not able to be tested

Science is *not* concerned with the supernatural. An explanation is *supernatural* if it cannot be tested. Many supernatural explanations involve magic or miracles. Supernatural explanations are not science because they cannot be tested.

Recall Activity

1. Science is *not* concerned with the _____.

2. An explanation is supernatural if it cannot be _____.

3. Are supernatural explanations science? Why or why not?_____

_____

Concept 6: Science and the Supernatural

Biologist Ernst Mayr made this statement about the differences between science and the supernatural: "Science does not invoke supernatural explanations or rely on revelation to understand how the universe operates." Scientific explanations require the support of facts. You can think of science and the supernatural as the two sides of a coin (**Figure 1.3**). You can only see one side of a coin at a time. In the same way, you can view science or the supernatural, but not both at the same time.

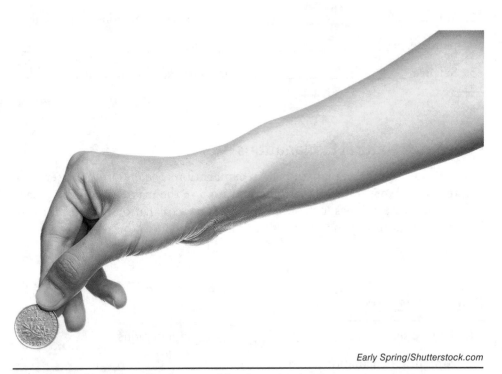

Early Spring/Shutterstock.com

Figure 1.3   You can only see one side of a coin at a time.

Recall Activity

1. Scientific explanations require the support of _____.

2. You can think of _____ and the _____ as the two sides of a coin.

3. You can only see _____ side(s) of a coin at a time.

Concept 7: Explaining Observations

When explaining observations, science seeks natural explanations instead of supernatural ones. An example of an observed phenomenon is lightning (**Figure 1.4**). A natural explanation of lightning is an electrical discharge between clouds or clouds and the earth. A supernatural explanation of lightning is the anger of the Norse god of lightning, Thor.

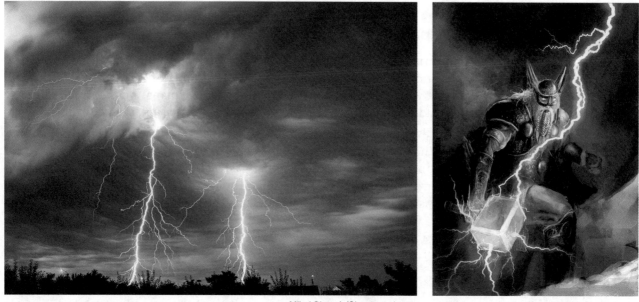

Mihai Simonia/Shutterstock.com   Fotokostic/Shutterstock.com

Figure 1.4 Lightning can be explained naturally or supernaturally.

Recall Activity

1. A(n) _____ explanation of lightning is an electrical discharge between clouds or clouds and the earth.

2. A(n) _____ explanation of lightning is the anger of the Norse god of lightning, Thor.

Concept 8: Acceptance Versus Belief

In science, people *accept* explanations rather than *believe* in them. This is because science is based on facts. Belief is based on feelings and opinions. It is not correct to say you believe in science because science is not based on your opinions or feelings. It is better to say that you accept or do not accept the evidence presented in a scientific explanation. Saying one does or does not believe in a scientific explanation shows a misunderstanding of science.

Recall Activity

1. Science is _____ on facts.

2. Is it correct to say you believe in science? Why or why not? _____

_____

Concept 9: Science Changes

As scientists gather facts and evidence, they become more certain of a scientific explanation. Scientific explanations are based on the evidence available today. As such, you can never be 100% certain that an explanation is correct. If, in the future, additional evidence leads to a better explanation, science will change.

For example, at one time, doctors thought that gastric ulcers (holes in the wall of the stomach) were caused by stress or spicy foods. In the 1980s, an Australian doctor gathered evidence that gastric ulcers were caused by a stomach infection by one species of bacteria. Today, doctors prescribe antibiotics to cure a gastric ulcer if a breath test detects the bacterium in a patient.

Recall Activity

1. Can you ever be 100% certain that a scientific explanation is correct? Why or why not? _____

_____

2. If additional evidence leads to a better explanation, science will _____.

Concept 10: Fields of Science

biology the science that studies life

genetics an area of biology that studies inheritance

cytology an area of biology that studies cells

histology an area of biology that studies tissues

There are many *fields*, or areas, of science—for example, physics, chemistry, geology, and biology. The fields of science are *interconnected*, meaning that knowledge in one field (such as chemistry) will aid in understanding another field (such as biology). This book is primarily concerned with the field of biology and its interconnected areas. *Biology* is the science that studies life. Interconnected areas within biology include *genetics* (the study of inheritance), *cytology* (the study of cells), *histology* (the study of tissues), and anatomy and physiology. *Anatomy* is the study of the parts of the body, and *physiology* explains the functions of these body parts.

anatomy an area of biology that studies the parts of the body

physiology an area of biology that studies the functions of body parts

Recall Activity

1. Physics, chemistry, geology, and biology are _____ of science.

2. Biology is the science that studies _____.

3. _____ is the study of the parts of the body, and _____ explains the functions of these body parts.

Section 1.2 Reinforcement

Answer the following questions using what you learned in this section.

1. A fact is a(n) _____ observation.

2. Which of the following are natural explanations?
   A. magic
   B. magnetism
   C. concentration
   D. miracles
   E. opposite charges

3. *True or False.* You can argue against a fact. _____

4. Science seeks natural _____ to phenomena.

5. Should one *accept* or *believe* the evidence presented in a scientific explanation? Explain.

   _____

   _____

6. Facts are used as _____ to support scientific explanations.

7. *True or False.* Science does not invoke supernatural explanations. _____

8. _____ explanations require the support of facts.

9. *True or False.* Scientific techniques are the scientific methods used to obtain opinions. _____

10. Unscramble the letters: raaltun. Define the word that is formed. _____

    _____

11. Does science use *natural* or *supernatural* explanations? Explain. _____

    _____

12. Why does it help to see the natural and supernatural as two sides of one coin? _____

    _____

13. Biology is the science that studies _____.

14. *True or False*. Facts are not opinions. _____

15. If, in the future, additional evidence leads to a better explanation, _____ will change.

16. _____ explanations are not science.

17. Facts are _____ of people and opinions.

18. As scientists gather facts, they become more _____ of a scientific explanation.

19. Unscramble the letters: neeccis. Define the word that is formed. _____

_____

20. *True or False*. A phenomenon is a physically observable fact or event. _____

21. Belief is based on _____ and _____.

22. *True or False*. If additional evidence leads to a better explanation, science will change. _____

23. Is science based on feelings or facts? Explain. _____

_____

24. An explanation is natural if it is _____ and _____.

25. Scientific explanations are based on the _____ available today.

26. Name and define the areas of biology. _____

_____

_____

Match the following terms with their definitions.

_____ 27. Observable and testable

_____ 28. A physically observable fact or event

_____ 29. Not testable

_____ 30. A confirmed observation

_____ 31. An area of biology that studies cells

_____ 32. An area of biology that studies inheritance

_____ 33. The science that studies life

_____ 34. An area of biology that studies the functions of body parts

_____ 35. An area of biology that studies body parts

_____ 36. An area of biology that studies tissues

A. phenomenon
B. fact
C. natural
D. supernatural
E. cytology
F. histology
G. genetics
H. biology
I. physiology
J. anatomy

Comprehensive Review (Chapter 1)

Answer the following question using what you have learned so far in this book.

37. Explain the practice of active learning. _____

_____

Section 1.3 Study Skills

As you enter the field of science, you will encounter new topics and vocabulary. Understanding these topics and vocabulary will prepare you for your future career. Learning and understanding scientific concepts and terms may be challenging, but having a strong set of study skills can set you up for success. In this section, you will learn about study skills vital to succeeding in science.

The terms below are some of those that will be introduced in Section 1.3. To become familiar with these terms, reproduce each word on the line beside it. Pronounce each term as you write it. You will learn the definitions of these words as you complete this section.

1. studying _____

2. terminology _____

3. attitude _____

4. mnemonic _____

Concept 1: Studying

The fact that you are here, reading this book, is quite a feat. If you are reading this book, you have already learned how to interpret the 26 symbols of the English language, construct words, communicate thoughts, and verbalize emotions. You have also learned how to listen, speak, write, calculate, and function in society. You learn every day of your life, as you study faces, directions, video games, and names. As with any subject or concept, if you want to learn science, you must study it. *Studying* is concentrated learning. It is the deliberate effort to make long-term memories about subject matter. Each section in this book provides an opportunity for you to study. As you work through each section, you are studying the content presented. You will develop the ability to study and learn. Thus, you can be successful in science.

studying concentrated learning; the deliberate effort to make long-term memories about subject matter

Recall Activity

1. Studying is concentrated _____.

2. As you work through each section in this book, you are _____.

3. Studying is the deliberate effort to make _____ memories about subject matter.

Concept 2: Understanding Terminology

The goal of this book is to help you achieve success and learn basic scientific concepts. Many students find that the biggest obstacle to success in science is the challenging scientific vocabulary (**Figure 1.5**). How can you learn science if you don't speak the language? The most basic skill you can master to ensure your success is understanding the words, also known as the *terminology*, of science. Once you understand scientific terminology, you can build on that knowledge to comprehend more complex scientific concepts.

terminology the words used in science

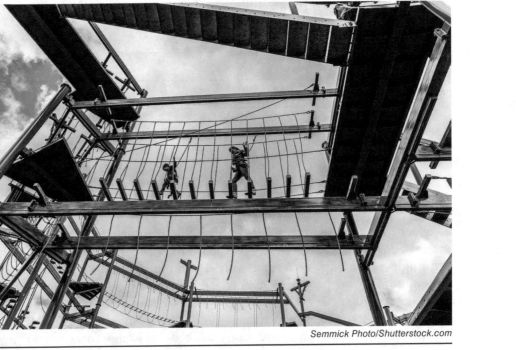

Semmick Photo/Shutterstock.com

Figure 1.5 Vocabulary is the biggest obstacle to learning science.

Recall Activity

1. The goal of this textbook is to help you achieve _____ and learn basic scientific concepts.

2. The biggest obstacle to your success in science is the challenging scientific _____.

Concept 3: Having a Good Attitude

When it comes to learning, attitude is everything. Your *attitude* is your way of feeling, thinking about, and viewing a situation. How should you view your efforts in a science class?

attitude a way of feeling, thinking about, and viewing a situation

When studying science, always remember that the science skills you gain will build a better future for you. How you view a science class or subject will, to a great degree, determine your success or failure. You can view studying as building your future success, concept by concept. Adjust your attitude to view basic science as a step to a better future.

Recall Activity

1. When it comes to learning, _____ is everything.

2. How you view a science class or subject will, to a great degree, determine your _____ or _____.

3. Adjust your _____ to view basic science as a step to a better future.

Concept 4: Thinking Positively

Your thinking will affect your success or failure in science. Students tend to like subjects they are good at and dislike subjects they do not understand. Do your best to think positively, even if you are studying a subject that challenges you. It's important to tell yourself, "I can do this," or "I will learn this," and avoid negative thinking.

Working through the sections in this book will help you understand basic science and will prepare you for future success in other science courses. Stay on task and concentrate on the material. You will grow to like science once you understand the basics.

Recall Activity

1. Students tend to _____ subjects they are good at and _____ subjects they do not understand.

2. Avoid _____ thinking.

3. You will grow to _____ science once you understand the basics.

Concept 5: Concentrating

Forget multitasking. In reality, you can do only one task well at a time. For success in science, concentrate on the material you are learning. Make the most of your study time by eliminating or ignoring distractions. Take out your earbuds and put away your phone while you are studying. Work through the concept or section at hand and ignore everything else. Wrestle your brain into focusing on the material. If you are having trouble concentrating, try varying your study location, time, duration, or method.

Recall Activity

1. In reality, you can do only _____ task(s) well at a time.

2. If you are having trouble concentrating, try _____ your study location, time, duration, or method.

Concept 6: Using Mnemonics

mnemonic a word, acronym, or phrase that can help you recall information

When studying, you can use mnemonics to remember terms and concepts. A *mnemonic* is a word, acronym, or phrase that can help you recall information. For example, when you need to remember a list of terms, you can construct a mnemonic with the first letter of each term. To remember the five types of white blood cells in the body (**b**asophils, **l**ymphocytes, **e**osinophils, **mono**cytes, and **n**eutrophils), you could remember the acronym *blemn*. Listed in order from most common in the body to least common, the five types of white blood cells are **n**eutrophils, **l**ymphocytes, **mono**cytes, **e**osinophils, and **b**asophils. To remember this order, you could memorize the phrase, "**N**ow **l**et's **m**ake **e**verything **b**etter."

Recall Activity

1. A(n) _____ is a word, acronym, or phrase that can help you recall information.

2. What word could you use to remember the five types of white blood cells? _____

Concept 7: Repetition, Repetition, Repetition

Repeatedly writing, reading, hearing, or speaking words will help you remember them. Varying reinforcement questions, such as groupings of different types of questions in a review activity, will also help you remember. As you work through each section, you are studying. In the margins of the text, you will see marginal definitions that identify and define the key vocabulary terms in each section. Review these definitions at least five times every day. Pronounce each word and definition. You can impress your friends and family by using these scientific words in conversation (**Figure 1.6**).

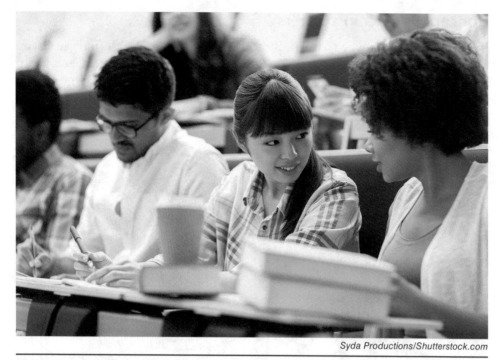

Syda Productions/Shutterstock.com

Figure 1.6 Use scientific words in conversations with your friends.

Recall Activity

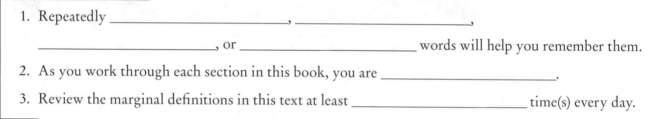

1. Repeatedly _____, _____,

   _____, or _____ words will help you remember them.

2. As you work through each section in this book, you are _____.

3. Review the marginal definitions in this text at least _____ time(s) every day.

Concept 8: Rewarding Yourself

As you study, planning rewards for yourself can motivate your learning. A reward can be anything you value. For example, do you value food? video games? sleep? exercise? daydreaming? When you're getting ready to learn, plan rewards at intervals such as completing a section, answering all of the questions in a reinforcement activity correctly, or getting an A on a test. Rewarding your efforts and celebrating your success will foster a positive attitude as you continue to study.

Recall Activity

1. A reward can be anything you _____.

2. When you're getting ready to learn, plan rewards at _____.

Concept 9: Teaching Others

Teaching is the best way to learn. By teaching a topic, you will find out if you actually understand it (**Figure 1.7**). Studying a topic in order to teach it can help motivate you to learn. Once you have mastered the material, find people who have no knowledge of the subject and teach the section to them. Repeat the terms and their definitions and explain the concepts of each section.

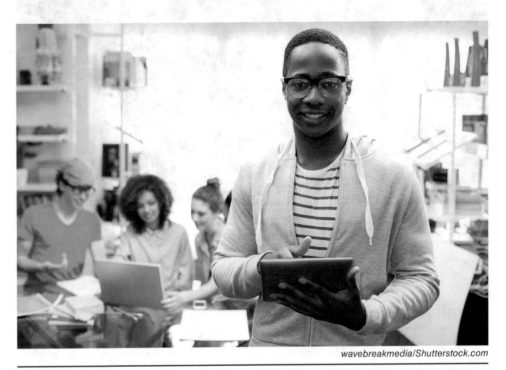

wavebreakmedia/Shutterstock.com

Figure 1.7 Teaching tests how well you know the material you have learned.

Recall Activity

1. _____ is the best way to learn.

2. Once you have _____ the material, teach the section to someone else.

Section 1.3 Reinforcement

Answer the following questions using what you learned in this section.

1. The goal of this book is to help you achieve _____.

2. Your _____ is your way of feeling, thinking about, and viewing a situation.

3. *True or False*. The biggest obstacle in learning science is understanding the words. _____

4. Write the letters backward: lufsseccus. Define the word that is formed. _____

_____

5. Which of the following will help you remember words?
   A. writing   C. speaking
   B. reading   D. All of the above.

6. Unscramble the letters: niteroptie. Define the word that is formed. _____
   _____

7. You can impress your friends and family by using _____ words in conversation.

8. What is a mnemonic? _____

9. *True or False.* You can concentrate on two or more tasks at one time. _____

10. As you work through each section in this book, you are _____.

11. When studying, devote your full _____ to the task at hand.

12. *True or False.* The most basic skill in learning science is understanding the terminology. _____

13. Once you have mastered material, identify people who have no _____ of the subject and explain the section to them.

14. Unscramble the letters: duitatte. Define the word that is formed._____
    _____

15. *True or False.* Teaching a section to someone will help you better understand the material. _____

16. Unscramble the letters: reinmtogylo. Define the word that is formed. _____
    _____

17. *True or False.* Students tend to like subjects at which they excel. _____

18. How many tasks can you do well at one time? _____

19. How you _____ a science class or subject will, to a great degree, determine your success or failure.

20. Repeatedly _____, _____,
    _____, or _____ words will help you remember them.

21. _____ your efforts and _____ your success will foster a positive attitude as you continue to study.

Comprehensive Review (Chapter 1)

Answer the following question using what you have learned so far in this book.

22. Explain the difference between natural and supernatural explanations. _____
    _____
    _____

Chapter 1 Review

Answer the following questions using what you learned in this chapter.

1. A fact is a confirmed _____.

2. Why should you check your answers to the questions in this book before moving on to the next section? _____

3. Your _____ is your way of feeling, thinking about, and viewing a situation.

4. Scientific explanations require the support of _____.

5. A person can stay focused on a task for about _____ minute(s).

6. *True or False.* Multitasking helps you achieve the best results._____

7. *True or False.* Each concept in this book progresses from simple to more complex._____

8. _____ are used as evidence to support scientific explanations.

9. A(n) _____ is a physically observable fact or event.

10. _____ is the deliberate effort to make long-term memories about subject matter.

11. Can science change? Why or why not? _____

12. *True or False.* Science builds upon itself. _____

13. Using your hands or feet while studying material is _____.

14. Are opinions scientific evidence? Why or why not?_____

_____

15. _____ seeks natural explanations to phenomena.

16. If you are having trouble concentrating, try varying your study _____,

_____, _____, or _____.

17. Why are supernatural explanations *not* considered science?_____

_____

18. An explanation is _____ if it is observable and testable.

19. *True or False.* When reading this book, it is recommended that you work for 20–30 minutes, and then reward yourself for completing a section by doing some type of physical activity._____

20. Most concepts in this book are not more than _____ sentence(s) in length.

21. Science seeks _____ explanations to phenomena.

22. Why is it not correct to say you believe in science?_____

_____

23. Why is it helpful to see the natural and the supernatural as two sides of one coin?_____

_____

24. *True or False.* The biggest obstacle in learning science is understanding the words. _____

25. Once you have mastered material, identify people who have no _____ of the subject and explain the section to them.

26. Which of the following are supernatural explanations?

   A. magic
   B. magnetism
   C. concentration
   D. miracles
   E. opposite charges

27. A(n) _____ can be anything you value.

28. _____ is the science that studies life.

29. Explain the difference between anatomy and physiology. _____

_____

Comprehensive Review (Chapter 1)

Using what you have learned so far in this book, match the following terms with their definitions.

_____ 30. Using your hands or feet while studying material

_____ 31. An explanation that is not testable

_____ 32. A word, acronym, or phrase that can help you recall information

_____ 33. Concentrated learning

_____ 34. To strengthen one's knowledge of material

_____ 35. A physically observable fact or event

_____ 36. Your way of feeling, thinking about, and viewing a situation

_____ 37. The words used in science

_____ 38. An explanation that is observable and testable

_____ 39. A confirmed observation

_____ 40. The body of knowledge and techniques that enables mankind to explain the natural world

_____ 41. An area of biology that studies inheritance

_____ 42. An area of biology that studies body parts

_____ 43. An area of biology that studies tissues

_____ 44. The science that studies life

_____ 45. An area of biology that studies the functions of body parts

_____ 46. An area of biology that studies cells

A. attitude
B. active learning
C. science
D. studying
E. natural
F. supernatural
G. reinforce
H. mnemonic
I. fact
J. phenomenon
K. terminology
L. biology
M. anatomy
N. genetics
O. cytology
P. physiology
Q. histology

Chapter 2
Scientific Vocabulary

Introduction

Reading scientific materials can be a daunting task. Understanding scientific words may seem like interpreting a different language. This chapter is your introduction to developing a scientific vocabulary. When you gain a firm grasp of scientific words, you will become equipped to understand all subjects in science. This chapter will teach you basic word parts, word disassembly, word assembly, and the contextual meanings of words. Each section will present basic word parts related to a specific topic. By working with the word parts, concept by concept, you will build your scientific vocabulary.

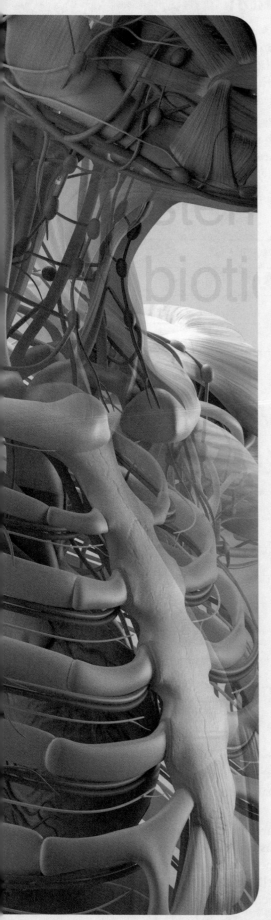

Anatomy Insider/Shutterstock.com

Objectives

After completing this chapter, you will be able to

- recognize word parts, including prefixes, combining forms, and suffixes
- understand word parts with opposite meanings
- create words using word parts related to directions
- know word parts related to numbers
- form words using word parts related to colors
- understand word parts related to sizes
- build words using word parts related to shapes
- know word parts related to locations
- understand word parts related to parts of the body

Key Terms

The following terms and word parts will be introduced and explained in Chapter 2. Read through the list to become familiar with the words.

a-	cyst	hydr/o	meso-	pseudo-
ab-	cyt/o	hyper-	micro-	quadri-
ad-	de-	hypo-	milli-	rect/o
af-	delt/o	-ia	mono-	ren/o
-al	derm/o	-ic	morph/o	root word
alb/o	di-	-ical	my/o	rubr/o
-algia	dis-	in-	neo-	semi-
an-	dors/o	infra-	neur/o	serrat/o
ana-	duct	inter-	-oid	spin
anti-	ecto-	intra-	-oma	-stasis
-ar	ef-	-ion	omni-	sten/o
arthr/o	endo-	-ist	-osis	strat/o
bi/o	enter/o	-itis	oste	sub-
bi-	epi-	kilo-	-ous	suffix
cardi/o	erythr/o	lat/o	peri-	supra-
centi-	ex-	later/o	-phage	tens
-ceps	gastr/o	leuk/o	-philic	tetra-
cerebr/o	-gen	-logist	-phobic	-tic
chlor/o	-genesis	-logy	physi/o	-tomy
coel/o	glob/o	lun	-plasm	tri-
combining	hem/o	lute/o	platy-	tub
form	hemi-	-lysis	-plegia	-ule
combining	hepat/o	macro-	poly-	ultra-
vowel	hetero-	medi/o	post-	-um
con-	hexa-	mega-	pre-	uni-
cortic/o	homo-	melan/o	prefix	ventr/o
cyan/o				

Section 2.1 Word Construction

Science has a language of its own, full of scientific words that may seem daunting. Learning the language of science, however, will open the door to understanding a multitude of science concepts. Scientific words follow predictable patterns of construction. By knowing how scientific words are structured, you can more easily understand them. In this section, you will learn how to dissect and build terminology using scientific word parts.

The terms below are some of those that will be introduced in Section 2.1. To become familiar with these terms, reproduce each word on the line beside it. Pronounce each term as you write it. You will learn the definitions of these words as you complete this section.

1. combining form _____
2. root word _____
3. combining vowel _____
4. prefix _____
5. suffix _____
6. bi/o _____
7. -tic _____
8. a- _____
9. physi/o _____
10. -logy _____
11. ana- _____
12. -tomy _____
13. anti- _____
14. -al _____
15. -ical _____
16. -ist _____
17. -logist _____

18. an- _____
19. neo- _____
20. pseudo- _____
21. cardi/o _____
22. cyt/o _____
23. derm/o _____
24. hydr/o _____
25. morph/o _____
26. -gen _____
27. -genesis _____
28. -ic _____
29. -lysis _____
30. -osis _____
31. -ous _____
32. -plasm _____
33. -stasis _____
34. -um _____

Concept 1: Scientific Words

Scientific words can be long and may be unfamiliar and hard to understand at first. Learning how to disassemble words, or break them into smaller parts, can help you interpret them.

Scientific words are descriptive of the structures or procedures to which they refer. For example, when the sternocleidomastoid muscles in your neck contract, your head nods toward your chest. Sternocleidomastoid muscles are named for the bones to which they are attached: the sternum (or *breastbone*), the clavicles (or *collarbones*), and the *mastoid* process of the temporal bones.

Sternocleidomastoid might look like an intimidating word, but the name is descriptive of where the muscles are located. When broken apart, the term can be easily interpreted. As you learn scientific terminology, do not be afraid of any word. Disassembling the word will help you understand it.

Recall Activity

1. Scientific words are _____ of the structures or procedures to which they refer.

2. _____ a word will help you understand it.

3. Sternocleidomastoid muscles are named for the _____ to which they are attached.

Concept 2: Word Parts

When you disassemble a scientific term, you are breaking the term into its component word parts. *Word parts* are small segments of a word. They include combining forms, suffixes, and prefixes (**Figure 2.1**).

- A *combining form* is a root word plus its combining vowel. The *root word* is the central component of a scientific term. The *combining vowel* is a vowel (usually *o*) that helps combine the root word with other word parts. Combining forms often refer to specific body parts. Prefixes, suffixes, and other combining forms attach to a combining form (or sometimes just to a root word) to create a scientific term.

- A *prefix* is a letter or group of letters preceding a combining form. Prefixes often describe time, location, or number.

- A *suffix* is a letter or group of letters following a combining form. Suffixes usually describe certain types of diseases or procedures.

Combining forms, prefixes, and suffixes make up many of the terms you will encounter in anatomy and physiology. Take the word *biotic* as an example. In biotic, the combining form *bi/o* means "life." The suffix *-tic* means "pertaining to." Thus, the term *biotic* means "pertaining to something that is alive" (for example, a bacterium or a human). If you attached the prefix *a-* (meaning "not") to the word *biotic*, this would form the word *abiotic*, which means "pertaining to something that is not alive" (for example, a rock).

combining form a root word plus its combining vowel

root word the central component of a scientific term; often refers to a specific body part

combining vowel a vowel that is attached to a root word when a term is assembled

prefix a letter or group of letters preceding a combining form; describes time, location, and number

suffix a letter or group of letters following a combining form; describes certain types of diseases or procedures

bi/o combining form meaning "life"

-tic suffix meaning "pertaining to"

a- prefix meaning "not"

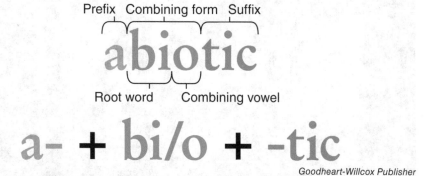

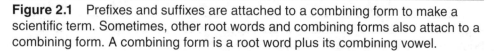

Goodheart-Willcox Publisher

Figure 2.1 Prefixes and suffixes are attached to a combining form to make a scientific term. Sometimes, other root words and combining forms also attach to a combining form. A combining form is a root word plus its combining vowel.

Recall Activity

1. Draw lines to connect each word part with its correct definition.

   prefix   a root word plus its combining vowel

   combining form   a letter or group of letters preceding a combining form

   suffix   a letter or group of letters following a combining form

2. The suffix of the term *abiotic* is _____.

3. The combining form *bi/o* means "_____."

4. The prefix of the term *abiotic* means "_____."

5. The word *abiotic* means "_____."

Concept 3: Word Disassembly

physi/o combining form meaning "function"

-logy suffix meaning "study of"

ana- prefix meaning "apart"

-tomy suffix meaning "to cut"

Using word parts, you can disassemble a word to understand its meaning. Once you become familiar with common word parts, you will be able to interpret a term's meaning even if you have never seen it before.

To disassemble a word, identify its word parts. For example, the term *physiology* can be broken into two word parts: the combining form *physi/o* (meaning "function") and the suffix *-logy* (meaning "study of"). Thus, *physiology* means "the study of function."

Some scientific terms do not contain a combining form; instead, they contain only prefixes and suffixes. For example, the word *anatomy* can be disassembled into the prefix *ana-* (meaning "apart") and the suffix *-tomy* (meaning "to cut"). The science of anatomy, or the science of "cutting a body apart," identifies the body's parts, including organs, tissues, and cells (**Figure 2.2**). Thus, human anatomy and physiology is the study of the parts of the human body and how the parts function.

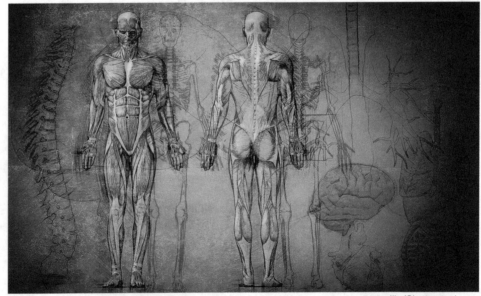

adike/Shutterstock.com

Figure 2.2 The study of anatomy developed through dissections of the human body. In these dissections, the human body was "cut apart."

Recall Activity

1. Disassemble the word *biology* by identifying its combining form and suffix._____

2. The combining form of *biology* means "_____," and the suffix of *biology* means "_____."

3. Using the word parts you know so far, infer what happens to the tonsils in a *tonsillotomy*. _____

_____

Concept 4: Word Assembly

Using word parts, you can also assemble scientific terms. Assembling scientific terms is good practice for memorizing word parts and for disassembling scientific words for their meanings. To assemble a scientific term, identify the word parts needed to create the correct meaning. Then attach the appropriate word parts to one another.

In this example, you will assemble a scientific term that means "pertaining to against life." First, identify the word parts you need to use. For "life," you can use the combining form *bi/o*. For "against," use the prefix *anti-*, and for "pertaining to," use the suffix *-tic*. First, add the prefix *anti-* to the combining form. Then add the suffix *-tic* to make the term *antibiotic*. Antibiotics are drugs that act against living organisms like bacteria.

anti- prefix meaning "against"

More word parts commonly used in word assembly are defined below.

Word Part	Meaning
-al	character of
-ical	character of
-ist	specialist
-logist	one who studies

Recall Activity

Use the word parts you have learned so far in this chapter to complete the following activities.

1. Assemble a word that means "one who studies life." _____

2. Assemble a word that means "one who studies function."_____

3. Assemble a word that means "specialist in cutting apart."_____

4. Assemble a word that means "character of the study of function." _____

Concept 5: Applying Word Disassembly and Assembly

As you learn the definitions of various word parts, you will be able to assemble and disassemble many scientific terms. Below are some word parts common among scientific terms. Learn the definitions of these word parts to better interpret and build scientific vocabulary. A comprehensive list of all the word parts introduced in this chapter can be found in Appendix A.

Word Part	Meaning
an-	without
neo-	new
pseudo-	false
cardi/o	heart
cyt/o	cell
derm/o	skin
hydr/o	water
morph/o	form
-gen	producer
-genesis	production
-ic	pertaining to
-lysis	breakdown
-osis	condition
-ous	nature of
-plasm	formation
-stasis	stay or stop
-um	structure

Recall Activity

Use the word parts you have learned so far in this chapter to complete the following activities.

1. Assemble a word that means "the study of cells." _____

2. Disassemble and define the word *dermolysis*. _____

3. Assemble a word that means "pertaining to a life form." _____

4. Disassemble and define the word *amorphous*. _____

5. Assemble a word that means "water producer." _____

6. Disassemble and define the word *cardium*. _____

7. Assemble a word that means "false form." _____

8. Disassemble and define the word *anhydrous*. _____

9. Assemble a word that means "stoppage of water." _____

10. Disassemble and define the word *hydromorphic*. _____

11. Assemble a word that means "new formation." _____

12. Disassemble and define the word *biogenesis*. _____

Concept 6: Word Context

In addition to disassembling words, understanding words in the context of a sentence will help you read and understand scientific terminology. When reading in context, you may only recognize a part of a word, but that should be enough for you to understand the word's meaning.

Recall Activity

Examine the italicized words to determine their meanings. Then use this knowledge to fill in the blanks and complete the sentence.

1. The *neonatal* unit at a hospital is for _____ born babies.

2. An overgrowth of connective tissue causes *cirrhosis*, a(n) _____ that affects the liver.

3. All *pseudostratified* cells rest on the basement membrane, an example of _____ layering.

Section 2.1 Reinforcement

Answer the following questions using what you learned in this section.

1. What does the word *cytolysis* mean? _____

2. If the root word *pod* means "foot," what scientific term would mean "false foot"? _____

3. A(n) _____ is a letter or group of letters preceding a combining form.

4. *True or False.* The combining form *morph/o* means "form." _____

5. Disassemble and define the term *pseudomorphic*. _____

   _____

6. Which of the following word parts means "function"?
   A. -logy   C. physi/o
   B. pseudo-   D. hydr/o

7. A hydrologist studies _____.

8. *True or False.* Anti- is to "against" what -*genesis* is to "form." _____

9. The word parts meaning "form" and "production" combine to form the word

   _____.

10. Which of the following word parts are misspelled?
    A. psuedo-   C. -plasm
    B. hedr/o   D. morf/o

11. Cytoplasm is a formation found inside _____.

12. *True or False.* The suffix -*plasm* means "new." _____

13. What is the root word of the term *neocytic*? _____

14. A morphologist studies _____.

15. What is the prefix in the term *antibacterial*? _____

16. *True or False*. The combining form *hydr/o* means "water." _____

17. Something that is antimorphic acts _____ a form.

18. The term *plasmic* means "_____."

19. Arrange these word parts in the order in which they typically appear in a term: combining form, prefix, and suffix. _____

Comprehensive Review (Chapters 1–2)

Answer the following questions using what you have learned so far in this book.

20. Why should you check your answers to the questions in this book before moving on to the next section?

_____

21. Identify the three types of word parts. _____

Section 2.2 Word Parts with Opposite Meanings

To disassemble and interpret scientific terms, you need a solid foundation of knowledge about word parts and their meanings. In the next few sections, you will learn the meanings of word parts related to several topics. In this section, you will learn about sets of opposite word parts.

The terms below are some of those that will be introduced in Section 2.2. To become familiar with these terms, reproduce each word on the line beside it. Pronounce each term as you write it. You will learn the definitions of these words as you complete this section.

1. ecto- _____   7. inter- _____

2. endo- _____   8. intra- _____

3. hetero- _____   9. post- _____

4. homo- _____   10. pre- _____

5. hyper- _____   11. -philic _____

6. hypo- _____   12. -phobic _____

Concept 1: Opposite Word Parts

Understanding opposite word parts will help you remember word part meanings and use them to interpret scientific terms. You will be able to compare scientific terms and determine their definitions. Below are some opposite word parts commonly used in scientific terminology.

Word Part	Meaning
ecto-	outside
endo-	inside
hetero-	different
homo-	same
hyper-	above; beyond
hypo-	below
inter-	between
intra-	within
post-	after
pre-	before
-philic	loving
-phobic	fearing

Recall Activity

1. Write the definition of each word part.

   pre- _____

   homo- _____

   post- _____

   -philic _____

   hyper- _____

   endo- _____

   -phobic _____

   hypo- _____

   ecto- _____

   hetero- _____

   intra- _____

   inter- _____

2. Write the corresponding word part next to its definition.

   inside _____

   below _____

   different _____

   loving _____

   before _____

within _____

outside _____

above; beyond _____

same _____

fearing _____

after _____

between _____

3. Draw lines to match the word parts with their opposites.

endo-   homo-

intra-   ecto-

hetero-   inter-

-philic   post-

pre-   -phobic

hyper-   hypo-

Concept 2: Assembling Terms

When you assemble terms using opposite word parts, you form scientific words that have opposite meanings. For example, the term *ectocytic* means "pertaining to outside the cell." The term *endocytic* means "pertaining to inside the cell" (**Figure 2.3**). The word parts *ecto-* and *endo-* have opposite meanings.

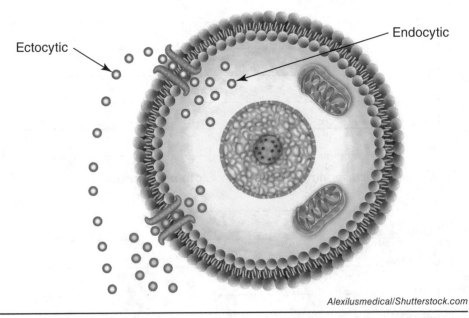

Ectocytic

Endocytic

Alexilusmedical/Shutterstock.com

Figure 2.3 Structures inside a cell are endocytic. Structures outside a cell are ectocytic.

Recall Activity

Use the word parts you have learned so far in this chapter to complete the following activities. You can easily review all of the word parts covered in this chapter by referencing Appendix A in the back of the book.

1. Assemble a word that means "water loving."_____

2. Assemble a word that means "below the skin."_____

3. Assemble a word that means "pertaining to within the cell."_____

4. Assemble a word that means "same form."_____

5. Assemble a word that means "the character of something inside the heart."_____

Concept 3: Disassembling Terms

Knowing word parts with opposite meanings can help you disassemble and interpret scientific words. If you understand the meanings of a pair of opposite word parts, you can easily and quickly interpret a scientific term.

Recall Activity

Use the word parts you have learned so far in this chapter to complete the following activities.

1. Disassemble and define the word *endocardiologist.* _____

2. Disassemble and define the word *cytophilic.* _____

3. Disassemble and define the word *heteromorph.* _____

4. Disassemble and define the word *hydrophobic.* _____

5. Disassemble and define the word *ectoderm.* _____

Concept 4: Using Context

Paying attention to the context of a term will help you interpret it. If you know the meanings of opposite word parts, using context to understand a term will be even easier. For example, if you know that the prefix *homo-* means "same," you can interpret the meaning of the term *homogenized*, even if you cannot fully disassemble the word. You can know that, if naturally occurring fat is uniformly distributed in homogenized milk, two samples taken from a gallon of homogenized milk will contain the same amount of fat.

Recall Activity

For each scenario, use contextual knowledge and knowledge of word parts to fill in the blanks and complete the sentence.

1. A basketball player is not able to play because he hyperextended his knee in a fall. This means his

   knee was extended _____ the normal range of motion.

2. Rabies is sometimes called *hydrophobia* because a rabid animal will _____ water.

3. Cerebrospinal fluid circulates through the interventricular foramen, meaning it flows _____ ventricles.

4. In an ectopic pregnancy, the embryo develops _____ the uterus.

Section 2.2 Reinforcement

Answer the following questions using what you learned in this section.

1. *True or False.* The prefix *inter-* means "between." _____

2. Which of the following word parts means "within"?
   A. homo-   C. pre-   E. intra-
   B. inter-   D. post-   F. hetero-

3. Write the letters backward: cibohp. Define the word part that is formed. _____

   _____

4. Unscramble the letters: eerhot. Define the word part that is formed. _____

   _____

5. The word part that means the opposite of *-philic* is _____ .

6. Which of the following word parts means "above"?
   A. post-   C. hyper-
   B. homo-   D. endo-

7. The prefix *pre-* means "before," and *post-* means "_____ ."

8. *True or False.* The prefixes *pre-* and *post-* have opposite meanings. _____

9. Write the letters backward: otce. Define the word part that is formed. _____

   _____

10. *True or False.* The prefix *hetero-* means "different." _____

11. The prefix *ecto-* means "_____ ."

12. The word part that means "between" is _____ .

13. Which of the following word parts means "same"?
    A. homo-   C. post-
    B. hetero-   D. -philic

14. _____ means "above," and _____ means "below."

15. The word part that means "loving" is _____ .

16. *True or False.* The prefix *hyper-* means "fearing." _____

17. The word part that means "within" is _____ .

18. Unscramble the letters: ratni. Define the word part that is formed._____

_____

19. *True or False.* The prefix *intra-* means "below." _____

20. The word part that means the opposite of *hyper-* is _____.

Comprehensive Review (Chapters 1–2)

Answer the following questions using what you have learned so far in this book.

21. The word part *-logist* means "_____."

22. What is the term for the body of knowledge and techniques that enables mankind to explain the natural world? _____

Section 2.3 Word Parts Related to Directions

Many word parts relate to a direction of movement or to a structure's placement as compared to other structures. Understanding these word parts will help you envision anatomical structures and movements. In this section, you will learn word parts related to directions.

The terms below are some of those that will be introduced in Section 2.3. To become familiar with these terms, reproduce each word on the line beside it. Pronounce each term as you write it. You will learn the definitions of these words as you complete this section.

1. ab-_____   9. ex- _____

2. ad-_____   10. in- _____

3. af- _____   11. sub-_____

4. ef- _____   12. supra-_____

5. con- _____   13. duct_____

6. dis- _____   14. -ion_____

7. infra- _____   15. tens_____

8. epi- _____

Concept 1: Direction Word Parts

Knowing the meanings of word parts related to directions will help you more easily construct and disassemble scientific terms. You will be able to recognize whether a movement occurs toward or away from an object, for example. Below are some direction word parts commonly used in scientific terminology.

Word Part	Meaning
ab-	away from
ad-	toward
af-	toward
ef-	away from
con-	together
dis-	apart
infra-	under
epi-	upon
ex-	out of
in-	into
sub-	below
supra-	above

Recall Activity

1. Draw lines to match the word parts with their meanings.

epi-	out of
dis-	above
ad-	away from
infra-	toward
ex-	into
con-	together
supra-	upon
ef-	under
in-	apart

2. Write the corresponding word part next to its definition. Some questions will have two answers.

below _____

together _____

out of _____

into _____

toward _____

away from _____

above _____

upon _____

apart _____

under _____

3. Write the definition of each word part.

dis- _____

sub- _____

in- _____

infra- _____

ef- _____

ab- _____

ad- _____

epi- _____

supra- _____

ex- _____

con- _____

af- _____

Concept 2: Assembling Terms

When you assemble terms using direction word parts, you form scientific words that refer to specific movements or locations. This is especially important in anatomy and physiology. For example, the term *abduction* is formed from the prefix *ab-*, the root word *duct* (meaning "to carry"), and the suffix *-ion* (meaning "process"). Thus, *abduction* means "the process of carrying away from the body" (**Figure 2.4**). Similarly, the term *extension* is formed from

duct root word meaning "to carry"; combining form *duct/o*

-ion suffix meaning "process"

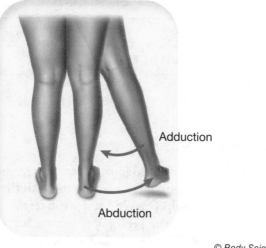

Adduction

Abduction

© Body Scientific International

Figure 2.4 Abduction describes movement away from the midline of the body. Adduction describes movement toward the midline of the body.

tens root word meaning "to stretch"; combining form *tens/o*

the prefix *ex-*, the root word *tens* (meaning "to stretch"), and the suffix *-ion*. *Extension* means "the process of stretching out from the body."

Recall Activity

Use the word parts you have learned so far in this chapter to complete the following activities. You can easily review all of the word parts covered in this chapter by referencing Appendix A in the back of the book.

1. Assemble a word that means "structure upon the heart." _____

2. Assemble a word that means "the process of stretching apart."_____

3. Assemble a word that means "the process of stretching out from the body beyond (the normal range of movement)."_____

4. Assemble a word that means "the process of carrying toward the body."_____

5. Assemble a word that means "the process of carrying together."_____

Concept 3: Disassembling Terms

When you know word parts with directional meanings, you can disassemble and interpret many scientific words. You can know the locations to which terms are referring and visualize directional movements.

Recall Activity

Use the word parts you have learned so far in this chapter to complete the following activities.

1. Disassemble and define the word *hypoextension.* _____

2. Disassemble and define the word *induction.* _____

3. Disassemble and define the word *supraduction.*_____

4. Disassemble and define the word *infracytology.*_____

5. Disassemble and define the word *subdermal.* _____

Concept 4: Using Context

Using context and your knowledge of word parts, you can interpret directional terms in scientific language. Learning to glean the meanings of scientific words from context will help you read scientific terms quickly and accurately. For example, knowing that the prefix *epi-* means "upon" can help you interpret the term *epineurium*. The epineurium is found upon the surface of a nerve.

Recall Activity

For each scenario, use contextual knowledge and knowledge of word parts to fill in the blanks and complete the sentence.

1. The peripheral nervous system includes efferent and afferent nerves. Efferent nerves move electrical impulses _____ the central nervous system. Afferent nerves move electrical impulses _____ the central nervous system.

2. The adductor muscle moves the leg _____ the body.

3. Breathing consists of inspiration and expiration. Expiration is breathing _____. Inspiration is breathing _____.

4. Submucosa is situated _____ the mucosa.

5. In dissection, a body is _____.

6. The supraorbital foramen is a hole in the bone _____ the eye.

7. The infratemporal fossa is a depression in the bone _____ the temple.

Section 2.3 Reinforcement

Answer the following questions using what you learned in this section.

1. *True or False.* The prefix *dis-* means "toward." _____

2. Which of the following word parts mean "toward"?
   A. ab-   C. epi-   E. ex-
   B. ad-   D. in-   F. af-

3. Write the letters backward: arfni. Define the word part that is formed. _____
   _____

4. The prefix *supra-* means "_____."

5. Which of the following word parts means the opposite of *ab-*?
   A. ex-   C. dis-   E. ad-
   B. in-   D. con-   F. supra-

6. Which of the following word parts means "into"?
   A. ex-   C. infra-   E. dis-
   B. in-   D. con-   F. ab-

7. Unscramble the letters: pusar. Define the word part that is formed. _____
   _____

8. *True or False.* Both *ad-* and *ab-* mean "toward." _____

9. Write the letters backward: sid. Define the word part that is formed. _____
   _____

10. *True or False.* The prefix *con-* means "apart." _____

11. Arrange these word parts in alphabetical order: epi-, ad-, ab-, supra-, dis-, con-, ef-, and af-._____

_____

12. Which of the following word parts means "upon"?

    A. epi-   C. con-   E. ab-

    B. dis-   D. ef-   F. ad-

13. The prefix _____ means "above."

14. The prefix *sub-* means "_____."

15. The prefixes _____ mean "toward."

16. *True or False.* The prefix *ad-* means "toward." _____

17. What is the definition of *ab-*? _____

18. The prefixes _____ mean "away from."

19. *True or False.* The prefixes *af-* and *ef-* have opposite meanings. _____

20. A submarine moves _____ water.

Comprehensive Review (Chapters 1–2)

Answer the following questions using what you have learned so far in this book.

21. *True or False.* The word *antibiotic* means "pertaining to against life." _____

22. Which of the following are natural explanations?

    A. magic   C. concentration   E. opposite charges

    B. magnetism   D. miracles

Section 2.4 Word Parts Related to Numbers

Some word parts indicate the number a word describes. In this section, you will learn about word parts that indicate numbers and amounts.

The terms below are some of those that will be introduced in Section 2.4. To become familiar with these terms, reproduce each word on the line beside it. Pronounce each term as you write it. You will learn the definitions of these words as you complete this section.

1. mono- _____   6. tri-_____

2. uni-_____   7. quadri- _____

3. di- _____   8. tetra- _____

4. bi- _____   9. hexa-_____

5. hemi- _____   10. omni-_____

11. poly-_____   13. -plegia _____

12. -ceps_____   14. cyst _____

Concept 1: Number Word Parts

Number word parts communicate whether there are two, three, one, or more of an object or structure. By learning these word parts, you can easily interpret the numbers indicated by scientific terms. Below are some number word parts commonly used in scientific terminology.

Word Part	Meaning
mono-	one
uni-	one
di-	two
bi-	two
hemi-	half
tri-	three
quadri-	four
tetra-	four
hexa-	six
omni-	all
poly-	many

Recall Activity

1. Write the corresponding word part next to its definition. Some questions will have two answers.

six _____

all _____

three _____

four _____

two _____

one _____

many _____

half _____

2. Draw lines to match the word parts with their meanings.

one	omni-
two	quadri-
three	di-
four	uni-
six	tri-
all	poly-
many	hexa-

3. Write the definition of each word part.

di- _____

uni- _____

poly- _____

mono- _____

tri- _____

quadri- _____

tetra- _____

omni- _____

bi- _____

hemi- _____

Concept 2: Assembling Terms

-ceps suffix meaning "heads"

-plegia suffix meaning "paralysis"

Using number word parts, you can assemble scientific terms that indicate numbers or amounts. For example, to describe a muscle with two heads (attachments), you would combine the prefix *bi-* with the suffix *-ceps* (meaning "heads") to make the scientific word *biceps*. The biceps, as shown in **Figure 2.5**, is a two-headed muscle. Similarly, if you wanted to describe the paralysis of one-half of the body, you would combine the prefix *hemi-* with the suffix *-plegia* (meaning "paralysis") to make the term *hemiplegia*.

Recall Activity

Use the word parts you have learned so far in this chapter to complete the following activities. You can easily review all of the word parts covered in this chapter by referencing Appendix A in the back of the book.

1. Assemble a word that means "three heads." _____

2. Assemble a word that means "one cell." _____

3. Assemble a word that means "paralysis of four parts." _____

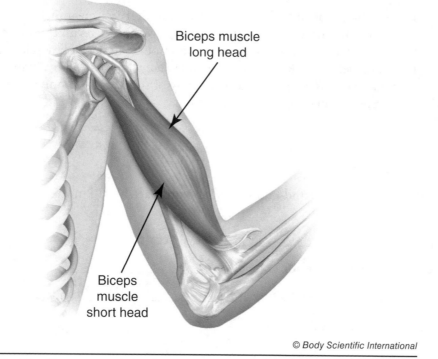

Biceps muscle
long head

Biceps
muscle
short head

© *Body Scientific International*

Figure 2.5 The biceps muscle has two heads.

4. Assemble a word that means "four heads." _____

5. Assemble a word that means "the study of all." _____

Concept 3: Disassembling Terms

Once you know number word parts, you can disassemble words indicating number with ease. Even if you don't know the exact meaning of a word, you will understand the number it communicates. For example, if you encounter the term *monocystic*, you will know the term describes one of something. The root word *cyst* means "cyst." A *cyst* is a liquid-filled sac. *Monocystic* describes one cyst.

cyst root word meaning "cyst"; combining form *cyst/o*

Recall Activity

Use the word parts you have learned so far in this chapter to complete the following activities.

1. Disassemble and define the word *unimorph*. _____

2. Disassemble and define the word *polycystic*. _____

3. Disassemble and define the word *diplegia*. _____

4. Disassemble and define the word *tetralogy*. _____

5. Disassemble and define the word *bicardial*. _____

Concept 4: Using Context

By reading terms in their context, you can interpret meanings even if you do not know all the word parts that make up a scientific term. If you know number word parts, you can understand the amounts described by scientific terms. For example, if you know that the prefix *poly-* means "many," you can interpret that the term *polymer* refers to many of something. A polymer is a chemical compound made of many molecules.

Recall Activity

For each scenario, use contextual knowledge and knowledge of word parts to fill in the blanks and complete the sentence.

1. Binocular microscopes have _____ eyepiece(s).

2. The triannual gallstone collectors convention is held _____ time(s) per year.

3. A glucose molecule is drawn as a hexagon, having _____ side(s).

4. A tetrapod has _____ feet.

Section 2.4 Reinforcement

Answer the following questions using what you learned in this section.

1. The prefix *poly-* means "_____."

2. Which of the following word parts mean "two"?
   A. omni-   C. di-   E. uni-
   B. mono-   D. tri-   F. bi-

3. Write the letters backward: artet. Define the word part that is formed. _____

   _____

4. The prefix *quadri-* means "_____."

5. Which of the following word parts are misspelled?
   A. omi-   C. du-   E. bi-
   B. mono-   D. tera-   F. quadri-

6. Which of the following word parts mean "one"?
   A. omni-   C. di-   E. uni-
   B. mono-   D. tri-   F. bi-

7. Unscramble the letters: yplo. Define the word part that is formed. _____

   _____

8. The prefixes *di-* and *bi-* both mean "_____."

9. Write the letters backward: onom. Define the word part that is formed. _____

   _____

10. *True or False.* The prefix *omni-* means "all." _____

11. A biplane has _____ wing(s).

12. Which of the following prefixes describes the largest number?
    A. di-   C. tri-   E. mono-
    B. bi-   D. hexa-   F. tetra-

13. Unscramble the letters: axhe. Define the word part that is formed. _____

    _____

14. Arrange these prefixes according to the numbers they describe (from smallest to largest): quadri-,
    di-, hexa-, mono-, and tri-.

    _____

15. The prefixes *uni-* and *mono-* both mean "_____."

16. *True or False.* The prefixes *tetra-* and *quadri-* both mean "five."_____

17. Arrange these prefixes according to the numbers they describe (from largest to smallest): tetra-,
    hexa-, uni-, bi-, and tri-.

    _____

18. Unscramble the letters: daqiru. Define the word part that is formed. _____

    _____

19. *True or False.* A polygon has one side. _____

20. Which of the following prefixes describes the smallest number?
    A. bi-   C. tri-   E. hexa-
    B. mono-   D. tetra-   F. omni-

21. The prefix *hemi-* means "_____."

Comprehensive Review (Chapters 1–2)

Answer the following questions using what you have learned so far in this book.

22. Your _____ is your way of feeling, thinking about, and viewing a situation.

23. The suffix *-philic* means "_____."

Section 2.5 Word Parts Related to Colors

Sometimes, when you read a scientific term, you can tell the color of the object
or structure being described. These scientific terms contain word parts related to
color. In this section, you will learn about some word parts that indicate color.

The following terms are some of those that will be introduced in Section 2.5.
To become familiar with these terms, reproduce each word on the line beside
it. Pronounce each term as you write it. You will learn the definitions of these
words as you complete this section.

1. alb/o _____   6. lute/o _____

2. chlor/o _____   7. melan/o _____

3. cyan/o _____   8. rubr/o _____

4. erythr/o _____   9. -oma _____

5. leuk/o _____

Concept 1: Color Word Parts

Color word parts indicate the color of an object or structure. A color word part, for example, can communicate that an object is red, blue, or green. Below are some color word parts commonly used in scientific terminology.

Word Part	Meaning
alb/o	white
chlor/o	green
cyan/o	blue
erythr/o	red
leuk/o	white
lute/o	yellow
melan/o	black
rubr/o	red

Recall Activity

1. Write the definition of each word part.

   cyan/o _____

   erythr/o _____

   chlor/o _____

   lute/o _____

   melan/o _____

   alb/o _____

   rubr/o _____

   leuk/o _____

2. Write the corresponding word part next to its definition. Some questions will have two answers.

   red _____

   blue _____

   white _____

   yellow _____

green_____

black_____

3. Draw lines to match the word parts with their meanings.

chlor/o	white
leuk/o	green
lute/o	red
rubr/o	blue
cyan/o	black
melan/o	yellow

Concept 2: Assembling Terms

If you know word parts that indicate color, you can construct many scientific terms describing colored structures or objects. For example, to describe a white tumor, combine the root word *leuk* and the suffix *-oma* (meaning "tumor") to make the word *leukoma*. To describe a condition of redness, combine the root word *erythr* with the suffix *-osis* (meaning "condition") to make the word *erythrosis*.

-oma suffix meaning "tumor"

Recall Activity

Use the word parts you have learned so far in this chapter to complete the following activities. You can easily review all of the word parts covered in this chapter by referencing Appendix A in the back of the book.

1. Assemble a word that means "condition of blueness." _____

2. Assemble a word that means "green fearing." _____

3. Assemble a word that means "black tumor." _____

4. Assemble a word that means "condition of white cells."_____

5. Assemble a word that means "breakdown of yellow (matter)." _____

Concept 3: Disassembling Terms

Disassembling scientific terms can help you interpret them. Using word parts, you can determine the color of the structure or object a scientific term is describing. For example, the word *erythrogenesis* can be broken into the combining form *erythr/o* and the suffix *-genesis* (meaning "production"). Erythrogenesis refers to the production of red blood cells (**Figure 2.6**).

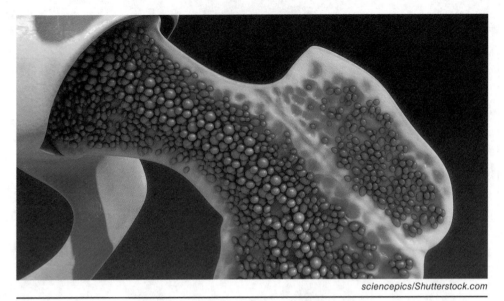

sciencepics/Shutterstock.com

Figure 2.6 Erythrogenesis, or red blood cell production, takes place in the bone marrow.

Recall Activity

Use the word parts you have learned so far in this chapter to complete the following activities.

1. Disassemble and define the word *leukosis*. _____

2. Disassemble and define the word *luteum*. _____

3. Disassemble and define the word *melanogenesis*. _____

4. Disassemble and define the word *cyanogen*. _____

5. Disassemble and define the word *erythrostasis*. _____

Concept 4: Using Context

Using context and color word parts, you can interpret many aspects of words you do not understand. This will make reading scientific terminology faster and easier. It will also help you understand other word parts. For example, if you know that the combining form *rubr/o* means "red," you can infer that *rubrospinal tracts* are associated with red cells.

Recall Activity

For each scenario, use contextual knowledge and knowledge of word parts to fill in the blanks and complete the sentence.

1. The albumin of an egg is _____ in color.

2. Melanin is _____ in color.

3. Regardless of race, the skin color of an albino person is _____.

4. Leaves are _____ in color due to chlorophyll.

Section 2.5 Reinforcement

Answer the following questions using what you learned in this section.

1. *True or False.* The combining forms *alb/o* and *melan/o* have opposite meanings. _____

2. Which of the following word parts mean "red"?
   A. rubr/o
   B. chlor/o
   C. erythr/o
   D. leuk/o

3. Write the letters backward: orolhc. Define the word part that is formed. _____

   _____

4. The combining form *cyan/o* means "_____."

5. Which of the following word parts are misspelled?
   A. cyan/o
   B. erthr/o
   C. chlor/o
   D. mela/o

6. Which of the following word parts means "white"?
   A. rubr/o
   B. cyan/o
   C. chlor/o
   D. erythr/o
   E. leuk/o
   F. melan/o

7. Arrange the following word parts in alphabetical order: rubr/o, cyan/o, chlor/o, erythr/o, leuk/o, and melan/o. _____

8. *True or False.* The combining forms *alb/o* and *cyan/o* both mean "white." _____

9. Write the letters backward: okuel. Define the word part that is formed. _____

   _____

10. *True or False.* The combining form *leuk/o* means "black." _____

11. The combining form *chlor/o* means "_____."

12. Which of the following word parts describes the darkest color?
    A. cyan/o
    B. rubr/o
    C. melan/o
    D. erythr/o
    E. alb/o
    F. leuk/o

13. The combining form _____ means "blue."

14. Unscramble the letters: noacy. Define the word part that is formed. _____

    _____

15. The word parts _____ mean "white."

16. *True or False.* Melanin is dark pigment. _____

17. The word parts _____ mean "red."

18. Unscramble the letters: aonelm. Define the word part that is formed. _____

    _____

19. *True or False.* The cells of green plants contain chlorophyll._____

20. Which of the following word parts describes the lightest color?
   A. erythr/o   C. cyan/o   E. rubr/o
   B. alb/o   D. melan/o   F. chlor/o

Comprehensive Review (Chapters 1–2)

Answer the following questions using what you have learned so far in this book.

21. *True or False.* Each concept, section, and chapter in this book progresses from simple to more complex. _____

22. Identify and define the prefix in the term *endometriosis.*_____

Section 2.6 Word Parts Related to Sizes

Sometimes scientific terms indicate the size of an object. In this section, you will learn about word parts related to size.

The terms below are some of those that will be introduced in Section 2.6. To become familiar with these terms, reproduce each word on the line beside it. Pronounce each term as you write it. You will learn the definitions of these words as you complete this section.

1. macro-_____   8. centi- _____

2. mega-_____   9. milli- _____

3. kilo- _____   10. -phage _____

4. ultra- _____   11. tub_____

5. semi-_____   12. lun_____

6. micro- _____   13. -ar _____

7. -ule _____

Concept 1: Size Word Parts

Word parts related to size describe the size of a measurement, object, or structure in relation to other measurements, objects, or structures. These word parts provide an easy way of judging the size or amount of an object. Below are some size word parts commonly used in scientific terminology. For the purpose of measurement, one unit refers to 1 meter, gram, liter, or degree Celsius. You will learn more about units of measurement in Chapter 4.

Word Part	Meaning
macro-	large
mega-	large
kilo-	1000 units

```
ultra- .........................beyond
semi- .........................half
micro- .........................small
-ule .........................small
centi- .........................¹⁄₁₀₀ of one unit
milli- .........................¹⁄₁₀₀₀ of one unit
```

Recall Activity

1. Write the definition of each word part.

   mega- _____

   milli- _____

   micro- _____

   semi- _____

   macro- _____

   kilo- _____

   ultra- _____

   -ule _____

   centi- _____

2. Write the corresponding word part next to its definition. Some questions will have two answers.

   1000 units _____

   small _____

   half _____

   large _____

   ¹⁄₁₀₀₀ of one unit _____

   beyond _____

   ¹⁄₁₀₀ of one unit _____

3. Draw lines to match the word parts with their meanings.

   mega-   small

   micro-   half

   semi-   large

   ultra-   beyond

   kilo-   ¹⁄₁₀₀₀ of one unit

   centi-   1000 units

   milli-   ¹⁄₁₀₀ of one unit

Concept 2: Assembling Terms

-phage suffix meaning "eat"

tub root word meaning "tube"; combining form *tub/o*

Using size word parts, you can assemble terms that describe the size of an object or structure. For example, to describe a large structure that eats or swallows another structure, combine the prefix *macro-* with the suffix *-phage* (meaning "eat") to make the word *macrophage* (**Figure 2.7**). To describe a small tube, combine the root word *tub* (meaning "tube") and the suffix *-ule* to make the word *tubule*.

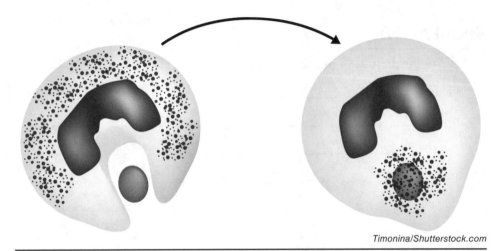

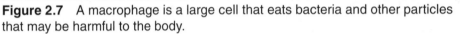

Timonina/Shutterstock.com

Figure 2.7 A macrophage is a large cell that eats bacteria and other particles that may be harmful to the body.

Recall Activity

Use the word parts you have learned so far in this chapter to complete the following activities. You can easily review all of the word parts covered in this chapter by referencing Appendix A in the back of the book.

1. Assemble a word that means "small eat (a small structure that eats another structure)." _____

2. Assemble a word that means "half water loving." _____

3. Assemble a word that means "condition of large cells." _____

4. Assemble a word that means "the study of large forms." _____

Concept 3: Disassembling Terms

lun root word meaning "crescent shape"; combining form *lun/o*

-ar suffix meaning "pertaining to"

By disassembling terms and identifying size word parts, you can determine the size of an object or structure. For example, the term *semilunar* can be broken into the prefix *semi-*, the root word *lun* (meaning "crescent shape"), and the suffix *-ar* (meaning "pertaining to"). Thus, *semilunar* means "pertaining to a half crescent shape."

Recall Activity

Use the word parts you have learned so far in this chapter to complete the following activities.

1. Disassemble and define the word *ultrahydrophobic*. _____

2. Disassemble and define the word *macrobiotic*. _____

3. Disassemble and define the word *microtension*. _____

4. Disassemble and define the word *lunule*. _____

Concept 4: Using Context

If you use context and know size word parts, you can interpret scientific terms, even if you do not know terms' exact meanings. For example, knowing that the prefix *macro-* means "large" can help you remember that your body requires large amounts of *macronutrients* (such as carbohydrates and proteins).

Recall Activity

For each scenario, use contextual knowledge and knowledge of word parts to fill in the blanks and complete the sentence.

1. Blood platelets develop from megakaryocytes, which are _____ in size.

2. A tubercule is a(n) _____ bone process.

3. A distance of 1 meter contains _____ centimeter(s).

4. An ultrasound, which produces sound waves _____ normal hearing, can diagnose an aneurysm.

5. In the condition microcardia, the heart is abnormally _____ in size.

6. A mass of 2 kilograms is equivalent to _____ gram(s).

7. A semicircular canal is shaped like _____ a circle.

8. An object's volume is 1 liter. This can also be written as _____ milliliter(s).

Section 2.6 Reinforcement

Answer the following questions using what you learned in this section.

1. *True or False*. The prefix *micro-* means "large." _____

2. Which of the following word parts means "half"?
   A. mega-
   B. semi-
   C. micro-
   D. ultra-

3. Write the letters backward: artlu. Define the word part that is formed. _____

_____

4. The suffix *-ule* means "_____."

5. Arrange these word parts in alphabetical order: mega-, semi-, micro-, ultra-, and macro-. _____

_____

6. Which of the following word parts mean "small"?

    A. mega-   C. micro-

    B. semi-   D. -ule

7. Unscramble the letters: eul. Define the word part that is formed. _____

_____

8. *True or False.* The prefix *micro-* describes an object smaller than the prefix *mega-*. _____

9. Write the letters backward: imes. Define the word part that is formed. _____

_____

10. Macrosis is a condition of a(n) _____ object.

11. Which of the following word parts means "beyond"?

    A. semi-   C. mega-

    B. macro-   D. ultra-

12. The prefixes _____ mean "large."

13. Micrology is the study of _____ objects.

14. *True or False.* The prefix *semi-* means "half." _____

15. The prefix *ultra-* means "_____."

16. *True or False.* The prefix *mega-* describes a small object. _____

17. Which of the following word parts are misspelled?

    A. utlra-   C. semmi-

    B. micro-   D. macro-

18. Unscramble the letters: corim. Define the word part that is formed. _____

_____

19. *True or False.* The prefix *ultra-* means "beyond." _____

20. The prefix *macro-* describes an object _____ than the suffix *-ule* does.

21. A microtome is a device for cutting extremely _____ sections of material.

Section 2.7 Word Parts Related to Shapes

Word parts can describe the shape of an object or structure. Knowing these word parts can help you imagine what an object or structure looks like. In this section, you will learn about word parts related to shapes.

The terms below are some of those that will be introduced in Section 2.7. To become familiar with these terms, reproduce each word on the line beside it. Pronounce each term as you write it. You will learn the definitions of these words as you complete this section.

1. platy- _____
2. coel/o _____
3. delt/o _____
4. glob/o _____
5. lat/o _____
6. rect/o _____

7. serrat/o _____
8. sten/o _____
9. strat/o _____
10. -oid _____
11. -ia _____

Concept 1: Shape Word Parts

Shape word parts indicate the general appearance of an object or structure. They can describe whether an object is narrow, triangular, or round. Below are some shape word parts commonly used in scientific terminology.

Word Part	Meaning
platy-	flat
coel/o	hollow
delt/o	triangular
glob/o	round
lat/o	wide
rect/o	straight
serrat/o	jagged
sten/o	narrow
strat/o	layer

Recall Activity

1. Write the definition of each word part.

    lat/o _____

    platy- _____

    serrat/o _____

    rect/o _____

    glob/o _____

    strat/o _____

    sten/o _____

    coel/o _____

    delt/o _____

2. Write the corresponding word part next to its definition.

    flat _____

    straight _____

    hollow _____

    layer _____

    narrow _____

    triangular _____

    wide _____

    jagged _____

    round _____

3. Draw lines to match the word parts with their meanings.

    lat/o   layer

    rect/o   hollow

    platy-   jagged

    glob/o   triangular

    coel/o   straight

    strat/o   flat

    delt/o   narrow

    serrat/o   wide

    sten/o   round

Concept 2: Assembling Terms

When you assemble terms using shape word parts, you make words that describe the shapes of objects or structures. For example, if you want to describe something resembling a globe, combine the root word *glob* and the suffix *-oid* (meaning "resembling") to make the word *globoid*.

-oid suffix meaning "resembling"

Recall Activity

Use the word parts you have learned so far in this chapter to complete the following activities. You can easily review all of the word parts covered in this chapter by referencing Appendix A in the back of the book.

1. Assemble a word that means "process of being jagged." _____

2. Assemble a word that means "resembling a triangle." _____

3. Assemble a word that means "condition of being narrow." _____

4. Assemble a word that means "straight structure." _____

Concept 3: Disassembling Terms

If a scientific term is formed from a shape word part, you can usually envision the shape of the object being described. For example, the term *stenocardia* can be disassembled into the combining form *sten/o*, the root word *cardi*, and the suffix *-ia* (meaning "condition"). *Stenocardia* means "condition of narrowing in the heart" (**Figure 2.8**).

-ia suffix meaning "condition"

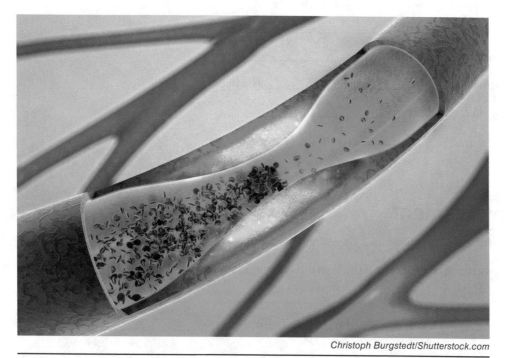

Christoph Burgstedt/Shutterstock.com

Figure 2.8 *Stenocardia* describes the narrowing of blood vessels in the heart. This often occurs due to buildup of plaque in the blood vessels. Stenocardia can cause *angina*, or a sensation of chest pain.

Recall Activity

Use the word parts you have learned so far in this chapter to complete the following activities.

1. Disassemble and define the word *stenosis*. _____

2. Disassemble and define the word *coelum*._____

3. Disassemble and define the word *stratum*. _____

4. Disassemble and define the word *platymorphia*. _____

Concept 4: Using Context

Using context and your knowledge of word parts, you can often infer the meaning of a scientific term even if you do not know its exact definition. Learning words from context can help expand your vocabulary. For example, knowing that the combining form *strat/o* means "layer," you can interpret that *stratified epithelium* consists of many layers.

Recall Activity

For each scenario, use contextual knowledge and knowledge of word parts to fill in the blanks and complete the sentence.

1. A globular protein is _____ in shape.

2. An acoelomate organism has no _____ body cavity.

3. The deltoid muscle is _____ in shape.

4. The serratus anterior muscle has a(n) _____ shape.

5. The shape of the rectus abdominis muscle is _____.

6. The latissimus dorsi muscle is _____ in shape.

7. The shape of the platysma muscle is _____.

8. Hemoglobin is _____ in shape.

Section 2.7 Reinforcement

Answer the following questions using what you learned in this section.

1. Write the letters backward: otarres. Define the word part that is formed. _____

   _____

2. Unscramble the letters: tplay. Define the word part that is formed._____

   _____

3. Identify the shape word part that is four letters long. _____

4. The combining form *coel/o* means "_____."

5. *True or False.* The prefix *platy-* means "flat." _____

6. Which of the following word parts means "straight"?
   A. platy-   C. glob/o
   B. rect/o   D. lat/o

7. *True or False.* The combining form *strat/o* means "layer." _____

8. Write the letters backward: onets. Define the word part that is formed. _____
   _____

9. *True or False.* Both *sten/o* and *strat/o* mean "round." _____

10. *Sten/o* is to "narrow" as _____ is to "wide."

11. Which of the following word parts are misspelled?
    A. glob/o   C. plati
    B. seratus/o   D. coel/o

12. Unscramble the letters: tloed. Define the word part that is formed. _____
    _____

13. Which of the following word parts means "narrow"?
    A. rect/o   C. serrat/o
    B. coel/o   D. sten/o

14. The combining form *glob/o* means "_____."

15. *True or False.* The combining form *delt/o* means "triangular." _____

16. Unscramble the letters: bloog. Define the word part that is formed. _____
    _____

17. *True or False.* The combining form *serrat/o* means "jagged." _____

18. Which of the following word parts means "layer"?
    A. sten/o   C. strat/o
    B. lat/o   D. coel/o

Comprehensive Review (Chapters 1–2)

Answer the following questions using what you have learned so far in this book.

19. Biology is the science that studies _____.

20. Identify and define the prefix of the term *hypersensitivity*. _____

Section 2.8 Word Parts Related to Locations

Word parts that relate to location describe the position of a structure or object. Many of these word parts describe location specifically on the human body and thus are important for comprehending anatomy and physiology. In this section, you will learn about word parts related to location.

The terms below are some of those that will be introduced in Section 2.8. To become familiar with these terms, reproduce each word on the line beside it. Pronounce each term as you write it. You will learn the definitions of these words as you complete this section.

1. de-_____
2. meso-_____
3. peri-_____
4. cortic/o_____
5. dors/o_____

6. later/o_____
7. medi/o_____
8. ventr/o_____
9. spin/o_____
10. oste/o_____

Concept 1: Location Word Parts

Word parts that describe location can help you identify the position of an object or structure in comparison to other structures and the human body. Below are some location word parts commonly used in scientific terminology.

Word Part	Meaning
de-	down from
meso-	middle
peri-	around
cortic/o	outer region
dors/o	back (of body)
later/o	side
medi/o	middle
ventr/o	belly side (of body)

Recall Activity

1. Write the definition of each word part.

ventr/o_____

peri-_____

medi/o_____

de-_____

dors/o_____

cortic/o_____

later/o _____

meso- _____

2. Write the corresponding word part next to its definition. Some questions will have two answers.

back (of body) _____

side _____

around _____

middle _____

belly side (of body) _____

down from _____

outer region _____

3. Draw lines to match the word parts with their meanings.

meso-	around
ventr/o	down from
dors/o	middle
cortic/o	back (of body)
later/o	belly side (of body)
peri-	side
de-	outer region

Concept 2: Assembling Terms

Using word parts related to location, you can describe the position of an object or structure on the human body. For example, to describe the back of the spine, combine the combining form *dors/o*, the root word *spin* (meaning "spine"), and the suffix *-al* to make the word *dorsospinal*. Dorsospinal means "character of the back of the spine" (**Figure 2.9**).

spin root word meaning "spine"; combining form *spin/o*

Recall Activity

Use the word parts you have learned so far in this chapter to complete the following activities. You can easily review all of the word parts covered in this chapter by referencing Appendix A in the back of the book.

1. Assemble a word that means "the structure around the heart." _____

2. Assemble a word that means "middle skin." _____

3. Assemble a word that means "character of the side." _____

4. Assemble a word that means "character of the side and belly of the body." _____

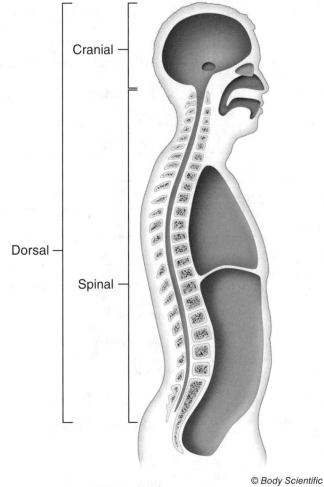

Cranial

Dorsal

Spinal

© Body Scientific International

Figure 2.9   The term *dorsospinal* refers to the back side of the spine.

Concept 3: Disassembling Terms

Disassembling terms and identifying their location word parts can help you envision placement on the body. For example, the word *periosteum* can be broken into the prefix *peri-*, the root word *oste* (meaning "bone"), and the suffix *-um*. The periosteum is the structure around a bone.

oste root word meaning "bone"; combining form *oste/o*

Recall Activity

Use the word parts you have learned so far in this chapter to complete the following activities.

1. Disassemble and define the word *periosteoma*._____

2. Disassemble and define the word *mesomorph*. _____

3. Disassemble and define the word *dorsal*._____

4. Disassemble and define the word *ventromedial*. _____

Concept 4: Using Context

If you use context and your knowledge of location word parts, you will be able to glean the meanings of many anatomical and scientific terms. You will be able to imagine structures on the body using just the terms and word parts you know. For example, knowing that the combining form *medi/o* means "middle," you can interpret that the *mediastinum* is a partition in the middle of two body cavities.

Recall Activity

For each scenario, use contextual knowledge and knowledge of word parts to fill in the blanks and complete the sentence.

1. Cerebrocortical matter is located in the _____ region of the brain.

2. The perimetrium is the outermost layer _____ the uterus.

3. The dorsal body cavity is located in the _____ part of the body.

4. Lateral ventricles are C-shaped chambers in the _____ of the brain.

5. The mesothelium is the _____ lining in a body cavity.

6. The ventral body cavity is located in the _____ part of the body.

7. Deglutition is the movement of food _____ the throat.

Section 2.8 Reinforcement

Answer the following questions using what you learned in this section.

1. *True or False.* Adrenocortical matter is located in the outer portion of the adrenal gland. _____

2. Which of the following word parts means "side"?
   A. medi/o
   B. later/o
   C. meso-
   D. ventr/o

3. Write the letters backward: ocitroc. Define the word part that is formed. _____
   _____

4. The combining form *ventr/o* means "_____."

5. Unscramble the letters: ripe. Define the word part that is formed._____
   _____

6. Which of the following word parts means "back (of the body)"?
   A. ventr/o
   B. later/o
   C. meso-
   D. dors/o

7. List the two location word parts that begin with the letter *m*._____

8. *True or False.* The prefix *de-* means "middle." _____

9. Unscramble the letters: reolat. Define the word part that is formed. _____

   _____

10. *True or False.* The prefix *meso-* means "middle," and the combining form *medi/o* means "side." _____

11. Write the letters backward: ortnev. Define the word part that is formed. _____

    _____

12. Which of the following word parts has the most letters?
    A. medi/o   C. meso-
    B. peri-   D. cortic/o

13. Unscramble the letters: diome. Define the word part that is formed. _____

    _____

14. The prefix *peri-* means "_____."

15. Identify and define the location word part in the term *corticosteroid*. _____

16. *True or False.* The prefix *de-* means "down from." _____

17. The word part _____ means "side."

18. Which of the following word parts mean "middle"?
    A. de-   C. peri-   E. medi/o
    B. meso-   D. ventr/o   F. later/o

19. *True or False.* The word parts *peri-* and *cortic/o* both mean "around." _____

20. A laterodeviation is a displacement to the _____.

Comprehensive Review (Chapters 1–2)

Answer the following questions using what you have learned so far in this book.

21. Abduction is movement _____ the midline of the body.

22. Should one *accept* or *believe* the evidence presented in a scientific explanation? Explain.

    _____

Section 2.9 Word Parts Related to the Body

Understanding word parts can help you comprehend anatomy and physiology. Some word parts pertain to specific body parts or areas of the body. In this section, you will learn about word parts that refer to body structures.

The following terms are some of those that will be introduced in Section 2.9. To become familiar with these terms, reproduce each word on the line beside it.

Pronounce each term as you write it. You will learn the definitions of these words as you complete this section.

1. arthr/o _____
2. cerebr/o _____
3. enter/o _____
4. gastr/o _____
5. hem/o _____
6. hepat/o _____

7. my/o _____
8. neur/o _____
9. ren/o _____
10. -algia _____
11. -itis _____

Concept 1: Body Word Parts

Word parts referring to specific body structures are used often in the study of anatomy and physiology. You have already learned some body word parts in this chapter. For example, you have learned that the combining form *cardi/o* means "heart," the combining form *derm/o* means "skin," and the combining form *oste/o* means "bone." Below are some other body word parts commonly used in scientific terminology.

Word Part	Meaning
arthr/o	joint
cerebr/o	brain
enter/o	intestine
gastr/o	stomach
hem/o	blood
hepat/o	liver
my/o	muscle
neur/o	nerve
ren/o	kidney

Recall Activity

1. Write the definition of each word part.

my/o _____

ren/o _____

gastr/o _____

arthr/o _____

enter/o _____

hepat/o _____

neur/o _____

hem/o _____

cerebr/o _____

2. Write the corresponding word part next to its definition.

kidney _____

stomach _____

blood _____

joint _____

nerve _____

muscle _____

brain _____

liver _____

intestine _____

3. Draw lines to match the word parts with their meanings.

neur/o	stomach
gastr/o	joint
hem/o	blood
my/o	liver
enter/o	kidney
hepat/o	brain
ren/o	intestine
cerebr/o	nerve
arthr/o	muscle

Concept 2: Assembling Terms

Using body word parts, you can assemble terms describing anatomical structures. You can also assemble terms that describe diseases or conditions related to certain body parts. For example, to describe pain in a nerve, combine the root word *neur* and the suffix *-algia* (meaning "pain") to form the word *neuralgia*.

-algia suffix meaning "pain"

Recall Activity

Use the word parts you have learned so far in this chapter to complete the following activities. You can easily review all of the word parts covered in this chapter by referencing Appendix A in the back of the book.

1. Assemble a word that means "the study of nerves." _____

2. Assemble a word that means "muscle production." _____

3. Assemble a word that means "pain in a joint." _____

4. Assemble a word that means "to cut into the intestine."_____

5. Assemble a word that means "breakdown of blood." _____

Concept 3: Disassembling Terms

When you encounter scientific vocabulary—especially vocabulary related to anatomy and diseases of the human body—you can determine the meaning of a word by disassembling it into its word parts. For example, the term *hepatitis* can be broken down into the root word *hepat* and the suffix *-itis* (meaning "inflammation"). Hepatitis describes the inflammation of the liver.

-itis suffix meaning "inflammation"

Recall Activity

Use the word parts you have learned so far in this chapter to complete the following activities.

1. Disassemble and define the word *arthrosis*. _____

2. Disassemble and define the word *myocytolysis*. _____

3. Disassemble and define the word *suprarenal*. _____

4. Disassemble and define the word *cerebroma*. _____

5. Disassemble and define the word *gastroenteritis*._____

6. Disassemble and define the word *hepatologist*._____

Concept 4: Using Context

Using context and knowledge of body word parts, you can interpret scientific terms more easily when learning about the human body. This skill will be important as you enter the study of anatomy and physiology. For example, if you know that the combining form *my/o* means "muscle," you can infer that the *epimysium*, a structure continuous with a tendon, is part of a muscle (**Figure 2.10**).

Recall Activity

For each scenario, use contextual knowledge and knowledge of word parts to fill in the blanks and complete the sentence.

1. The cerebrum consists of two hemispheres. The cerebrum is part of the _____.

2. Renal failure, a major cause of death, is failure of the _____.

3. Arthrodesis is a surgical procedure involving a(n) _____.

4. Gastric glands secrete gastric juice in the _____.

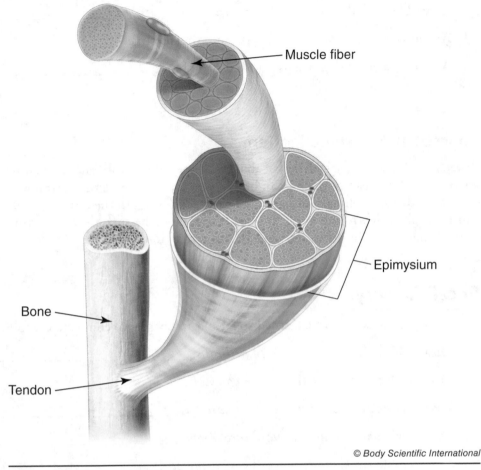

Muscle fiber

Epimysium

Bone

Tendon

© Body Scientific International

Figure 2.10 The epimysium is part of a muscle.

Section 2.9 Reinforcement

Answer the following questions using what you learned in this section.

1. Unscramble the letters: treeon. Define the word part that is formed. _____

   _____

2. Which of the following word parts means "blood"?

   A. gastr/o   C. cardi/o

   B. hem/o   D. my/o

3. Write the letters backward: otapeh. Define the word part that is formed._____

   _____

4. The combining form *ren/o* means "_____."

5. Arrange the following word parts in alphabetical order: gastr/o, neur/o, ren/o, hepat/o, hem/o, and my/o. _____

6. Which of the following word parts means "stomach"?

   A. hem/o   C. my/o   E. neur/o

   B. gastr/o   D. hepat/o   F. enter/o

7. Unscramble the letters: brcoeer. Define the word part that is formed. _____

_____

8. *True or False.* Hepatocytes are found in the liver. _____

9. Write the letters backward: oruen. Define the word part that is formed. _____

_____

10. *True or False.* The combining form *hem/o* means "blood." _____

11. "Heart" is to *cardi/o* as "stomach" is to _____.

12. Which of the following word parts means "joint"?
    A. oste/o   C. ren/o   E. arthr/o
    B. gastr/o   D. neur/o   F. cerebr/o

13. Which of the following word parts has the most letters?
    A. gastr/o   C. ren/o   E. neur/o
    B. cerebr/o   D. arthr/o   F. oste/o

14. *True or False.* The combining form *hepat/o* means "blood."_____

15. The combining form _____ means "brain."

16. *True or False.* The combining form *arthr/o* means "bone." _____

17. Which of the following word parts means "intestine"?
    A. hem/o   C. enter/o
    B. gastr/o   D. hepat/o

18. Which part of the body does a gastrologist study? _____

19. *True or False.* The combining form *enter/o* means "stomach."_____

20. Which of the following word parts are misspelled?
    A. ren/o   C. my/o   E. anthr/o
    B. neurm/o   D. hetap/o   F. hem/o

Comprehensive Review (Chapters 1–2)

Answer the following questions using what you have learned so far in this book.

21. *True or False.* The prefix *pseudo-* means "true."_____

22. How many tasks can you do well at one time?_____

Chapter 2 Review

Answer the following questions using what you learned in this chapter.

1. Identify and define the combining form of the term *biography*. _____

2. The root word of the term *dimorphous* is _____.

3. Identify and define the suffix of the term *homeostasis*. _____

4. Disassemble and define the word *bilateral*. _____

5. The suffix -*lysis* means "_____."

6. Disassemble and define the word *amorphous*. _____

7. Hepatitis describes an inflammation of the _____.

8. *True or False.* The suffix -*plasm* means "producer." _____

9. Which of the following word parts are misspelled?
   A. -phillic   C. anthr/o
   B. hyper-   D. -phobic

10. The prefix *hypo-* means "_____."

11. A postmenopausal condition occurs _____ menopause.

12. Which of the following word parts means the opposite of "below"?
    A. hyper-   C. pre-
    B. hypo-   D. post-

13. The prefix *inter-* means "_____."

14. The combining form *bi/o* means "_____."

15. Assemble a word that means "condition inside the heart." _____

16. Identify and define the combining form of the term *physiology*. _____

17. Which of the following word parts means "above"?
    A. dis-   C. ef-   E. ad-
    B. con-   D. ab-   F. supra-

18. The prefix *dis-* means "_____."

19. Identify and define the root word of the term *dehydration*. _____

20. Disassemble and define the word *hemicerebrum*. _____

21. Which of the following word parts represents the largest value?
    A. uni-   C. bi-
    B. tri-   D. di-

22. Cerebrospinal fluid circulates in the spinal cord and in the _____.

23. Which of the following word parts means "under"?
    A. infra-   C. ab-
    B. inter-   D. ad-

24. Which two word parts mean "one"? _____

25. If an embryo is triploblastic, how many cell layers does it have? _____

26. In polycythemia, the bone marrow makes too _____ red blood cells.

27. Identify the two word parts that mean "four." _____

28. Erythroblasts are _____ in color.

29. Which of the following word parts means "black"?
   A. lute/o   C. rubr/o
   B. melan/o   D. alb/o

30. The word parts *micro-* and *-ule* both mean "_____."

31. A hemisphere is _____ of a sphere.

32. *True or False.* The combining form *cortic/o* means "core." _____

33. Which of the following word parts means "belly side (of body)"?
   A. ventr/o   C. meso-
   B. dors/o   D. medi/o

34. Assemble a word that means "the study of the stomach and intestine." _____

35. The combining form _____ means "round."

36. The combining form *delt/o* means "_____."

37. The term *osteoarthritis* describes the inflammation of the _____ and

   _____.

Comprehensive Review (Chapters 1–2)

Using what you have learned so far in this book, match the following terms with their definitions.

_____ 38. A combining form that means "back (of the body)"

_____ 39. The science that studies life

_____ 40. A suffix that means "character of"

_____ 41. A prefix that means "against"

_____ 42. A prefix that means "six"

_____ 43. A combining form that means "green"

_____ 44. A physically observable fact or event

_____ 45. A combining form that means "kidney"

_____ 46. A word or phrase that can help you recall information

_____ 47. A prefix that means "out of"

_____ 48. An area of biology that studies cells

A. mnemonic
B. chlor/o
C. dors/o
D. -al
E. biology
F. hexa-
G. ren/o
H. ex-
I. phenomenon
J. anti-
K. cytology

Chapter 3
Scientific Methods

Introduction

Your understanding of the natural world is based in science. Science is key to comprehending phenomena around you and to learning about chemistry, biology, and anatomy and physiology. Scientific methods are pathways to understanding the world. There is no one single scientific method. In this chapter, you will learn about two: the experimental scientific method and the diagnostic scientific method. In this chapter, you will also learn about how facts are used in science and scientific laws and theories.

Objectives

After completing this chapter, you will be able to

- understand that science is a part of everyday life
- know that there is not just one scientific method
- list the steps in the experimental scientific method
- recognize the components of a hypothesis
- know how to conduct an experiment
- list the steps in the diagnostic scientific method
- understand how to gather and sift facts
- explain how to make a diagnosis
- understand the importance of facts, scientific laws, and scientific theories
- identify the parts of a scientific article

Key Terms

The following terms and phrases will be introduced and explained in Chapter 3. Read through the list to become familiar with the words.

analysis	experimental scientific method
anemia	humane
constant	hypothesis
control group	independent variable
decide	kidney stone
dehydration	literature
dependent variable	OHEAD
diabetes	scientific law
diagnose	scientific method
diagnostic scientific method	scientific theory
evidence	sift
experiment	subject
experimental group	

Section 3.1 Science Is Part of Everyday Life

As you have learned, *science* is the body of knowledge and techniques (scientific methods) that enables mankind to explain the natural world. Science seeks *natural* explanations, or explanations that are observable and testable. Science is not concerned with the supernatural. Science and its methods are part of everyday life. They involve your observations and the conclusions you draw based on those observations. In this section, you will explore the role that science plays in everyday life experiences and will be introduced to the concept of scientific methods.

The terms below are some of those that will be introduced in Section 3.1. To become familiar with these terms, reproduce each word on the line beside it. Pronounce each term as you write it. You will learn the definitions of these words as you complete this section.

1. scientific method _____

2. evidence _____

Concept 1: An Everyday Problem

Science is how you understand the natural world based on the evidence you have today. You use the methods of science all the time. You start with an everyday problem. As an example, your jeep will not start. You turn the key, and the starter does not turn the engine over. You wonder, *What is the cause of this problem? How can I figure out how to get my jeep to start?* As you consider the problem, you begin to think about possible explanations. In science, you only consider natural (testable and observable) explanations.

Recall Activity

1. In science, you only consider _____ explanations.

2. Read the following explanations for your jeep not starting. Circle the natural explanations and draw boxes around the supernatural explanations.

   A. The battery is dead.

   B. Gremlins stole the magic from the jeep.

   C. The jeep decided not to start today.

   D. The starter switch wire is broken.

Concept 2: Possible Cause

After considering some natural explanations for your jeep not starting, you choose one natural explanation to explore. Since the engine will not start and you don't hear the starter turning the engine over, the battery may be dead. So you test the jeep battery. The results of the test will determine what you do next.

Recall Activity

1. The results of the _____ will determine what you do next.

2. After considering some natural explanations for your jeep not starting, you choose _____ natural explanation(s) to explore.

Concept 3: Test Results

You test the jeep battery by measuring the voltage reading between the positive and negative posts. A dead battery would have a reading of less than 12 volts (V). The jeep's battery reading in **Figure 3.1** is 12.3 V, so the battery is not dead. The battery is not causing the problem.

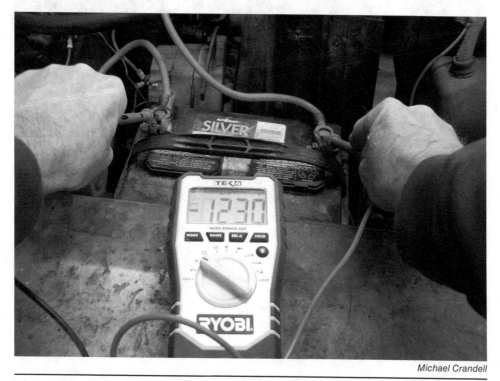

Michael Crandell

Figure 3.1 This test shows that the battery is not dead.

Recall Activity

1. A dead battery would have a reading of less than 12 V. Because the jeep's battery reading is 12.3 V, the battery _____ dead.

2. The battery is tested by measuring the _____ reading between the positive and negative posts.

Concept 4: New Possible Cause

While the jeep battery is not causing the problem, an inspection of the battery cables reveals that the negative cable is loose. The loose negative cable means that the vehicle electrical system is not complete and may be causing the jeep to not start. Tightening the cable completes the vehicle electrical system (**Figure 3.2**). The jeep starts.

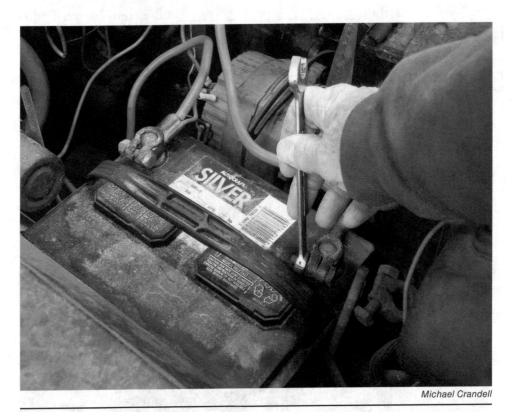

Michael Crandell

Figure 3.2 Tightening the loose cable solves the problem.

Recall Activity

1. An inspection of the battery cables finds that the negative cable is _____.

2. _____ the cable completes the vehicle electrical system.

Concept 5: Steps in Everyday Science

In concepts 1–4, you used a logical sequence of steps to solve an everyday problem. You observed a problem, predicted a possible solution to the problem, tested the possible solution, and evaluated the results of the test. When the first solution didn't work, you tried another solution.

Recall Activity

1. In concepts 1–4, you used a(n) _____ sequence of steps to solve an everyday problem.

2. When the first solution didn't work, you tried _____ solution.

3. After observing a problem, you _____ a possible solution to the problem and then _____ the possible solution.

Concept 6: Scientific Method

In solving the everyday problem of your jeep not starting, you used a scientific technique, or a *scientific method*. Scientific methods are logical processes that enable mankind to solve problems and answer questions about the natural world.

Science is approachable by many pathways. Scientific methods test a statement with facts, but there is no one single scientific method. Instead, science utilizes different types of *evidence* (facts that relate to a possible cause) from many sources to answer a variety of questions. All scientific methods are logical processes that enable mankind to evaluate the natural world.

scientific method a logical process for solving problems and answering questions about the natural world

evidence facts that relate to a possible cause

Recall Activity

1. Scientific methods are _____ processes.

2. Science utilizes different types of _____ from many sources.

3. Science is approachable by many _____.

Concept 7: Testing with Facts

Using scientific methods, scientists propose an answer to a question or a solution to a problem. Then they test the proposal with *facts* (confirmed observations). The proposal is rejected if any fact contradicts the proposal. If facts support the proposal, more facts are gathered. If no facts contradict the answer or solution, scientists are more certain that the proposal is correct.

Fitting facts together is like assembling a jigsaw puzzle (**Figure 3.3**). More facts give you a clearer view. If a fact contradicts a proposal, the proposal must be rejected and modified to test again.

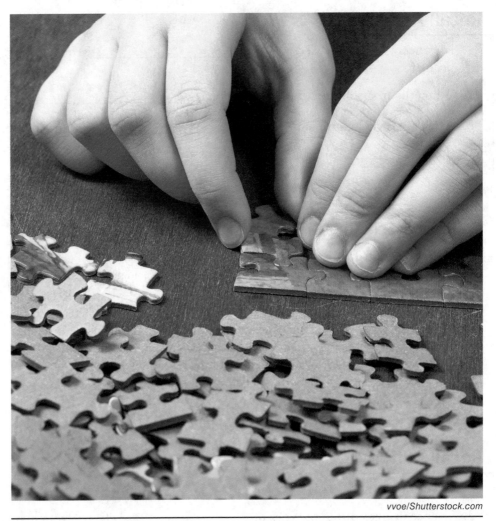

vvoe/Shutterstock.com

Figure 3.3 When you assemble a jigsaw puzzle, fitting more pieces together gives you a better view of the whole picture.

Recall Activity

1. Scientists test a proposed solution with _____.

2. If a fact contradicts a proposal, the proposal must be _____ and _____ to test again.

3. Fitting facts together is like assembling a(n) _____.

Section 3.1 Reinforcement

Answer the following questions using what you learned in this section.

1. *True or False.* There is one universal scientific method. _____

2. Scientists propose a(n) _____ to a question or a solution to a problem.

3. *True or False.* Scientists test a proposal with facts. _____

4. If facts support a proposal, more _____ are gathered.

5. Fitting _____ together is like assembling a jigsaw puzzle.

6. Scientific methods are the _____ processes that enable mankind to solve problems.

7. *True or False.* Science is how you understand the natural world. _____

8. What does a scientist do if a first solution to a problem doesn't work?_____

_____

9. A proposal is _____ if any fact contradicts the proposal.

10. Unscramble the letters: temdoh. Define the word that is formed._____

_____

11. *True or False.* You use the methods of science all the time. _____

12. Unscramble the letters: needvice. Define the word that is formed. _____

_____

13. *True or False.* More facts give you a clearer view. _____

14. All scientific methods are _____ processes that enable mankind to evaluate the natural world.

15. A logical process to evaluate the natural world is known as a(n) _____.

Comprehensive Review (Chapters 1–3)

Answer the following questions using what you have learned so far in this book.

16. Which of the following combining forms means "red"?
    A. lute/o
    B. melan/o
    C. rubr/o
    D. alb/o

17. Science utilizes different types of _____, or facts that relate to a possible cause.

18. _____ is the body of knowledge and techniques that enables mankind to explain the natural world.

Section 3.2 The Experimental Scientific Method Pathway

There are many scientific methods, all of which use evidence to evaluate the natural world. In this section, you will learn about one scientific method: the experimental scientific method.

The terms below are some of those that will be introduced in Section 3.2. To become familiar with these terms, reproduce each word on the line beside it. Pronounce each term as you write it. You will learn the definitions of these words as you complete this section.

1. experimental scientific method _____

2. OHEAD _____

3. hypothesis _____

4. independent variable _____

5. dependent variable _____

6. experiment _____

7. control group _____

8. experimental group _____

9. constant _____

10. analysis _____

11. decide _____

Concept 1: Steps in the Experimental Scientific Method

experimental scientific method a scientific method that formulates a prediction and then tests the prediction to obtain data

OHEAD an acronym for the five steps of the experimental scientific method: observation, hypothesis, experiment, analysis, and decide

The *experimental scientific method* formulates a prediction and then tests the prediction to obtain data. There are five steps in the experimental scientific method. You can easily remember them using the acronym *OHEAD*. The five steps are

- Observation
- Hypothesis
- Experiment
- Analysis
- Decide

The first step in the experimental scientific method is observation. In this case, an *observation* is based on the phenomenon that you have witnessed, detected, or read about.

Recall Activity

1. A(n) _____ is based on a phenomenon that you have witnessed, detected, or read about.

2. OHEAD stands for _____, _____,

_____, _____, and _____.

Concept 2: Hypothesis

The second step in the experimental scientific method is *hypothesis*. You may do research to obtain facts so your hypothesis aligns with what is already known. A *hypothesis* is a prediction about the outcome of an experiment. A hypothesis is also an "if/then" statement. You predict that *if* you do *this*, *then* *that* will happen. In a hypothesis, you are trying to connect the facts of the "this" portion of the hypothesis to the facts of the "that" portion.

Here is an example of a hypothesis: If laboratory rats are fed a diet that has 25% more calories than their existing diet, then their body weights will increase by at least 15%. The hypothesis is trying to prove the relationship between increased calorie intake ("this") and weight gain ("that").

hypothesis a prediction about the outcome of an experiment

Recall Activity

1. A hypothesis is a(n) _____ about the outcome of an experiment.

2. In a hypothesis, you predict that *if* you do _____ , *then* _____ will happen.

Concept 3: Variables

There are two *variables*, or changeable parts, in a hypothesis: the independent variable and the dependent variable. The *independent variable* is the "if" part of the hypothesis. It is manipulated to see if the *dependent variable* (the "then" part of the hypothesis) changes. In a hypothesis, you are predicting that change in the dependent variable depends on change in the independent variable.

independent variable the "if" part of a hypothesis; is manipulated to see if the dependent variable changes

dependent variable the "then" part of a hypothesis; hypothesized to depend on change in the independent variable

Recall Activity

1. The two variables in a hypothesis are the _____ variable and the _____ variable.

2. In a hypothesis, you are predicting that change in the _____ variable depends on change in the _____ variable.

3. The _____ variable is manipulated.

4. The "then" portion of a hypothesis is the _____ variable.

5. The _____ portion of a hypothesis is the independent variable.

experiment a test of a hypothesis

control group the part of an experiment that does *not* receive the independent variable

experimental group the part of an experiment that *does* receive the independent variable

constant an untested factor that could affect the dependent variable; is kept the same across all groups in an experiment

Concept 4: Experiment

The third step in the experimental scientific method is *experiment*. An *experiment* tests a hypothesis to find out if the independent variable will cause the predicted results in the dependent variable.

An experiment has a control group, an experimental group, and constants. The *control group* is the part of an experiment that does *not* receive the independent variable. The *experimental group* is the part of an experiment that *does* receive the independent variable. *Constants* are untested factors that could affect the dependent variable. These factors are kept the same across both groups in an experiment. At the end of an experiment, you compare the results from the experimental group to the results from the control group.

Recall Activity

1. A(n) _____ tests a hypothesis.

2. An experiment has a(n) _____ group, a(n) _____ group, and _____.

3. What is the difference between the experimental group and the control group? _____

_____

4. Which groups in an experiment have constants? _____

Concept 5: Analysis

analysis the step of the experimental scientific method in which data from the experiment is examined

In the *analysis* step of the experimental scientific method, the data from the experiment is examined. Because the only difference between the experimental group and control group is the independent variable, any difference between the experimental and control groups must be due to the independent variable. The data is examined to answer this question: *Did the independent variable cause the predicted change in the dependent variable?*

Recall Activity

1. Data is examined in the _____ step of the experimental scientific method.

2. Differences between the _____ and _____ groups must be due to the independent variable.

3. What question does the analysis of experimental data seek to answer? _____

_____

Concept 6: Decide

In the last step of the experimental scientific method, you *decide* to accept or reject the hypothesis. If data from the experiment shows the predicted change in the dependent variable, you accept the hypothesis. If data does *not* show the predicted change in the dependent variable, you reject the hypothesis. If you accept the hypothesis, you accept that the independent variable caused change in the dependent variable. If you reject the hypothesis, you do not accept that the independent variable caused change in the dependent variable.

decide the fifth step in the experimental scientific method in which one accepts or rejects the hypothesis

Recall Activity

1. In the last step of the experimental scientific method, you _____ to accept or reject the hypothesis.

2. If data does not show the predicted change, you _____ the hypothesis.

3. If data does show the predicted change, you _____ the hypothesis.

Concept 7: Beyond the Five Steps

The fifth step of the experimental scientific method is not the end of testing a hypothesis. If you accept the hypothesis, you do the experiment again to see if the results are the same. If you reject the hypothesis, you devise a new hypothesis and test that. If, after several repeated experiments, the experiment results are consistent, the results can be published. Concept 6 of Section 3.6 discusses publication in a scientific journal.

Recall Activity

1. If you _____ the hypothesis, you do the experiment again.

2. If you _____ the hypothesis, you devise a new hypothesis and test that.

Section 3.2 Reinforcement

Answer the following questions using what you learned in this section.

1. A hypothesis _____ that *if* you do *this*, *then that* will happen.

2. The "if" portion of a hypothesis is the _____ variable.

3. A(n) _____ is based on a phenomenon that you have witnessed, detected, or read about.

4. In the last step of the experimental scientific method, you decide to _____ or _____ the hypothesis.

5. *True or False.* The experimental group has constants. _____

6. Constants are _____ factors.

7. If you reject the hypothesis, you devise a new _____ and test that.

8. The second step of the experimental scientific method is _____.

9. In a hypothesis, you are predicting that change in the dependent variable _____ on change in the independent variable.

10. In the _____ step, the data from an experiment is examined.

11. *True or False.* If you accept the hypothesis, you do the experiment again. _____

12. The control and experimental groups in an experiment have exactly the same _____.

13. A(n) _____ is a prediction about the outcome of an experiment.

14. An experiment tests a(n) _____.

15. *True or False.* In an experiment, the control group receives the independent variable. _____

16. The "then" portion of a hypothesis is the _____ variable.

17. Unscramble the letters: hosisyphet. Define the word that is formed. _____ _____

18. In the last step of the experimental scientific method, you decide to accept or reject the _____.

19. The third step of the experimental scientific method is _____.

20. *True or False.* If you accept the hypothesis, you are done experimenting. _____

Match the following terms with their definitions.

_____ 21. The step in the experimental scientific method that tests the hypothesis

_____ 22. The group in an experiment that does not receive the independent variable

_____ 23. Untested factors that both the groups in an experiment have

_____ 24. A prediction about the outcome of an experiment

_____ 25. The "if" part of a hypothesis

_____ 26. The "then" part of a hypothesis

A. hypothesis
B. independent variable
C. constants
D. experiment
E. dependent variable
F. control group

Comprehensive Review (Chapters 1–3)

Answer the following questions using what you have learned so far in this book.

27. The prefix in the word *abiotic* means "_____."

28. The plural form of *phenomenon* is _____.

29. Science utilizes different types of _____ from many sources.

Section 3.3 The Experimental Scientific Method in Action

Now that you have learned about the experimental scientific method, this section will demonstrate the experimental scientific method in action as you analyze an experiment about fat gain in rats.

The terms below are some of those that will be introduced in Section 3.3. To become familiar with these terms, reproduce each word on the line beside it. Pronounce each term as you write it. You will learn the definitions of these words as you complete this section.

1. subject _____

2. humane _____

Concept 1: Make an Observation

The first step in the experimental scientific method is observation. For this example, you observe that people eating a high-fat diet seem to have more fat than people eating a low-fat diet. You know that eating excess calories will cause an increase in fat, but does a high-fat diet itself cause a gain of fat? You will use the experimental scientific method to answer this question. Since you cannot experiment on humans, you will use rats as your test *subjects* (the organisms on which you are experimenting). You will follow accepted criteria for the *humane* care, or the kind and ethical care, of lab rats during the experiment (**Figure 3.4**).

subject the organism on which you are experimenting

humane kind and ethical

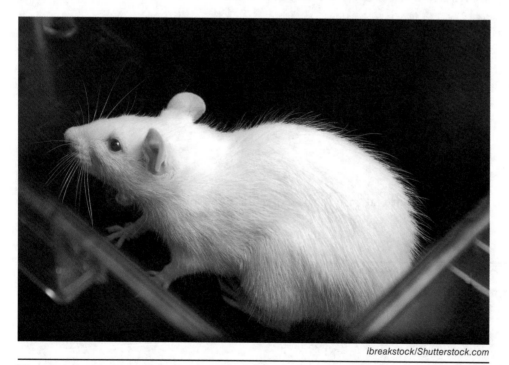

ibreakstock/Shutterstock.com

Figure 3.4 You will perform your experiment on rats.

Recall Activity

1. You observe that people eating a high-fat diet seem to _____ than people eating a low-fat diet.

2. You will follow accepted criteria for the _____ care of lab rats during your experiment.

Concept 2: Develop a Hypothesis

As you have learned, a hypothesis is a prediction about the outcome of an experiment. You are interested in the effects of a high-fat diet on gain of fat. In this experiment, the high-fat diet is the independent variable. Gain of fat is the dependent variable. Here is your hypothesis: If rats are fed a high-fat diet, then they will gain more fat.

Recall Activity

1. In your experiment, the _____ is the independent variable.

2. A hypothesis is a(n) _____ about the outcome of an experiment.

3. Gain of fat is the _____ variable.

Concept 3: Perform an Experiment

An experiment tests a hypothesis. In this experiment, you are going to feed two groups of rats: an experimental group and a control group. The experimental group will be fed a high-fat diet, and the control group will be fed a low-fat diet. The experiment will last 80 days. After that time, you will compare fat gain in the experimental group to fat gain in the control group.

Recall Activity

1. After the experiment, you will compare fat gain in the experimental group to fat gain in the _____ group.

2. An experiment _____ a hypothesis.

3. The _____ group will be fed a high-fat diet.

4. The _____ group will be fed a low-fat diet.

Concept 4: The Control Group

The control group is the standard for comparison. It does *not* receive the independent variable. Because you know that excess calories cause an increase in fat, you will feed rats in the control group a low-fat diet that has the same number of calories as the high-fat diet.

Recall Activity

1. The control group does not receive the _____ variable.

2. The rats in the control group will eat a low-fat diet that has the same number of _____ as the high-fat diet.

Concept 5: Understanding Constants

Constants are untested factors that could affect the dependent variable. Because you are only testing the independent variable, you must keep all constants the same for the experimental group and the control group. After the experiment, you will compare the results obtained with the independent variable to the results obtained without the independent variable. If all constants are the same, any differences *must* be caused by the independent variable because the independent variable is the only different factor.

Recall Activity

1. _____ are untested factors that could affect the dependent variable.

2. If all constants are the same, any differences must be caused by the _____ variable.

Concept 6: Regulating Constants

In developing your experiment, you must make sure that constants are the same in the control group and the experimental group. To do this, you regulate the following constant factors:

- The rats are selected at random from a genetically diverse population of 65- to 70-day-old rats weighing 250–350 grams (g) each.
- The rats are kept in identical individual cages and are held at a uniform temperature of 22°C with 12 hours of light and 12 hours of darkness. Both groups of rats are fed at the beginning of the dark cycle.

- The high-fat diet contains 20 g fat/100 g food. The low-fat diet contains 4 g fat/100 g food, but contains the same number of calories as the high-fat diet.
- The amount of fat in each rat will be measured the same way for the experimental group and the control group.

By ensuring these factors are constant for the control group and the experimental group, you can be more confident that any differences in the groups of rats after the experiment are due to the independent variable.

Recall Activity

1. The rat cages are held at a(n) _____ temperature of 22°C.

2. The rats are selected at _____ from a genetically diverse population.

3. Both groups of rats are fed at the beginning of the _____ cycle.

4. Constants are the _____ in the control group and the experimental group.

Concept 7: Analyze the Data

After performing the experiment, you collect the data shown in **Figure 3.5**. The data shows that the rats in the experimental group have more grams of fat per 100 g body weight.

Experimental Group	Control Group
13.4 g/100 g body weight	7.8 g/100 g body weight
11.6 g/100 g body weight	8.5 g/100 g body weight
13.1 g/100 g body weight	8.0 g/100 g body weight
13.4 g/100 g body weight	9.8 g/100 g body weight
12.5 g/100 g body weight	8.9 g/100 g body weight

Figure 3.5 The results from the experiment are recorded in grams per 100 g body weight.

Recall Activity

1. Add the values for the rats in the experimental group: _____ g/500 g body weight.

2. Add the values for the rats in the control group: _____ g/500 g body weight.

3. Divide the total value for the rats in the experimental group by 5: _____ g/100 g body weight.

4. Divide the total value for the rats in the control group by 5: _____ g/100 g body weight.

Concept 8: Accept or Reject the Hypothesis

If the data from your experiment supports your hypothesis, you accept the hypothesis. If the data does *not* support your hypothesis, you reject the hypothesis.

Recall Activity

1. Write the hypothesis for this experiment. _____
   _____

2. Did the experimental group have more fat than the control group? _____

3. Do you accept or reject the hypothesis? Explain. _____
   _____

4. What two facts are connected by these results? _____
   _____

Section 3.3 Reinforcement

Answer the following questions using what you learned in this section.

1. All constants are _____ for the experimental and control groups.

2. In this experiment, you used rats as your test _____.

3. In the experiment, you observed that people eating a high-fat diet seem to _____ than people eating a low-fat diet.

4. *True or False.* A hypothesis is a prediction about the outcome of an experiment. _____

5. Unscramble the letters: laasysni. Define the word that is formed. _____
   _____

6. An experiment only tests the _____ variable.

7. If the data does not support your hypothesis, you _____ the hypothesis.

8. The data from the experiment was measured in grams/_____ g body weight.

9. *True or False.* Controls are untested factors that could affect the dependent variable. _____

10. Before the experiment, you knew that excess calories cause an increase in _____.

11. _____ rats are fed a high-fat diet, _____ they will gain more fat.

12. Noticing that people who eat a lot of fat gain fat is an example of a(n) _____.

13. The control group does not receive the _____ variable.

14. *True or False.* Only the control rat group was fed at the beginning of the dark cycle. _____

15. Unscramble the letters: assnnttoc. Define the word that is formed. _____

_____

16. In an experiment, the _____ is the standard for comparison.

17. The feeding time, the ages of the rats, and temperature were _____ in the experiment.

18. *True or False.* All rats were fed the same number of calories. _____

19. Constants are _____ factors that could affect the dependent variable.

20. In the experiment, gain of fat was the _____ variable.

Comprehensive Review (Chapters 1–3)

Answer the following questions using what you have learned so far in this book.

21. A(n) _____ is a prediction about the outcome of an experiment.

22. Which combining form means "layer"? _____

23. A(n) _____ explanation of lightning is an electrical discharge between clouds or clouds and the earth.

Section 3.4 The Diagnostic Scientific Method Pathway

Another type of scientific method is the diagnostic scientific method. The diagnostic scientific method seeks to diagnose an ailment. In this section, you will learn about the steps in the diagnostic scientific method.

The terms below are some of those that will be introduced in Section 3.4. To become familiar with these terms, reproduce each word on the line beside it. Pronounce each term as you write it. You will learn the definitions of these words as you complete this section.

1. diagnostic scientific method _____

2. sift _____

3. diagnose _____

Concept 1: Steps in the Diagnostic Scientific Method

If a patient presents with an ailment, the task of the healthcare professional is to determine the cause of and treatment for the ailment. To do this, you use the diagnostic scientific method. The *diagnostic scientific method* gathers facts from two sources: patient history and a physical exam of the patient. There are four steps in the diagnostic scientific method:

- Facts
- Sift
- Test
- Diagnose

diagnostic scientific method a scientific method that collects facts from patient history and a physical exam of the patient; has four steps (facts, sift, test, and diagnose)

In the diagnostic scientific method, facts are sifted to determine possible causes of an ailment. These causes are ranked from *most likely* to *least likely*. Tests are performed to confirm if the most likely cause is the actual reason for the ailment. If the most likely cause is not supported, the next most likely cause is tested. Testing continues until a diagnosis is reached.

Recall Activity

1. If a patient presents with an ailment, the task of the healthcare professional is to determine the

_____ and _____ the ailment.

2. The diagnostic scientific method gathers facts from _____ and

_____.

3. List the steps of the diagnostic scientific method. _____

Concept 2: Obtain Facts from Patient History

In the diagnostic scientific method, the first source of facts is *patient history*. Patient history often includes

- the time line of the patient's current ailment
- any past ailments the patient has had
- the patient's family history of disease
- any prescription and nonprescription drugs the patient is taking
- the location, nature, and rating of the patient's pain
- the age of the patient

Often patient history is obtained by asking a patient to fill out a questionnaire with yes-or-no answers.

Recall Activity

1. In the diagnostic scientific method, the first source of facts is _____.

2. Patient history is obtained by asking a patient to fill out a(n) _____ with yes-or-no answers.

Concept 3: Obtain Facts from a Physical Exam

The diagnostic scientific method also uses facts obtained by examining a patient. Some checks performed in a physical exam include measuring height and weight; obtaining vital signs (blood pressure, temperature, pulse, and respiratory rate); searching the surface of the body, including the legs and feet; listening to heartbeat; tapping on the chest and abdomen; and looking at the eyes and ears.

Recall Activity

1. The diagnostic scientific method also uses facts obtained by _____ a patient.

2. What vital signs are checked in a physical exam?_____

_____

Concept 4: Sift Facts

sift to sort facts in order to propose the most likely cause

The second step in the diagnostic scientific method is sifting facts. A healthcare professional *sifts* facts when he or she sorts through the collected facts to propose the most likely cause of a patient's ailment (**Figure 3.6**).

If a fact contradicts a cause, that cause is rejected. If more facts support a proposed cause, this makes that cause more likely. If facts support two or more causes, the healthcare professional ranks the causes from *most likely* to *least likely*. For example, a patient with a family history of heart disease may be more likely to suffer from heart disease than someone without a family history of heart disease.

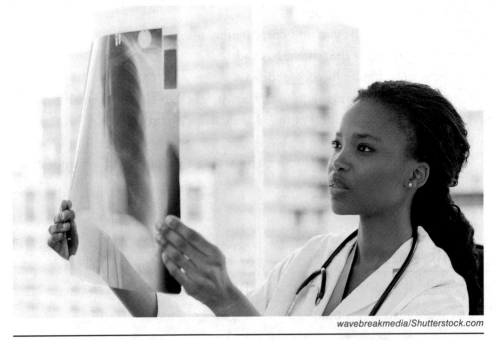

wavebreakmedia/Shutterstock.com

Figure 3.6 Sifting requires sorting through possible causes of an ailment.

Recall Activity

1. A healthcare professional _____ facts when he or she sorts through the collected facts to propose the most likely cause of a patient's ailment.

2. If more facts support a proposed cause, this makes that cause more _____.

3. If facts support two or more causes, the healthcare professional _____ the causes from most likely to least likely.

4. A healthcare professional obtains the following facts from the patient history and physical exam of a patient. Each number in the following results represents a different cause. Based on these facts, sort the possible causes from most likely to least likely.

Fact from patient history—2, 3, 5	Fact from physical exam—3, 5
Fact from patient history—4, 5	Fact from physical exam—3, 4, 5
Fact from patient history—1, 2, 3	Fact from physical exam—2, 3

_____

_____

Concept 5: Perform Tests

After sifting facts, the next step is to perform tests to confirm the most likely cause. Specific tests for a cause include collecting a urine, blood, or tissue (biopsy) sample for microscopic or chemical examination; passing sound waves through the body to make an image of internal structures (ultrasound); and passing a series of X-ray beams through the body to make images (CT scan). There are also many other types of tests.

Recall Activity

1. Collecting a tissue sample is also called a(n) _____.

2. A(n) _____ passes sound waves through the body to make an image of internal structures.

3. A(n) _____ passes a series of X-ray beams through the body to make images.

Concept 6: Diagnose

The purpose of a test is to confirm the proposed cause. If tests show that the proposed cause is present, you can *diagnose*, or identify and confirm the proposed cause of, an ailment. If tests cannot confirm that the proposed cause is present, then the proposed cause must be rejected and the next most likely cause tested until a diagnosis is reached.

diagnose to identify and confirm the proposed cause of an ailment

The probability that a confirmed diagnosis is the actual reason for an ailment is not 100%. There is always some degree of uncertainty in science, although more facts make a proposed cause more certain. A confirmed diagnosis allows a healthcare professional to determine proper treatment.

Recall Activity

1. The purpose of a test is to _____ the proposed cause.

2. If tests show that a proposed cause is present, you can _____ an ailment.

3. The probability that a confirmed diagnosis is the actual reason for an ailment is not

   _____.

4. There is always some degree of _____ in science.

5. More facts make a proposed cause more _____.

Section 3.4 Reinforcement

Answer the following questions using what you learned in this section.

1. The purpose of a test is to confirm the proposed _____.

2. More _____ supporting a proposed cause make that cause more likely.

3. *True or False.* A CT scan is a test. _____

4. List the steps of the diagnostic scientific method. _____

5. The first step of the diagnostic scientific method is _____.

6. More _____ make a proposed cause more certain.

7. *True or False.* In the diagnostic scientific method, you should continue testing until a diagnosis is reached. _____

8. Possible causes should be ranked from _____ likely to

   _____ likely.

9. If the most likely cause is not proven, the next most _____ cause is tested.

10. If a fact contradicts a cause, that cause is _____.

11. In the diagnostic scientific method, you should continue testing until a(n)

    _____ is reached.

12. *True or False.* There is always some degree of uncertainty in science. _____

13. _____ is sorting through collected facts to propose the most likely cause of the ailment.

14. Blood pressure is a(n) _____ sign.

15. The purpose of a(n) _____ is to confirm the proposed cause.

16. Passing sound waves through the body to make an image of internal structures is called a(n) _____.

17. *True or False.* In the diagnostic scientific method, test follows diagnosis. _____

18. The _____ scientific method gathers facts from two sources.

19. The two sources of facts in the diagnostic scientific method are _____ and _____.

20. There is always _____ degree of uncertainty in science.

21. To _____ is to sort through collected facts.

22. To _____ is to confirm the cause of an ailment.

Comprehensive Review (Chapters 1–3)

Answer the following questions using what you have learned so far in this book.

23. What color is a leukocyte? _____

24. *True or False.* The experimental group does not receive the independent variable. _____

25. The most basic skill in learning science is _____ the words.

Section 3.5 The Diagnostic Scientific Method in Action

The diagnostic scientific method is used to diagnose the cause of an ailment. This section will demonstrate the diagnostic scientific method in action. You will look at two ailments and the steps to diagnose each.

The terms below are some of those that will be introduced in Section 3.5. To become familiar with these terms, reproduce each word on the line beside it. Pronounce each term as you write it. You will learn the definitions of these words as you complete this section.

1. diabetes _____

2. anemia _____

3. dehydration _____

4. kidney stone _____

Concept 1: Case 1—Gathering Facts from Patient History

Presume that you are a healthcare professional. A patient comes into your office complaining of fatigue and thirst. The patient filled out the patient history shown in **Figure 3.7**. Your first step in the diagnostic scientific method is to gather facts from the patient history.

Patient History			
Age:	21	**Sex:**	Female
Prescription and nonprescription drugs you take regularly:	None		
What is your medical problem?	Tired, thirsty, always going to the bathroom		
How long has this problem existed?	About six weeks		

Have you ever had any of these conditions? Check all that apply to you.

❏ Heart attack   ❏ Mononucleosis
❏ Rheumatic fever   ❏ Nervous problems
❏ Heart murmur   ❏ Anemia
❏ Arterial disease   ❏ Thyroid problems
❏ Varicose veins   ❏ Pneumonia
❏ Arthritis   ❏ Bronchitis
❏ Diabetes   ❏ Asthma
❏ Phlebitis   ❏ Abnormal X-ray
❏ Autoimmune disease   ❏ Lung disease
❏ Epilepsy   ❏ Back injury
❏ Stroke   ❏ Kidney stones
❏ Diphtheria   ❏ Jaundice
❏ Scarlet fever

Check any that apply to your blood relatives (siblings, parents, aunts and uncles, grandparents).

☑ Heart attacks under age 50   ❏ Congenital heart disease
❏ Strokes under age 50   ❏ Heart operations
☑ High blood pressure   ❏ Kidney stones
☑ High cholesterol   ☑ Obesity (by 20 or more pounds)
☑ Diabetes   ❏ Leukemia or cancer under age 60
❏ Hay fever or asthma

Figure 3.7 This patient history details the patient's medical history and family history of disease.

Recall Activity

1. List the age and sex of the patient. _____

2. What is the patient's medical problem? _____

3. What conditions are present among the patient's blood relatives?_____

_____

Concept 2: Case 1—Gathering Facts from the Patient Exam

Next, you perform a physical exam to gather more facts about the patient. The patient is 5 feet 6 inches tall and weighs 175 pounds. She has a temperature of 37°C, a blood pressure of 140/95, and a heart rate of 80 beats per minute. The patient presents with fatigue, constant hunger and thirst, frequent urination, and numbness in the feet. A physical exam finds that the patient has dark patches of skin on her neck, has no pain, and has no swelling. Her heartbeat is normal.

Recall Activity

1. What is the patient's blood pressure reading? _____

2. A physical exam finds that the patient has _____ of skin on her neck.

Concept 3: Case 1—Sifting Facts

As you sift facts, you consider possible causes of the patient's ailment. The patient's fatigue, hunger, thirst, and frequent urination lead you to conclude the most likely cause is type 1 or type 2 diabetes. In *diabetes*, a person's body is unable to control levels of sugar in the blood. Due to the age of the patient, the absence of a history of autoimmune disease, and the dark patches of skin, type 2 diabetes is more likely than type 1 diabetes. Some less likely causes are *anemia* (a condition in which the blood cannot carry enough oxygen) due to the constant fatigue symptom or a cardiovascular system disease due to the numbness in the feet.

diabetes a condition in which a person's body is unable to control levels of sugar in the blood

anemia a condition in which the blood cannot carry enough oxygen

Recall Activity

1. What symptoms suggest that diabetes is the cause? _____

_____

2. Some less likely causes are _____ or a(n) _____.

Concept 4: Case 1—Performing Tests

Your next step is to test the most likely cause of the patient's ailment. To do this, you order a hemoglobin A1C test to determine the amount of sugar in the blood. The test results are 7.0%.

Recall Activity

1. The hemoglobin A1C test determines the amount of _____ in the blood.

2. The test results are _____.

Concept 5: Case 1—Making a Diagnosis

You review your test to make a diagnosis. If the hemoglobin A1C test results are 6.5% or greater, diabetes is the confirmed diagnosis. Test results between 5.7% and 6.4% signal prediabetes, and normal results would be between 4% and 5.6%.

Recall Activity

1. What were the results of the hemoglobin A1C test? _____

2. What is the confirmed diagnosis? _____

Concept 6: Case 2—Gathering Facts from Patient History

Imagine that another patient enters your office. This patient complains of vomiting and belly pain. The patient filled out the patient history shown in **Figure 3.8**. Your first step is to gather facts from this history.

Recall Activity

1. List the age and sex of the patient. _____

2. What is the patient's medical problem? _____

3. What conditions are present among the patient's blood relatives? _____

_____

Concept 7: Case 2—Gathering Facts from the Patient Exam

Next, you perform a physical exam of the patient. The patient is 6 feet tall and weighs 170 pounds. He has a temperature of 37.9°C, a blood pressure of 130/85, and a heart rate of 75 beats per minute. The patient presents with severe abdominal pain. On a scale of 1–10, he rates the pain at 4 and up to 8 at times. The pain is not constant, and the abdomen is tender to the touch. The patient's ankles, feet, and abdomen are not swollen. Pinching the skin on the back of the patient's hand creates a tent of skin that slowly sinks to normal, indicating *dehydration* (lack of water in body tissues). The patient says he has been vomiting.

dehydration lack of water in body tissues

Patient History			
Age:	*18*	**Sex:**	*Male*

Prescription and nonprescription drugs you take regularly:	*None*
What is your medical problem?	*Vomiting and belly pain*
How long has this problem existed?	*Since yesterday*

Have you ever had any of these conditions? Check all that apply to you.

❑ Heart attack	❑ Mononucleosis
❑ Rheumatic fever	❑ Nervous problems
❑ Heart murmur	❑ Anemia
❑ Arterial disease	❑ Thyroid problems
❑ Varicose veins	❑ Pneumonia
❑ Arthritis	❑ Bronchitis
❑ Diabetes	❑ Asthma
❑ Phlebitis	❑ Abnormal X-ray
❑ Autoimmune disease	❑ Lung disease
❑ Epilepsy	❑ Back injury
❑ Stroke	❑ Kidney stones
❑ Diphtheria	❑ Jaundice
❑ Scarlet fever	

Check any that apply to your blood relatives (siblings, parents, aunts and uncles, grandparents).

❑ Heart attacks under age 50	❑ Congenital heart disease
❑ Strokes under age 50	❑ Heart operations
❑ High blood pressure	☑ Kidney stones
☑ High cholesterol	❑ Obesity (by 20 or more pounds)
❑ Diabetes	❑ Leukemia or cancer under age 60
❑ Hay fever or asthma	

Figure 3.8 This patient history is for a patient complaining of vomiting and belly pain.

Recall Activity

1. What is the patient's blood pressure reading? _____

2. Pinching the skin is used to test for _____.

Concept 8: Case 2—Sifting Facts

As you sift the gathered facts, the patient's abdominal pain, fever, and vomiting lead you to suspect *kidney stones* (rock-like structures that form in the urinary system)

kidney stone a rock-like structure that forms in the urinary system

or appendicitis (inflammation of the appendix). Symptoms of kidney stones include pain below the ribs on the back or side, waves of pain, nausea, vomiting, fever, chills, and painful urination. Symptoms of appendicitis include abdominal pain, fever, loss of appetite, nausea, and vomiting. Less likely causes include gastroenteritis and colitis. Due to the family history of kidney stones, you decide to test for kidney stones first.

Recall Activity

1. The two most likely causes are _____ and _____.

2. The two less likely causes are _____ and _____.

Concept 9: Case 2—Performing Tests

To test for kidney stones, you order a CT scan. The CT scan reveals a kidney stone in the left kidney (**Figure 3.9**).

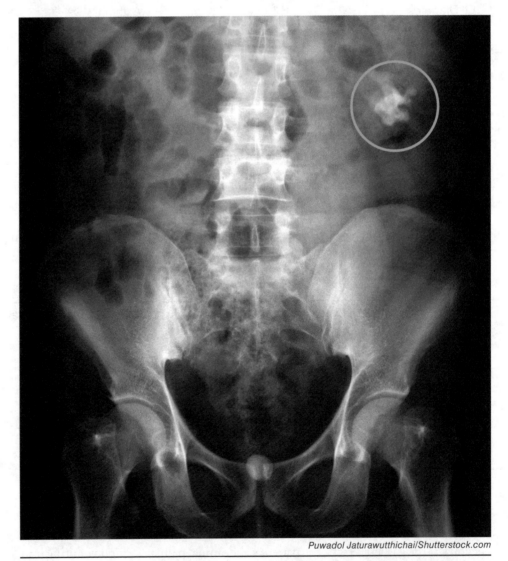

Puwadol Jaturawutthichai/Shutterstock.com

Figure 3.9 A kidney stone is shown in the left kidney (on the right side of the image).

Recall Activity

1. You order a(n) _____ scan to check for kidney stones.

2. What are the results of the CT scan? _____

Concept 10: Case 2—Making a Diagnosis

Your test revealed a kidney stone in the patient's left kidney. This supports the possible cause of kidney stones. You review your test to make a diagnosis.

Recall Activity

1. What is the confirmed diagnosis? _____

2. If the CT scan had *not* shown kidney stones, what would have been tested for next?

   _____

3. If the possible cause in question 2 could not be confirmed, what else would be tested for?

   _____

Section 3.5 Reinforcement

Answer the following questions using what you learned in this section.

1. The _____ test determines the amount of sugar in the blood.

2. What are the symptoms of diabetes? _____

   _____

3. *True or False.* A CT scan can check for kidney stones. _____

4. What symptoms do kidney stones and appendicitis have in common? _____

   _____

5. Which of the following A1C results is normal?
   A. 7.5%   C. 4.5%
   B. 6.4%   D. 6.6%

6. The two types of diabetes are _____ and _____.

7. What two sources of facts does the diagnostic scientific method consider? _____

   _____

8. *True or False.* An A1C test result of 6.3% is prediabetic. _____

9. A(n) _____ is used to test for kidney stones.

10. *True or False*. Fever is a symptom of kidney stones and appendicitis._____

11. 130/80 is a reading of _____.

12. *True or False*. In anemia, the blood cannot carry enough oxygen. _____

13. Unscramble the letters: ngsidosai. Define the word that is formed. _____

_____

14. The third step in the diagnostic scientific method is _____.

15. *True or False*. A CT scan checks for diabetes. _____

16. An A1C test result of 5.5% is _____.

17. Pain is rated on a scale from 1 to _____.

18. Unscramble the letters: menfidroc. Define the word that is formed. _____

_____

19. In case 2, was pain constant with the kidney stone?_____

20. _____ the skin is used to test for dehydration.

Comprehensive Review (Chapters 1–3)

Answer the following questions using what you have learned so far in this book.

21. What does the combining form *arthr/o* mean? _____

22. A(n) _____ explanation of lightning is the anger of the Norse god of lightning, Thor.

23. The first step of the experimental scientific method is _____.

Section 3.6 Laws and Theories

The scientific body of knowledge includes laws and theories that seek to explain the natural world. In this section, you will learn about scientific laws and scientific theories. You will also learn about scientific articles.

The terms below are some of those that will be introduced in Section 3.6. To become familiar with these terms, reproduce each word on the line beside it. Pronounce each term as you write it. You will learn the definitions of these words as you complete this section.

1. scientific law _____

2. scientific theory _____

3. literature _____

Concept 1: Scientific Laws

The scientific body of knowledge includes scientific laws. A *scientific law* is a general statement of fact. By accumulating enough facts, scientists develop an expectation of results. Scientific laws give you the expectation that a certain phenomenon will cause a known result. In this way, scientific laws tell you that the natural world is predictable.

An example of a scientific law is the Law of Segregation, formulated by Gregor Mendel after years of experiments and data gathered from pea plants. The Law of Segregation states that an individual possesses a pair of factors for a trait, but passes on only one factor during reproduction.

scientific law a general statement of fact that encourages the expectation of a result

Recall Activity

1. A scientific _____ is a general statement of fact.

2. By accumulating enough facts, scientists develop a(n) _____ of results.

3. Scientific laws tell you that the natural world is _____.

Concept 2: Scientific Theories

A *scientific theory* is the best explanation today of why a phenomenon occurs. Whereas a scientific law tells you *what* you can expect to happen, a scientific theory tells you *why* the result occurs. Scientific theories are the basis for mankind's understanding of the natural world. Do not confuse a scientific theory with the common use of the word *theory*. In common usage, a theory could be an unsubstantiated hunch or guess. Scientific theories, on the other hand, are based on the best evidence today.

scientific theory the best explanation today of why a phenomenon occurs

Recall Activity

1. A scientific _____ is the best explanation today of why a phenomenon occurs.

2. Scientific theories are the basis for mankind's _____ of the natural world.

3. Scientific theories are based on the best _____ today.

Concept 3: Facts, Laws, and Theories

To distinguish among scientific facts, laws, and theories, you can think of the following example from the science of physics. If you hold a brick in your hand and release it, the brick will fall to the ground (**Figure 3.10**). The brick falling to the ground after release is a *fact*. You could do this many times, and it has been done many more times. The brick always falls to the ground after release.

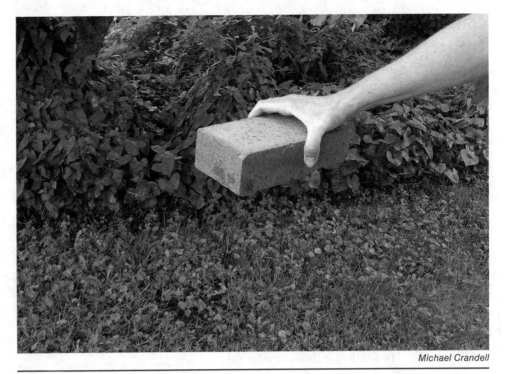

Michael Crandell

Figure 3.10 A brick falls to the ground after release.

The *law* of gravity is a general statement of the observation that many objects fall. You expect that when you hold an object above the ground and release it, the object will fall to the ground. The *theory* of gravity, the attraction of the earth for an object, explains why the object falls. This is the best explanation based on evidence today.

Recall Activity

1. The brick falling to the ground after release is a(n) _____.

2. The _____ of gravity is a general statement of the observation that many objects fall.

3. The _____ of gravity explains why the object falls.

Concept 4: The Hierarchy of Facts, Laws, and Theories

A *hierarchy* is a ranking system. For example, in the military, a hierarchy exists among privates, sergeants, and generals. The private is the lowest rank, and the general is the highest. In science, there is a hierarchy among facts, laws, and theories (**Figure 3.11**). Facts have the lowest rank. This does not mean facts are unimportant, but one fact by itself does not tell you much. Scientific laws, supported by many facts, provide expectations. They have the middle rank. Scientific theories have the highest rank because scientific theories tell you why a phenomenon or phenomena occurred. Scientific theories enable mankind to understand the natural world.

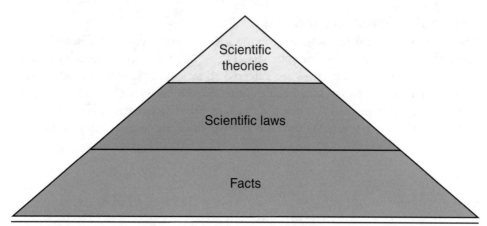

Figure 3.11 This hierarchy ranks facts, laws, and theories by importance.

Recall Activity

1. Scientific _____, supported by many facts, provide expectations.

2. One _____ by itself does not tell you much.

3. Scientific _____ enable mankind to understand the natural world.

Concept 5: Proving Laws and Theories False

Scientific laws and scientific theories can be proven false. Contradicting evidence will cause the rejection of a scientific law or scientific theory. This is not likely to happen because scientific theories and scientific laws have substantial supporting evidence. If this were to happen, however, the rejected scientific law or scientific theory could be modified to fit all the evidence (new and old).

For example, Gregor Mendel's Law of Independent Assortment stated that, preceding reproduction, the selection of one gene for each trait was not influenced by selection for a gene from any other trait. With additional study, however, it was found that genes located near one another on the same chromosome do not show independent assortment. A modified way to state the law is that chromosomes, not genes, show independent assortment.

Recall Activity

1. A scientific law or scientific theory _____ be proven false.

2. _____ evidence will cause the rejection of a scientific law or scientific theory.

3. A rejected scientific law or scientific theory can be _____ to fit all the evidence.

Concept 6: Scientific Journals

Scientists build on other scientists' work. As scientists conduct research, they share their results in scientific journals. These journals contain articles written by scientists. Scientific articles are referred to as *literature*, and to have an article accepted to appear in a scientific journal is to be *published*. The scientific community can read and critique the work of other scientists. When writing an article for a journal, scientists use facts published in previous articles as support.

Recall Activity

1. Scientific articles are referred to as _____.

2. Scientists _____ on other scientists' work.

3. To have an article accepted to appear in a scientific journal is to be _____.

Concept 7: Scientific Articles

Scientific articles published in scientific journals follow a standard format. They contain an abstract, an introduction, a materials and methods section, a results section, a discussion section, and a literature cited section. The *abstract* is a brief summary of the article so readers can quickly determine if the article is worth reading in entirety. The *introduction* gives the background and observations that lead to the topic of the article. The *materials and methods section* details the experiment so other scientists can repeat it, and the *results section* lists the outcomes of the experiment. The *discussion section* weaves together results of the experiment with other experiments to explain what the results mean. Finally, the *literature cited section* lists the sources of supporting facts.

Recall Activity

1. The _____ is a brief summary of the article.

2. The _____ section details the experiment so other scientists can repeat it.

3. The literature cited section lists the sources of _____ facts.

Section 3.6 Reinforcement

Answer the following questions using what you learned in this section.

1. A scientific _____ tells you why a result occurs.

2. A scientific law is a general statement of _____.

3. The _____ section of a scientific article lists the sources of supporting facts.

4. _____ build on other scientists' work.

5. Can scientific laws be proven false? Explain._____
_____

6. A scientific theory is the best _____ today for why a phenomenon occurs.

7. *True or False.* A scientific law or scientific theory cannot be proven false. _____

8. A(n) _____ is a ranking system.

9. Which section of a scientific article lists the outcomes of an experiment?_____

10. An abstract is a brief _____ of a scientific article.

11. In the hierarchy of facts, scientific laws, and scientific theories, which ranks highest?
_____

12. *True or False.* Scientific laws tell you that the natural world is predictable. _____

13. Scientific _____ are the basis for mankind's understanding of the natural world.

14. The _____ of a scientific article gives the background and observations that lead to the topic of the article.

15. *True or False.* Contradicting evidence will cause the rejection of a scientific law. _____

16. Scientists use facts published in previous articles as _____.

17. Why do facts rank lower than scientific laws and theories?_____
_____

18. Scientific _____ are referred to as *literature.*

19. The summary of a scientific article is the _____.

20. The _____ section of a scientific article lists the outcomes of the experiment.

21. In your own words, explain what a scientific theory is. _____
_____

22. A(n) _____ is a general statement of fact.

Comprehensive Review (Chapters 1–3)

Answer the following questions using what you have learned so far in this book.

23. What does the prefix *peri-* mean?_____

24. Physics, chemistry, geology, and biology are _____ of science.

25. The diagnostic scientific method considers two sources of facts: _____ and
_____.

Chapter 3 Review

Answer the following questions using what you learned in this chapter.

1. *True or False.* There is only one scientific method. _____

2. Scientists test a proposal with _____.

3. In the _____ step of the experimental scientific method, the data resulting from the experiment is examined.

4. The _____ group does not receive the independent variable.

5. The _____ portion of a hypothesis is the dependent variable.

6. _____ are untested factors in an experiment.

7. In the diagnostic scientific method, the first source of _____ is patient history.

8. The steps of the diagnostic scientific method are _____, sift, test, and _____.

9. Scientists continue testing until a(n) _____ is reached.

10. Scientific laws tell you that the _____ world is predictable.

11. Arrange these from highest to lowest rank: scientific law, scientific theory, and fact. _____

    _____

12. An abstract is a brief summary of a(n) _____.

13. In the last stage of the experimental scientific method, you decide to _____

    or _____ the hypothesis.

14. If data from your experiment supports your hypothesis, you _____ the hypothesis.

15. If a fact contradicts a cause, the cause is _____.

16. What are the two variables in an experiment?_____

    _____

17. List the steps in the experimental scientific method. _____

    _____

18. A logical process used to evaluate the natural world is known as a(n) _____.

19. The _____ section of a scientific article lists the sources of supporting facts.

20. Constants are untested factors that could affect the _____ variable.

21. In the following hypothesis, identify the independent and dependent variables: If water is kept below 0°C, it will freeze. _____

    _____

22. *True or False.* Science utilizes different types of evidence from just one source._____

23. Which of the following has the highest rank?
   A. scientific law   C. scientific theory
   B. fact

24. The _____ portion of a hypothesis is the dependent variable.

25. Explain the difference between the experimental group and the control group. _____
   _____

26. The "if" portion of a hypothesis is the _____ variable.

27. *True or False.* Scientific laws and theories can be proven false. _____

28. If all constants in an experiment are the same, any differences *must* be caused by the
   _____ variable.

29. List the sections of a scientific article. _____
   _____

30. As scientists conduct research, they share their results in _____.

Comprehensive Review (Chapters 1–3)

Using what you have learned so far in this book, match the following terms with their definitions.

_____ 31. A prefix that means "below"

_____ 32. A general statement of fact

_____ 33. A combining form that means "bone"

_____ 34. A prefix that means "middle"

_____ 35. A combining form that means "blue"

_____ 36. A prefix that means "four"

_____ 37. The study of cells

_____ 38. A combining form that means "brain"

_____ 39. A prefix that means "after"

_____ 40. The science that studies life

_____ 41. A combining form that means "kidney"

_____ 42. A combining form that means "intestine"

_____ 43. A combining form that means "narrow"

_____ 44. A confirmed observation

_____ 45. A prefix that means "flat"

A. cerebr/o
B. scientific law
C. biology
D. cyan/o
E. sub-
F. post-
G. oste/o
H. cytology
I. meso-
J. quadri-
K. platy-
L. enter/o
M. sten/o
N. fact
O. ren/o

Chapter 4
Math and Measurement

Introduction

All areas of science utilize math. Knowledge of fractions, decimals, and percentages is important for understanding measurement and conversion. Scientific fields use a system of measurement known as the *metric system*. Medical measurements such as height, weight, and body temperature are recorded in metric units. This chapter will introduce the metric units you need to know to work in science. You will learn to measure length (meters) and calculate the surface areas and volumes of rectangular and circular objects. You will also learn how to measure liquid volume (liters), mass (grams), and temperature (degrees Celsius).

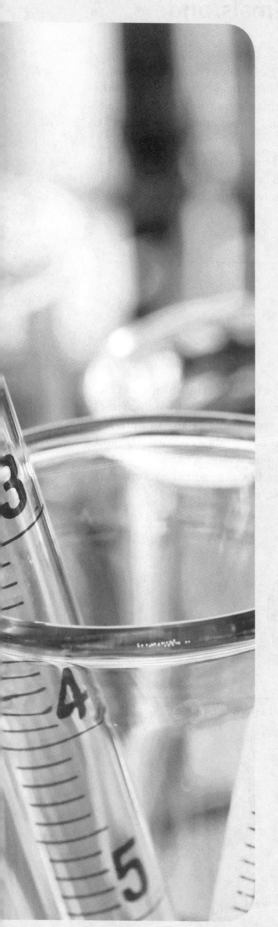

Objectives

After completing this chapter, you will be able to

- understand fractions, decimals, and percentages
- recognize and convert metric units of measurement
- take linear measurements in millimeters or centimeters
- calculate the surface area of a rectangle or circle
- calculate the dry volume of a cube or cylinder
- measure liquid volume in milliliters
- measure temperature in degrees Celsius
- measure mass in grams
- explain the concepts of concentration, pressure, and rate
- convert between metric and English measurements
- read and create graphs

Key Terms

The following terms and phrases will be introduced and explained in Chapter 4. Read through the list to become familiar with the words.

bar graph	mass
cell	meniscus
centimeter	meter
concentration	meter stick
conversion	metric system
conversion factor	milliliter
coordinate pair	millimeter
cubic unit	percentage
decimal	pi
degree Celsius	platform balance
diameter	pressure
dry volume	radius
electronic balance	rate
English system of measurement	ratio
	ruler
fraction	solute
graduated cylinder	solvent
gram	square unit
graph	surface area
line graph	weight
linear	x-axis
liquid volume	y-axis
liter	

Section 4.1 Fractions, Decimals, and Percentages

Math skills are important to your understanding of biology and anatomy and physiology. While you may know the basic mathematical operations of addition, subtraction, multiplication, and division, this section will introduce the concepts of fractions, decimals, and percentages. These concepts are key to taking and converting measurements.

The terms below are some of those that will be introduced in Section 4.1. To become familiar with these terms, reproduce each word on the line beside it. Pronounce each term as you write it. You will learn the definitions of these words as you complete this section.

1. fraction _____

2. decimal _____

3. percentage _____

Concept 1: Fractions

fraction a part of a whole number

A *fraction* represents a part of a whole number. In a fraction, the number on top (*numerator*) represents the part, and the number on the bottom (*denominator*) represents the whole number or the total number of parts. For an example, see **Figure 4.1**. The circle in Figure 4.1 is divided into two parts—one teal part and one purple part. To refer to one part of the circle, you would write ½. The total number of parts in the circle (2) is written on the bottom, and the number of parts being referred to (1) is written on the top. In Figure 4.1, ½ of the circle is teal, and ½ of the circle is purple.

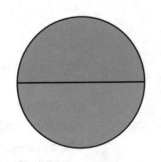

Figure 4.1 One-half of the circle is teal, and ½ of the circle is purple.

Recall Activity

1. View the circle to the right. Into how many parts is the circle divided? _____

2. In the circle to the right, _____ parts are yellow, so

   _____/_____ of the circle is yellow.

3. In the circle to the right, _____ part is green, so

   _____/_____ of the circle is green.

Concept 2: Decimals

Decimals are numbers that represent values containing fractions. In a decimal, a *decimal point* marks the divide between a whole number (a value equal to or greater than 0; for example, 2 or 65) and a fractional value of 1 (for example, ½ or 0.5). Numbers to the *left* of a decimal point are whole numbers; numbers to the *right* of a decimal point are a fraction of 1 (**Figure 4.2**).

decimal a number that represents a value containing a fraction

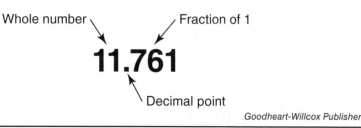

Figure 4.2 The decimal point divides the whole number from the fraction of 1.

If there is one number on the right of a decimal point, this represents *tenths* of 1 (for example, 0.2 or ²⁄₁₀). Two numbers on the right of a decimal point represent *hundredths* of 1 (for example, 0.35 or ³⁵⁄₁₀₀). Three numbers on the right of a decimal point represent *thousandths* of 1 (for example, 0.431 or ⁴³¹⁄₁₀₀₀). If you envision decimals as fractions, you can determine how large decimals are in comparison to other numbers. For example, 1 is greater than ¹⁄₁₀ (0.1), and ¹⁄₁₀₀₀ (0.001) is smaller than ¹⁄₁₀₀ (0.01).

Recall Activity

1. Arrange these numbers from smallest to largest: 0.001, 1, 0.01, 10, 1000, and 0.1. _____

   _____

2. Count the number of zeroes in the following numbers. Write the number of zeroes in the blank beside each number. For numbers less than 1, do not count zeroes to the left of the decimal point.

   100 _____   1 _____

   1000 _____   0.001 _____

   10 _____   0.01 _____

3. Draw a circle around the largest number and draw a square around the smallest number in the following list: 10, 1000, 1, 0.01, 0.1, 0.001, and 100.

4. Write ²⁄₁₀₀₀ as a decimal. _____

5. Write 0.67 as a fraction. _____

Concept 3: Converting Fractions into Decimals

To convert a fraction into a decimal, simply divide the fraction's numerator (number on top) by its denominator (number on the bottom). If you converted ¼ into a decimal, you would divide 1 by 4 for a decimal value of 0.25.

Recall Activity

1. Convert ⅕ into a decimal. _____

2. Convert ⁵⁄₁₀ into a decimal. _____

3. Convert ⅞ into a decimal. _____

Concept 4: Rounding

When you convert fractions into decimals, you can round the decimal. To round, look at the first number to the right of the place to which you are rounding. If that number is 5 or is greater than 5, round *up* to the next number. If that number is less than 5, the number to which you are rounding stays the same. For example, if you were converting ⅓ into a fraction, you would divide 1 by 3. To round the value to the second decimal place, you would look at the third decimal place. Because the third decimal place has a value of 3, you would round the number to 0.33.

Recall Activity

1. Round 2.765 to the first decimal place. _____

2. Round 92.98977 to the nearest whole number. _____

3. Round 0.239 to the second decimal place. _____

4. Round 0.6755 to the third decimal place. _____

5. Round 28.0855 to the nearest whole number. _____

Concept 5: Percentages

Like fractions, *percentages* also describe a part of a whole number. Percentages describe the number of parts out of 100 parts. In percentages, the total of 100 parts is written as 100%.

percentage a number of parts out of 100 parts

To calculate a percentage, first write the part of the total as a fraction. For example, if there are 40 parts out of a total of 80 parts, write this as $^{40}/_{80}$. Next, divide the numerator by the denominator. This should yield the decimal value of the fraction. Finally, multiply the decimal value by 100. In the example of $^{40}/_{80}$, $40 \div 80 = 0.5$, and $0.5 \times 100 = 50\%$.

Recall Activity

1. You have 30 parts out of 100 parts. Calculate the percentage. _____

2. You have 10 parts out of 40 parts. Calculate the percentage._____

3. You have 80 parts out of 200 parts. Calculate the percentage. _____

4. Convert the decimal 0.75 into a percentage. _____

5. What percentage of the circle below is yellow?_____

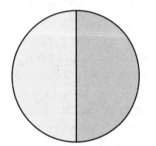

6. Calculate the following percentages for the circle to the right.

   percent that is yellow: _____

   percent that is green: _____

   percent of the whole circle (yellow or green): _____

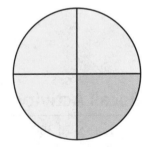

Concept 6: Calculating Percentages from Data

Percentages often communicate data from studies and surveys. To calculate percentages from any data, find the total and divide the parts by the total.

Read the following data as an example. A group of researchers conducted a study that included 100 people. Out of the 100 people, 48 people thought the world was flat, 42 people thought the world was round, and 10 people had no opinion. Based on this data, you can calculate that 48% of people thought the world was flat ($^{48}/_{100} = 0.48$; $0.48 \times 100 = 48\%$). Forty-two percent of people thought the world was round ($^{42}/_{100} = 0.42$; $0.42 \times 100 = 42\%$), and 10% of people had no opinion ($^{10}/_{100} = 0.01$; $0.01 \times 100 = 10\%$).

Recall Activity

Use the following survey data to answer questions 1–4: Thirty-two people believe that the sun rotates around the earth. Sixteen people believe that the earth rotates around the sun. Two people do not believe in any rotation involving the sun and the earth.

1. What is the total number of people surveyed? _____

2. What percentage of people believes the sun rotates around the earth? _____

3. What percentage of people believes the earth rotates around the sun? _____

4. What percentage of people does not believe in any rotation involving the sun and earth? _____

Concept 7: Converting Percentages into Other Numbers

To convert a percentage into a decimal and then into the number value of the percentage, reverse the equation for calculating percentage. First, divide the percentage by 100. This gives you the decimal value. Then multiply the decimal by the total number of parts. For example, suppose you earned a grade of 88% on a test with 50 questions. To determine how many questions you got correct, divide 88% by 100, yielding 0.88. Then multiply 0.88 by the total number of questions (50). You got 44 questions correct on the test.

If you want to find the total number of parts and you have a percentage and the number value of the percentage, begin by dividing the percentage by 100. This gives you the decimal value. Then divide the number value of the percentage by the decimal value. For example, 100 calories is 5% of the total calories an adult should consume in one day. In this example, 5% is the percentage, and 100 calories is the number value of the percentage. To calculate the total number of calories an adult requires in one day, divide 5% by 100, yielding 0.05. Then divide 100 calories by 0.05. Two thousand calories are required for an adult in one day.

Recall Activity

1. If 15% of 300 people voted "yes," how many people voted "yes"? _____

2. If you got 75% of 200 total questions correct, how many questions did you get correct? _____

3. The illustration below shows nutrition information for one serving of cereal. Complete the following calculations based on the illustration.

Nutrition Highlights

Calories	Saturated Fat	Sodium	Sugars	Fiber	Calcium
100	**0g**	**160mg**	**1g**	**3g**	**100mg**
5%	0%	7%		11%	10%

Amount and % Daily Value per serving

total daily value for sodium: _____

total daily value for fiber: _____

total daily value for calcium: _____

Section 4.1 Reinforcement

Answer the following questions using what you learned in this section.

1. Convert $^{16}\!/_{48}$ into a percentage. _____

2. Arrange these fractions from smallest to largest: ½, ⅜, and ¼. _____

3. *True or False.* Fifty percent is the same as ½. _____

4. A circle is ⅛ red, and the rest is blue. What fraction of the circle is blue? _____

5. If 75 people voted "yes," and 50 people voted "no," how many people voted? _____

6. If 12% of 200 people are right-handed, how many people are right-handed? _____

7. If 25% of 300 people have hitchhiker's thumb, how many people have hitchhiker's thumb? _____

8. A circle is ¼ blue, and the rest is red. What percentage of the circle is red? _____

9. *True or False.* Fifteen percent is the same as ¼. _____

10. Unscramble the letters: ragetepnec. Define the word that is formed. _____

_____

11. In a survey about whether students wanted to do more dissection in a general biology lab class, 40% of students said "yes," and the rest said "no." What percentage said "no"? _____

12. Convert $^{50}\!/_{250}$ into a percentage. _____

13. A circle is divided into 16 parts, and 7 parts are blue. What fraction of the circle is blue? _____

14. In a survey to determine if A&P tests were too hard, 40 students or 80% of the class said "yes." How many students are in the class? _____

15. *True or False.* One-fourth is the same as 33%. _____

16. Two students failed the first A&P exam, and 18 students passed it. What percentage of the class failed the exam? _____

17. A circle is ¾ blue, and the rest is red. What percentage of the circle is red? _____

18. If 15 people said "yes," and 45 people said "no," what percentage of the people said "yes"? _____

19. One-fourth of a circle is red, and the rest is blue. What fraction of the circle is blue? _____

20. Arrange these fractions from largest to smallest: ¼, ⅜, ⅛, ½, and ⅝. _____

_____

21. If a circle is divided into six equal parts, each part represents _____/_____ of the circle.

22. If a rectangle is divided into eight equal parts, three of which are shaded, what fraction of the rectangle is shaded? What fraction of the rectangle is not shaded?

_____

23. What is a fraction? _____

24. A(n) _____ is the number of parts out of 100 parts.

Comprehensive Review (Chapters 1–4)

Answer the following questions using what you have learned so far in this book.

25. How are fractions and percentages different? _____

_____

26. The prefix of the term *dimorphous* is _____.

27. The second step of the experimental scientific method is _____.

28. What is the difference between anatomy and physiology?_____

_____

Section 4.2 The Metric System

metric system the international system of measurement for science and healthcare fields

Now that you have learned about fractions, decimals, and percentages, you are ready to learn about the metric system of measurement. The *metric system* is the international system of measurement for science and healthcare fields. This system of measurement was established by Gabriel Mouton in 1670 and uses metric units to measure length, volume, temperature, and mass.

The terms below are some of those that will be introduced in Section 4.2. To become familiar with these terms, reproduce each word on the line beside it. Pronounce each term as you write it. You will learn the definitions of these words as you complete this section.

1. metric system _____
2. meter _____
3. gram_____

4. liter _____
5. degree Celsius_____
6. conversion _____

Concept 1: Powers of 10

The metric system is based on *powers of 10*. This means that conversions between similar units can be done by multiplying or dividing measurements by 10. Some U.S. currency is also based on powers of 10. For example, one dollar is the same amount of money as 10 dimes (1×10) or 100 pennies ($1 \times 10 \times 10$). One dime is the same amount of money as 10 pennies (1×10).

To convert between similar units based on powers of 10, use multiplication and division. In the example of the dollar, dime, and penny, the largest unit is the dollar, the next largest is the dime, and the smallest unit is the penny. To convert a larger unit into a smaller unit, use *multiplication*. For example, to determine how many dimes are in two dollars, multiply the number of dollars by the number of dimes per dollar (2 dollars × 10 dimes/dollar = 20 dimes). To convert this amount into an even smaller unit (pennies), multiply the number of dimes by the number of pennies per dime (20 dimes × 10 pennies/dime = 200 pennies).

To convert a smaller unit into a larger unit, use *division*. To determine how many dimes are equal to 300 pennies, divide the number of pennies by the number of pennies per dime (300 pennies ÷ 10 pennies/dime = 30 dimes). To convert this amount into an even larger unit (dollars), divide the number of dimes by the number of dimes per dollar (30 dimes ÷ 10 dimes/dollar = 3 dollars).

Recall Activity

1. One dollar is equal to _____ pennies.

2. Ten dimes is equal to _____ dollar(s).

3. There are _____ dimes in one dollar.

4. One dime is worth _____ pennies.

5. Two dollars is equal to _____ pennies.

6. If you have 15 dimes, how many dollars do you have? _____

7. Twelve dimes is equal to _____ pennies.

8. One hundred pennies is equal to _____ dollar.

9. How many pennies are in $6.92? _____

Concept 2: Moving the Decimal Point

When multiplying and dividing based on powers of 10, you can take a shortcut by *moving the decimal point*. Multiplying by a whole number makes a number larger. When multiplying a number by 10, move the decimal point one place to the *right*. This makes the number larger. Dividing by a whole number makes a number smaller. When dividing a number by 10, move the decimal point one place to the *left*. This makes the number smaller.

To easily multiply and divide by other powers of 10 (for example, 100 and 1000), count the number of zeroes and then move the decimal point that number of spaces. To multiply or divide by 10, move the decimal point one space because 10 has one zero. To multiply or divide by 100, move the decimal point two spaces because 100 has two zeroes. To multiply or divide by 1000, move the decimal point three places because 1000 has three zeroes.

Recall Activity

1. Does multiplying by a whole number make a number larger or smaller? _____

2. _____ by a whole number makes a number smaller.

3. Moving the decimal point to the _____ makes a number larger, and moving the decimal point to the _____ makes a number smaller.

4. To _____ by 10, move the decimal point one place to the right.

5. To divide a number by 10, move the decimal point one place to the _____.

6. For each operation, circle the number of spaces and the direction in which the decimal point moves.

multiply by 100	1/2/3/4	left/right
divide by 1000	1/2/3/4	left/right
multiply by 1000	1/2/3/4	left/right
divide by 100	1/2/3/4	left/right

7. Change each number to 1 by moving the decimal point the appropriate number of spaces. Circle *left* or *right* to indicate the direction the decimal point moved, and on the lines provided, write how many places you moved the decimal point.

1000	left/right	_____
100	left/right	_____
10	left/right	_____
1	left/right	_____
0.001	left/right	_____
0.1	left/right	_____
0.01	left/right	_____

Concept 3: Metric Units

meter the metric unit of length

gram the metric unit of mass or weight

liter the metric unit of volume

degree Celsius the metric unit of temperature

The standard units of the metric system are the *meter*, the *gram*, the *liter*, and the *degree Celsius*. **Figure 4.3** shows the metric units, their abbreviations, and what they measure.

Metric Unit	Abbreviation	Type of Measurement
meter	m	length
gram	g	mass or weight
liter	L	volume
degree Celsius	°C	temperature

Figure 4.3 The four metric units are the meter, gram, liter, and degree Celsius.

The prefixes *milli-*, *centi-*, and *kilo-* are important for measuring with metric units. These prefixes are used for measurements larger or smaller than one unit (**Figure 4.4**). One unit might be 1 meter, gram, liter, or degree Celsius. For example, there are 1000 milliliters (mL) in 1 liter (L), 100 centimeters (cm) in 1 meter (m), and 1000 meters (m) in 1 kilometer (km).

Prefix	Abbreviation	Equivalency
milli-	m	There are 1000 milli- in one unit.
centi-	c	There are 100 centi- in one unit.
kilo-	k	There are 1000 units in one kilo-.

Figure 4.4 These three prefixes indicate measurements larger or smaller than one unit.

Recall Activity

1. The metric unit of length is the _____.

2. The metric unit of weight is the _____.

3. The metric unit of volume is the _____.

4. The metric unit of temperature is the _____.

5. There are 1000 _____ in 1 liter.

6. There are 100 _____ in 1 gram.

7. Draw a circle around the smallest unit of measurement and a square around the largest: centimeter, kilometer, and millimeter.

8. Circle the larger unit of measurement in each pair.

   meter/millimeter   milligram/gram

   centimeter/millimeter   kilogram/milligram

   kilogram/gram   milliliter/liter

9. Circle the smaller unit of measurement in each pair.

   gram/milligram   centimeter/millimeter

   liter/milliliter   kilogram/milligram

Concept 4: Conversion Direction

conversion changing a measurement from one unit to another unit

Conversion means changing a measurement from one unit to another unit. For example, a conversion might change a measurement in millimeters to a measurement in centimeters. The first step in conversion is knowing whether you are changing from a larger unit to a smaller unit or from a smaller unit to a larger unit. If you are converting a larger unit to a smaller unit, use multiplication. If you are converting a smaller unit to a larger unit, use division. As you have learned, you can also multiply and divide by powers of 10 by moving the decimal point to the left or right.

Recall Activity

1. For each conversion, write in the blank *large to small* or *small to large*.

   milli- to centi-_____   millimeters to meters _____

   milli- to kilo- _____   meters to centimeters_____

   centi- to kilo- _____   liters to milliliters _____

   kilo- to milli- _____   centimeters to meters_____

   kilo- to centi- _____   grams to kilograms_____

2. For each conversion, write *multiply* or *divide* in the blank.

   grams to milligrams _____   millimeters to meters_____

   milliliters to liters _____   kilometers to centimeters_____

   grams to kilograms _____   centimeters to millimeters _____

3. For each conversion, circle the direction the decimal point should be moved.

meters to millimeters	left/right
milliliters to liters	left/right
kilograms to grams	left/right
liters to milliliters	left/right
centimeters to meters	left/right
centimeters to millimeters	left/right

Concept 5: Converting Between Metric Units

Once you know the direction of a conversion, you can convert units by multiplying or dividing by the correct power of 10. The following is a brief overview of common conversions and their operations:

- To convert milli- to the unit, divide by 1000.
- To convert centi- to the unit, divide by 100.

- To convert kilo- to units, multiply by 1000.
- To convert units to milli-, multiply by 1000.
- To convert units to centi-, multiply by 100.
- To convert units to kilo-, divide by 1000.

Recall Activity

1. For each conversion, circle *large to small* or *small to large*.

millimeters to meters	large to small/small to large
liters to milliliters	large to small/small to large
meters to centimeters	large to small/small to large
centimeters to meters	large to small/small to large
grams to kilograms	large to small/small to large
millimeters to kilometers	large to small/small to large

2. For each conversion, circle *multiply* or *divide*, circle whether the unit should be multiplied or divided by *100* or *1000*, and indicate if the decimal point should be moved *left* or *right*.

grams to milligrams	multiply/divide	100/1000	left/right
milliliters to liters	multiply/divide	100/1000	left/right
meters to millimeters	multiply/divide	100/1000	left/right
millimeters to meters	multiply/divide	100/1000	left/right
kilograms to grams	multiply/divide	100/1000	left/right
grams to kilograms	multiply/divide	100/1000	left/right

3. Convert 100 grams into kilograms. _____

4. Convert 10 liters into milliliters. _____

5. Convert 1 centimeter into millimeters. _____

6. Convert 10 centimeters into meters. _____

7. Convert 100 kilograms into grams. _____

Section 4.2 Reinforcement

Answer the following questions using what you learned in this section.

1. Which of the following is the largest measurement?
   A. 10 mm
   B. 1 cm
   C. 1 m
   D. 0.1 m

2. To convert 0.001 to 1, move the decimal to the _____.

3. *True or False.* The metric unit of volume is the meter. _____

4. There are _____ milliliters in 1 liter.

5. Arrange these measurements from smallest to largest: 1 mm, 7 cm, 6 mm, 1 cm, and 0.5 mm.

   _____

6. Convert 50 cm into meters. _____

7. There are _____ grams in 1 kilogram.

8. Which of the following is the smallest measurement?
   A. 16 mm   C. 0.2 m   E. 0.2 cm
   B. 2 cm   D. 1.7 cm   F. 4 cm

9. Moving the decimal point one place to the left makes a number _____.

10. There are _____ centimeters in 1 meter.

11. Convert 17 mm into cm. _____

12. Convert 1.5 liters into milliliters. _____

13. *True or False.* To multiply by 10, move the decimal point one place to the right. _____

14. Write the letters backward: retil. Define the word that is formed. _____

    _____

15. *True or False.* A volume of 0.01 L is the same as 100 mL. _____

16. Arrange these numbers from smallest to largest: 4 L, 1000 mL, 200 mL, 2.4 L, and 0.3 L.

    _____

17. There are _____ millimeters in 1 meter.

18. Which of the following are *not* measurements of length?
    A. grams   C. degrees Celsius   E. liters
    B. millimeters   D. meters   F. milliliters

19. The metric unit of weight is the _____.

20. Arrange these measurements from largest to smallest: 1.7 cm, 16 mm, 0.15 m, 20 cm, and 186 mm.

    _____

21. Convert 3 cm into millimeters. _____

22. There are _____ milligrams in 1 gram.

23. *True or False.* To divide by 10, move the decimal point two spaces to the left. _____

24. Which of the following values is the heaviest?
    A. 0.01 kg   C. 10 mg
    B. 1 mg   D. 100 mg

25. *True or False.* Twelve grams is the same as 1200 kg. _____

Match the following terms with their definitions.

_____ 26. The metric unit of volume

_____ 27. The prefix for ¹⁄₁₀₀ of a unit

_____ 28. The metric unit of temperature

_____ 29. The prefix for 1000 units

_____ 30. The prefix for ¹⁄₁₀₀₀ of a unit

_____ 31. The metric unit of mass or weight

_____ 32. The metric unit of length

A. meter

B. milli-

C. liter

D. centi-

E. gram

F. degree Celsius

G. kilo-

Comprehensive Review (Chapters 1–4)

Answer the following questions using what you have learned so far in this book.

33. The prefix of the term *endoplasmic* means "_____."

34. Convert 0.31 into a fraction._____

35. *True or False.* Facts are not opinions. _____

36. The control group in an experiment does not receive the _____ variable.

Section 4.3 Linear Measurements

In this section, you will learn about linear measurements. Linear measurements are measurements of length. The metric unit of length is the meter, and length is measured using a meter stick or a ruler.

The terms below are some of those that will be introduced in Section 4.3. To become familiar with these terms, reproduce each word on the line beside it. Pronounce each term as you write it. You will learn the definitions of these words as you complete this section.

1. linear _____

2. meter stick _____

3. ruler _____

4. centimeter _____

5. millimeter _____

Concept 1: Meters

The term *linear* refers to a straight line. Linear measurements determine the length of an object. As you have learned, the metric unit of length is the meter (m). A *meter stick* is used to take linear measurements (**Figure 4.5**). The meter stick is 1 meter in length. A *ruler* can also be used to take linear measurements. A ruler is 30 cm in length.

linear straight line

meter stick a tool for taking linear measurements; is 1 meter in length

ruler a tool for taking linear measurements; is 30 cm in length

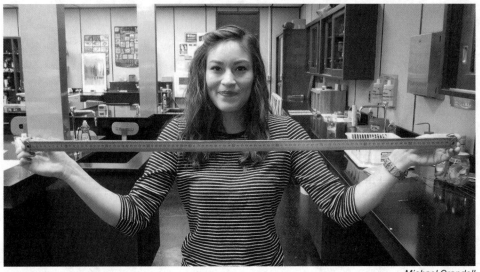

Michael Crandell

Figure 4.5 A meter stick is the length of 1 meter.

Recall Activity

1. The metric unit for linear measurements is the _____.

2. The term *linear* refers to a straight _____.

3. A meter stick is _____ meter(s) in length.

4. A ruler is _____ cm in length.

Concept 2: Centimeters and Millimeters

centimeter ¹⁄₁₀₀ of a meter
millimeter ¹⁄₁₀₀₀ of a meter

Linear measurements are also taken in *centimeters* (cm) and *millimeters* (mm). These units of measurement are smaller than the meter. There are 100 centimeters in 1 meter and 1000 millimeters in 1 meter. There are 10 millimeters in 1 centimeter. In **Figure 4.6**, all of the circled numbers indicate centimeters on a meter stick. The meter stick contains 100 centimeters (cm). The small lines between the centimeters are millimeters (mm). There are 10 millimeters per centimeter.

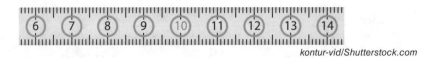

kontur-vid/Shutterstock.com

Figure 4.6 The circled numbers are centimeters, and the lines between the numbers are millimeters.

Recall Activity

1. The number 8 on the meter stick represents _____ cm or _____ mm.

2. The meter stick contains _____ mm, _____ cm, or _____ m.

Concept 3: Reading Linear Measurements

To read a meter stick, find the number to the left of the measurement and then count the number of lines between the number and the measurement. In **Figure 4.7**, the arrow represents a measurement. The number to the left of the arrow is 10, representing 10 centimeters. There are five lines between the number 10 and the arrow, representing 5 millimeters. Thus, the arrow is at a measurement of 10 cm plus 5 mm. The reading is 105 mm, 10.5 cm, or 0.105 m.

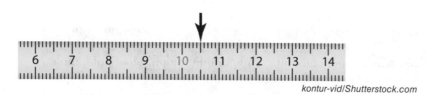

kontur-vid/Shutterstock.com

Figure 4.7   The reading is 10 cm plus 5 mm, or 10.5 cm.

Figure 4.8 and **Figure 4.9** show the linear measurements of some other common items. Figure 4.8 shows a dime and a nickel. A dime is about 1 mm thick; a nickel is about 2 mm thick. Figure 4.9 shows a large paper clip about 1 cm wide.

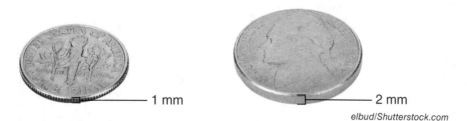

elbud/Shutterstock.com

Figure 4.8   A dime is about 1 mm thick, and a nickel is 2 mm thick.

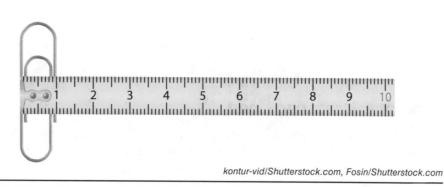

kontur-vid/Shutterstock.com, Fosin/Shutterstock.com

Figure 4.9   A big paper clip is 1 cm wide.

Recall Activity

1. Read the measurement depicted below. How long is the paper sheet in centimeters?_____

kontur-vid/Shutterstock.com

2. Read the measurement depicted below. How long is the paper sheet in centimeters?_____

kontur-vid/Shutterstock.com

3. In the space below, draw a meter stick up to 10 cm. Label the centimeters and millimeters in your drawing.

Concept 4: Measuring Lines

Using the skills you learned in Concept 3, you can begin measuring lines. Use a meter stick or ruler to measure lines. When you write a measurement, be sure to include the units (mm, cm, or m). Without a unit, a measurement is useless.

Recall Activity

1. Using a ruler or meter stick, measure and record the length of the line below in mm.

    ──────────────   Measurement _____

2. Using a ruler or meter stick, measure and record the length of the line below in cm.

    ────────────────────   Measurement _____

3. Using a ruler or meter stick, measure and record the length of the line below in mm.

    ──   Measurement _____

4. In the space below, draw a line that is 5.4 cm in length.

5. In the space below, draw a line that is 32 mm in length.

Section 4.3 Reinforcement

Answer the following questions using what you learned in this section.

1. Which of the following is the largest unit of measurement?
   A. millimeter
   B. meter
   C. centimeter
   D. kilometer

2. The line below is _____ cm in length.

    ────────────

3. Convert the measurement from question 2 into meters. _____

4. There are _____ meters in 1 kilometer.

5. The line below is _____ millimeter(s) in length.

_____

6. A millimeter is 1/_____ of a meter.

7. *True or False.* You must multiply to convert km to m. _____

8. A millimeter is 1/_____ of a centimeter.

9. A centimeter is 1/_____ of a meter.

10. To convert millimeters to centimeters, _____ by 10.

11. There are _____ centimeters in 1 meter.

12. The line below is _____ cm in length.

_____

13. There are _____ millimeters in 1 meter.

14. Which of the following is the smallest unit of measurement?
    A. millimeter   C. meter
    B. kilometer   D. centimeter

15. *True or False.* There are 100,000 cm in 1 km. _____

16. Convert 0.65 m into cm. _____

17. A meter is 1/_____ of a kilometer.

18. There are _____ millimeters in 1 centimeter.

19. *True or False.* There are 100 centimeters in 1 millimeter. _____

20. Convert 124 cm into m. _____

Comprehensive Review (Chapters 1–4)

Answer the following questions using what you have learned so far in this book.

21. An erythrocyte is _____ in color.

22. The metric unit of temperature is the _____.

23. If all constants in an experiment are the same, any differences *must* be caused by the _____ variable.

24. *True or False.* Scientific techniques are the scientific methods used to obtain opinions. _____

Section 4.4 Surface Area

Using linear measurements, you can calculate the surface areas of objects. *Surface area* is the total area of the outer surface of an object. In this section, you will learn about using measurements to calculate the surface areas of rectangles, cubes, circles, tubes, and cylinders.

surface area the total area of the outer surface of an object

The terms below are some of those that will be introduced in Section 4.4. To become familiar with these terms, reproduce each word on the line beside it. Pronounce each term as you write it. You will learn the definitions of these words as you complete this section.

1. surface area _____
2. square unit _____
3. radius _____

4. diameter _____
5. pi _____

Concept 1: Measuring the Width and Height of a Rectangle or Square

To calculate the surface area of a rectangle or square, first measure the rectangle's width and height. A rectangle's *width* is its length across. A rectangle's *height* is its length up and down (**Figure 4.10**). In a square, width and height should be equal.

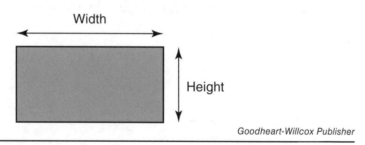

Goodheart-Willcox Publisher

Figure 4.10 Width and height are used to calculate surface area.

Recall Activity

1. Measure the width of the rectangle in Figure 4.10 using both millimeters and centimeters. Record the measurements. _____

2. Measure the height of the rectangle in Figure 4.10 using both millimeters and centimeters. Record the measurements. _____

Concept 2: Calculating the Surface Area of a Rectangle or Square

Multiplying width and height determines the surface area of a rectangle or square. In **Figure 4.11**, the width of the rectangle is 5 cm, and the height is 4 cm. To determine the surface area, multiply 5 cm by 4 cm for a surface area of 20 cm².

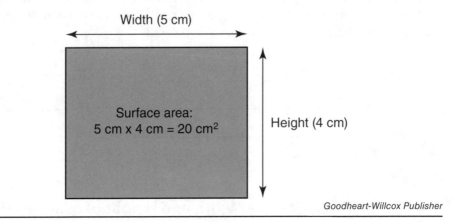

Width (5 cm)

Surface area:
5 cm x 4 cm = 20 cm²

Height (4 cm)

Goodheart-Willcox Publisher

Figure 4.11 Both the measurements and the units should be multiplied when determining surface area.

square unit a unit of measurement that results when two measurements of the same unit are multiplied together

When you multiply width (cm) and height (cm), you are also multiplying cm by cm. Multiplying the same units of measurement yields *square units* (units²). In this example, cm × cm = cm², which are also called *square centimeters*. The ² is shorthand for one unit multiplied by the same unit.

Recall Activity

1. Multiplying width by height determines the _____ of a rectangle or square.

2. cm × cm = _____

3. Measure the rectangle below and calculate the surface area in square centimeters.

Width: _____

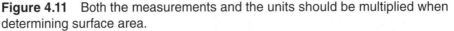

Surface area: _____   Height: _____

Concept 3: Calculating the Surface Area of a Cube

Remember that surface area is the area of the *outer surface* of an object. When calculating the surface area of a three-dimensional object, such as a cube, you are calculating the area of the object's outer surfaces.

A *cube* is a three-dimensional object made of six square surfaces (**Figure 4.12**). To calculate the surface area of a cube, add together the areas for each side of the cube. You will have six numbers to add together, because there are six sides to a cube. Because the sides of a cube are squares and all have the same area, you can also figure surface area by multiplying the area of one side of the cube by 6. To calculate the area of one side of the cube, multiply the side's width by its height.

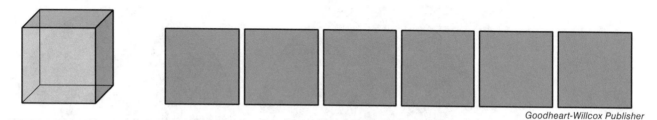

Goodheart-Willcox Publisher

Figure 4.12 The area of each side is equal to the other sides.

Recall Activity

1. Measure the width and height of each side of the cube below. Record your measurements in centimeters. Then calculate the surface area of the cube.

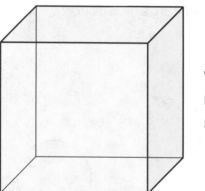

Width: _____

Height: _____

Surface area: _____

2. In the space below, carefully measure and draw a cube. Each side of the cube should have a height of 1 cm and a width of 1 cm. What is the surface area of the cube?

Concept 4: Measuring the Radius and Diameter of a Circle

radius the measurement from one edge of a circle to the center; half the distance across a circle

diameter the longest measurement across a circle

To calculate the surface area of a circle, you need to measure the circle's radius. The *radius* is the measurement from one edge of the circle to the center (half the distance across a circle). The radius of a circle is ½ the *diameter* (the longest measurement across the circle). To figure a circle's radius from its diameter, simply divide the diameter by 2 (**Figure 4.13**).

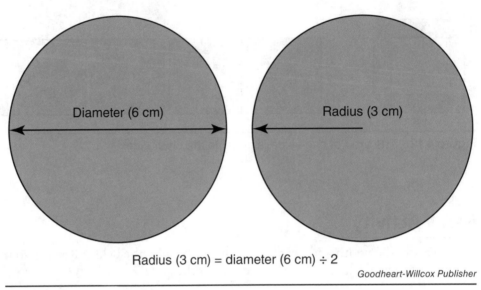

Radius (3 cm) = diameter (6 cm) ÷ 2

Goodheart-Willcox Publisher

Figure 4.13 A circle's radius is ½ its diameter.

Recall Activity

1. In the circles below, draw and label the radius and diameter.

2. The diameter of a circle is the _____ measurement across the circle.

3. The _____ is the measurement from one edge of the circle to the center.

4. The radius of a circle is _____ the diameter.

5. Measure the diameter of a penny in mm and convert into cm. Then calculate the radius.

    diameter: _____

    radius: _____

6. Measure the diameter of a nickel in mm and convert into cm. Then calculate the radius.

    diameter: _____

    radius: _____

Concept 5: Calculating the Surface Area of a Circle

The surface area of a circle is figured using the circle's radius and the value pi. *Pi* is a constant value, not a measurement. Pi has no units. Use the number 3.14 for the value of pi.

pi the value 3.14; used for calculating the surface area of a circle

The formula for calculating the surface area of a circle is $3.14 \times r^2$. The *r* represents the circle's radius, and r^2 can also be written as $r \times r$ (the radius of the circle multiplied by the radius of the circle). As an example, see the circle in **Figure 4.14**. The circle is 28 mm in diameter, so the radius is 14 mm (28 mm ÷ 2). To calculate the surface area of the circle, multiply 3.14 by the radius squared: $3.14 \times 14 \text{ mm} \times 14 \text{ mm} = 615 \text{ mm}^2$. Notice that you also multiply the units in this equation (mm × mm = mm²).

Radius: 28 mm ÷ 2 = 14 mm

Surface area: 3.14 × 14 mm × 14 mm = 615 mm²

Diameter (28 mm)

Figure 4.14 The surface area of this circle is expressed in mm². If measurements were in centimeters, surface area would be expressed in cm².

Recall Activity

1. A circle has a diameter of 22 cm. The radius of the circle is _____ cm.

2. Calculate the surface area of the circle below. Show your work by writing out the formula with the correct values.

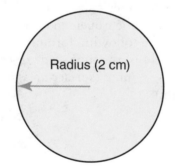
Radius (2 cm)

Surface area: _____

3. Calculate the surface area of the circle below. Show your work by writing out the formula with the correct values.

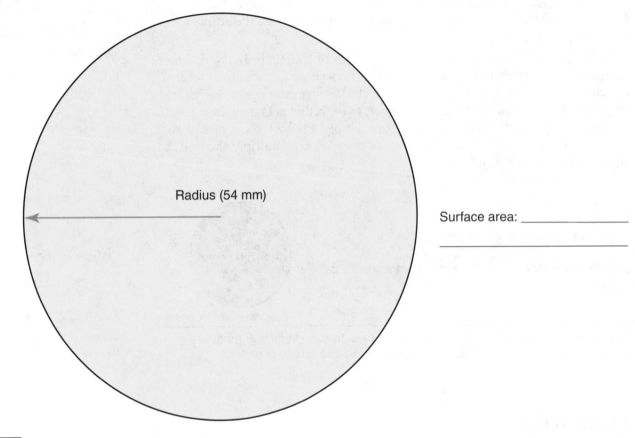

Radius (54 mm)

Surface area: _____

_____

Concept 6: Calculating the Surface Area of a Tube

Imagine a tube as an open-ended pipe. To calculate the surface area of a tube, first measure the radius of one of the tube's open ends and the height of the tube's side (**Figure 4.15**). Then use the following formula: surface area = 2 × radius of the tube's top × 3.14 × height of the tube's side. Include the units in the formula so it looks like this: _____ mm² (surface area) = 2 × _____ mm (radius) × 3.14 × _____ mm (height).

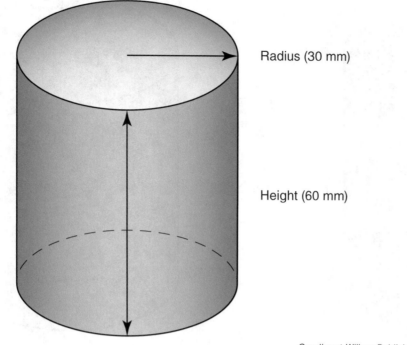

Radius (30 mm)

Height (60 mm)

Goodheart-Willcox Publisher

Figure 4.15 From this perspective, the radius is measured as halfway across the longest distance of the circle. A tube's radius and height are used in calculating surface area.

Recall Activity

View Figure 4.15 to answer the following questions.

1. What is the radius of the tube? _____

2. What is the diameter of the tube?_____

3. What is the height of the tube? _____

4. Calculate the surface area of the tube. _____

Concept 7: Calculating the Surface Area of a Cylinder

A cylinder is like a tube, except that it has a top and a bottom. To calculate the surface area of a cylinder, first determine the surface area of the tube. Then, using the equation to calculate surface area for a circle, calculate the surface areas of the cylinder's top and bottom. Finally, add these three surface areas together.

As an example, see the cylinder in **Figure 4.16**. The top of the cylinder has a radius of 3 cm, and the cylinder's height is 6 cm. First, calculate the surface area of the tube: 2×3 cm (radius) $\times 3.14 \times 6$ cm (height) = 113 cm². Then calculate the surface area of the cylinder's top or bottom: 3.14×3 cm (radius) $\times 3$ cm (radius) = 28 cm². Finally, add the surface area of the tube, the surface area of the top, and the surface area of the bottom: 113 cm² + 28 cm² + 28 cm² = 169 cm².

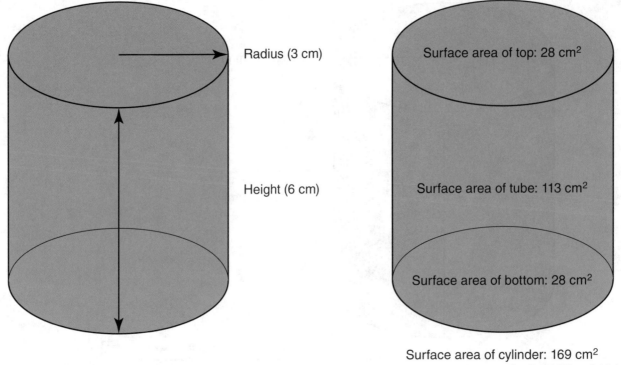

Radius (3 cm)

Height (6 cm)

Surface area of top: 28 cm²

Surface area of tube: 113 cm²

Surface area of bottom: 28 cm²

Surface area of cylinder: 169 cm²

Goodheart-Willcox Publisher

Figure 4.16 A cylinder is composed of one tube and two circles (one top and one bottom).

Recall Activity

1. What three values should you add to calculate the surface area of a cylinder?_____

_____

2. Measure the cylinder to the right using centimeters. Then calculate the following values, showing your work.

   surface area of the tube: _____

   surface area of the top:_____

   surface area of the bottom: _____

   surface area of the cylinder:_____

   Radius: _____

   Height: _____

3. Construct a cylinder by stacking five quarters. Then complete the following measurements and calculations.

Measure the diameter of a quarter in cm. _____

Calculate the radius in cm. _____

Measure the height of the five-quarter stack in cm. _____

Determine the surface area of the cylinder in cm². _____

Section 4.4 Reinforcement

Answer the following questions using what you learned in this section.

1. Write the letters backward: suidar. Define the word that is formed. _____

   _____

2. *True or False.* The surface area of a cube is width × height × 4. _____

3. Which of the following are *not* units of surface area?
   A. cm
   B. mm³
   C. cm²
   D. mm
   E. mm²
   F. cm³

4. A rectangle has a width of 4 cm and a height of 6 cm. What is the surface area? _____

5. What is the value of pi?_____

6. The area of a rectangle is the _____ multiplied by the height.

7. A circle has a diameter of 20 cm. What is the surface area?_____

8. Which measurement is larger: the diameter or the radius?_____

9. The formula 3.14 × r² calculates the area of a(n) _____.

10. Unscramble the letters: aaer. Define the word that is formed. _____

    _____

11. If the radius of a circle is 25 mm, the diameter of the circle is _____ mm.

12. *True or False.* Pi has units._____

13. Which of the following are square units?
    A. cm²
    B. mm³
    C. mm²
    D. cm

14. A circle with a diameter of 16 mm has a radius of _____ mm.

15. *True or False.* Surface area is measured in square units. _____

16. A cylinder has a diameter of 12 cm and a height of 50 cm. Calculate the surface area of the cylinder.

    _____

17. If the diameter of a circle is 120 cm, the radius is _____ cm.

18. How many sides are in a cube? _____

19. Unscramble the letters: eerdamit. Define the word that is formed. _____

_____

20. A cube has a width of 5 cm and a height of 5 cm. Calculate the surface area of the cube._____

Match the following terms with their definitions.

_____ 21. Half the distance across a circle

_____ 22. The longest distance across a circle   B. diameter

_____ 23. The total area of an object's outer surfaces   C. radius

A. surface area

Comprehensive Review (Chapters 1–4)

Answer the following questions using what you have learned so far in this book.

24. Thirty centimeters is equal to _____ millimeters.

25. *True or False.* The prefix *sub-* means "below." _____

26. A scientific law is a general statement of _____.

27. *True or False.* Students tend to like subjects at which they excel. _____

Section 4.5 Dry Volume

The surface area of a three-dimensional object relates to its dry volume. In this section, you will learn about calculating dry volume, the ratio between dry volume and surface area, and cell volume.

The terms below are some of those that will be introduced in Section 4.5. To become familiar with these terms, reproduce each word on the line beside it. Pronounce each term as you write it. You will learn the definitions of these words as you complete this section.

1. dry volume _____   3. ratio _____

2. cubic unit _____   4. cell_____

Concept 1: Calculating the Dry Volume of a Cube

dry volume the amount of space in a three-dimensional object

Dry volume is the amount of space in a three-dimensional object. It is calculated using linear measurements. To calculate the volume of a cube, multiply the depth, width, and height. For the cube in **Figure 4.17**, calculate dry volume as follows: 4 cm (depth) × 4 cm (width) × 4 cm (height) = 64 cm³ (volume). In this example, the unit for volume is cm³, or *cubic centimeters* (abbreviated as cc).

These are *cubic units* (units³) of measurement because three measurements of the same unit are multiplied together.

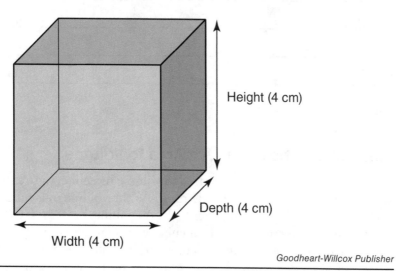

Height (4 cm)

Depth (4 cm)

Width (4 cm)

Goodheart-Willcox Publisher

Figure 4.17 To calculate the dry volume of a cube, measure height, depth, and width.

Recall Activity

1. What three measurements are multiplied together to calculate volume? _____

   _____

2. _____ units of measurement are created by multiplying three measurements of the same unit together.

3. The abbreviation for _____ is cc.

4. Cubic centimeters measure _____.

5. Measure the cube below and calculate its dry volume.

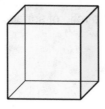

Height: _____

Depth: _2 cm_

Width: _____

Dry volume: _____

Concept 2: Ratios

A *ratio* is a comparison of numbers. For example, the ratio 2:1 expresses that there are two of the first number for every one of the second number. If you have 20 units of A and 10 units of B, you can write the comparison as the ratio 20:10. A ratio can be simplified by dividing the first number in the ratio by the second number. For example, in the ratio 20:10, divide 20 by 10, simplifying the ratio to 2:1. Similarly, you can simplify the ratio 6:8 by dividing 6 by 8, yielding a simplified ratio of 0.75:1.

Recall Activity

1. Simplify the ratio 81:9. _____

2. Simplify the ratio 150:25. _____

3. Simplify the ratio 6:2. _____

4. Simplify the ratio 15:10. _____

Concept 3: Ratio of Surface Area to Volume

To calculate the ratio of surface area to volume in a cube, figure the surface area and volume and then simplify the ratio. As the volume in a cube increases, the surface-area-to-volume ratio decreases. As volume decreases, the surface-area-to-volume ratio increases. Thus, a cube with a large volume has a smaller surface-area-to-volume ratio than a cube with a small volume.

As an example, see the cube in **Figure 4.18**. First, calculate the cube's total surface area: 3 cm × 3 cm = 9 cm² per side, and 9 cm² per side × 6 = 54 cm². Next, calculate the cube's dry volume: 3 cm × 3 cm × 3 cm = 27 cm³. The ratio of surface area to volume is 54:27, which can be simplified to 2:1. This ratio tells us that, for every one unit of volume, there are two units of surface area.

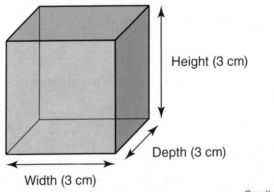

Height (3 cm)

Depth (3 cm)

Width (3 cm)

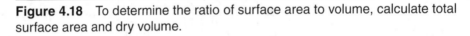

Figure 4.18 To determine the ratio of surface area to volume, calculate total surface area and dry volume.

Compare this to the larger cube in **Figure 4.19**. First, calculate the cube's total surface area: 12 cm × 12 cm = 144 cm², and 144 cm² × 6 = 864 cm². Then calculate the cube's dry volume: 12 cm × 12 cm × 12 cm = 1728 cm³. The ratio of surface area to volume is 864:1728, which can be simplified to 0.5:1. This tells us that, for every one unit of volume, there is one-half unit of surface area. The ratio of surface area to dry volume is greater in the small cube than in the large cube.

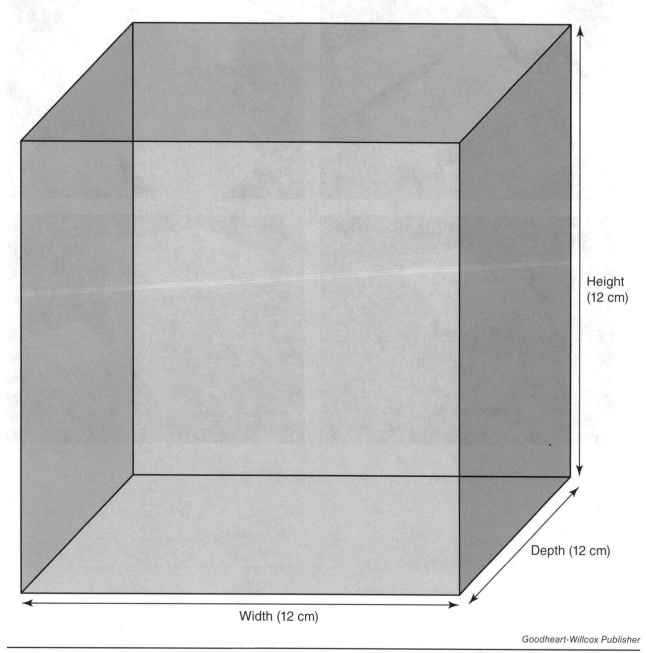

Height (12 cm)

Depth (12 cm)

Width (12 cm)

Goodheart-Willcox Publisher

Figure 4.19 A large cube, such as this one, has a smaller ratio of surface area to volume than a smaller cube.

Recall Activity

1. For this activity, see the layout below for creating a cube. Draw layouts for two cubes: one measuring 3 cm × 3 cm × 3 cm and one measuring 6 cm × 6 cm × 6 cm. Cut out the cube sides, folding them to create one large and one small cube.

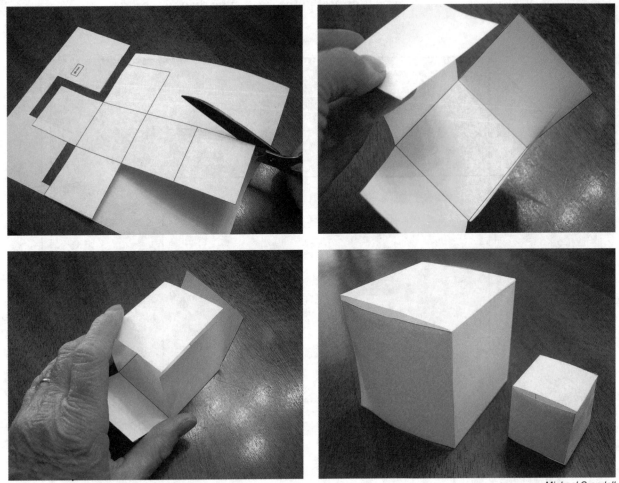

Michael Crandell

After you have cut out the cubes, calculate the following:

Large cube

surface area:_____   dry volume:_____

ratio of surface area to dry volume:_____

How many units of surface area are there for each unit of volume?_____

Small cube

surface area:_____   dry volume:_____

ratio of surface area to dry volume:_____

How many units of surface area are there for each unit of volume?_____

2. Which cube, small or large, has more surface area per unit of volume? _____

3. Will the surface-area-to-dry-volume ratio for a 1 cm × 1 cm × 1 cm cube be larger or smaller than the ratio of surface area to volume for a 3 cm × 3 cm × 3 cm cube? _____

4. Calculate the surface-area-to-volume ratio for a 1 cm × 1 cm × 1 cm cube. _____

_____

5. How many units of surface area are there for each unit of volume in the following cubes? Refer to the calculations you have already done in this concept.

large (216 cm³) cube: _____

small (27 cm³) cube: _____

smallest (1 cm³) cube: _____

Concept 4: Cells and the Ratio of Surface Area to Volume

Calculating the surface-area-to-volume ratios of different sizes of cubes helps explain why *cells*, the basic units of life, are so small. Your body is composed of trillions of microscopic cells. These cells make up body tissues and organs, carry oxygen and other substances through your body, and are involved in the reproduction of life.

cell the basic unit of life

Raw materials enter your cells, and products and waste exit your cells. As a result, the volume inside each cell is very busy processing materials and producing waste. These raw materials, products, and waste move through the surface area, or the plasma membrane, of a cell (**Figure 4.20**). A larger cell with a large volume requires the movement of more materials through the plasma membrane than a smaller cell. Thus, a cell cannot be any larger than the surface area required to move the materials that keep it alive.

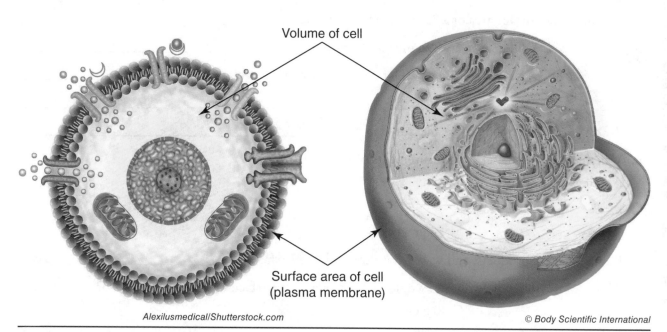

Volume of cell

Surface area of cell
(plasma membrane)

Alexilusmedical/Shutterstock.com

© Body Scientific International

Figure 4.20 The image on the left is a two-dimensional cross-section of a cell showing the exchange of raw materials and products across the plasma membrane. The image on the right is a three-dimensional illustration of a cell showing the plasma membrane, which represents the surface area of the cell.

This explains why cells are so small. Cells are small because smaller volumes (small cubes or small cells) have a large enough surface-area-to-volume ratio to allow the sufficient exchange of raw materials, products, and waste.

Recall Activity

1. _____ enter your cells, and _____ and
   _____ exit your cells.

2. What part of the cell do raw materials, products, and waste move through? _____

   _____

3. The plasma membrane is the _____ area of the cell.

4. Cells are _____ because smaller volumes have a large surface-area-to-volume ratio.

5. A(n) _____ surface-area-to-volume ratio allows the sufficient exchange of raw materials, products, and waste.

Section 4.5 Reinforcement

Answer the following questions using what you learned in this section.

1. Which of the following volumes would yield the greatest surface-area-to-volume ratio?
   A. 4 cm³   C. 0.8 cm³
   B. 0.5 cm³   D. 3.3 cm³

2. Calculate the surface area of a 2 cm × 2 cm × 2 cm cube. _____

3. *True or False.* Volume is measured in square units. _____

4. Write the letters backward: emulov. Define the word that is formed. _____

   _____

5. *True or False.* Square units are measured in cc. _____

6. Which of the following are measurements of volume?
   A. cm³   C. cm²
   B. cc   D. cm

7. _____ enter a cell.

8. Raw materials, products, and waste move through the surface _____ of a cell.

9. Which of the following volumes would yield the smallest surface-area-to-volume ratio?
   A. 1.9 cm³   C. 0.5 cm³
   B. 18 cm³   D. 7 cm³

10. Unscramble the letters: bicuc. Define the word that is formed. _____

    _____

11. *True or False.* Cubic units are used to measure volume. _____

12. The square centimeter is a unit of _____.

13. *True or False.* A cube with a large volume will have a greater surface-area-to-volume ratio than a cube with a small volume. _____

14. Products and _____ exit a cell.

15. Would a large cube or a small cube have a smaller surface-area-to-volume ratio? _____

    _____

16. Unscramble the letters: lomvue. Define the word that is formed. _____

    _____

17. Which of the following volumes would yield the smallest surface-area-to-volume ratio?
    A. 4 cm^3 C. 0.8 cm^3
    B. 0.5 cm^3 D. 3.3 cm^3

18. Your body is made up of trillions of _____ cells.

19. *True or False.* Materials must enter and leave a cell. _____

20. The cubic centimeter is a unit of _____.

Comprehensive Review (Chapters 1–4)

Answer the following questions using what you have learned so far in this book.

21. Three dollars is equal to _____ dimes.

22. The combining form _____ means "narrow."

23. *True or False.* Teaching a section to someone will help you better understand the material. _____

24. Scientific _____ are mankind's basis for understanding the natural world.

Section 4.6 Liquid Volume and Temperature

The metric units for liquid volume and temperature are liters or milliliters and degrees Celsius. In this section, you will learn about calculating and measuring liquid volume and temperature.

   The following terms are some of those that will be introduced in Section 4.6. To become familiar with these terms, reproduce each word on the line beside it. Pronounce each term as you write it. You will learn the definitions of these words as you complete this section.

1. liquid volume _____   3. graduated cylinder _____

2. milliliter _____   4. meniscus _____

Concept 1: Cubic Centimeters and Milliliters

liquid volume the amount of liquid in a three-dimensional object

milliliter $\frac{1}{1000}$ of a liter

Liquid volume is the amount of liquid in a three-dimensional object, usually a cylinder. Whereas dry volume is measured in cubic centimeters, liquid volume is measured using *milliliters* (mL) or liters (L). There are 1000 cubic centimeters in 1 liter, and there are 1000 milliliters in 1 liter (L). Therefore, the volume contained in 1 cubic centimeter (cc or cm^3) is equal to the volume contained in 1 milliliter (mL).

Recall Activity

1. Convert 10 cc into mL. _____

2. The volume contained in 1 cc is _____ the volume contained in 1 mL.

Concept 2: Reading a Meniscus

graduated cylinder a narrow cylinder with milliliter increments; used for measuring liquid volume

meniscus the semicircular surface of liquid in a cylinder

Liquid volume can be measured using a *graduated cylinder*, a narrow cylinder with milliliter increments. When liquid fills and climbs up the side of the graduated cylinder, a meniscus will form. The *meniscus* is the semicircular surface of liquid in a cylinder. To determine the volume of liquid, read the cylinder at the *bottom* of the meniscus (**Figure 4.21**).

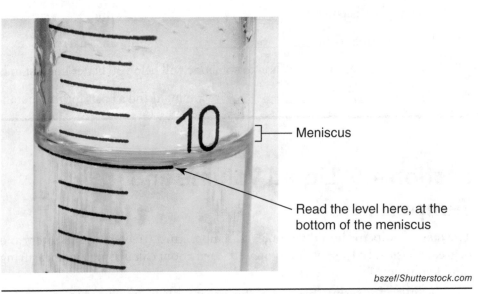

Meniscus

Read the level here, at the bottom of the meniscus

bszef/Shutterstock.com

Figure 4.21 To measure liquid volume, read the measurement at the bottom of the meniscus.

Recall that a graduated cylinder is marked in milliliter increments. This means that each number on the cylinder marks the number of milliliters. The volume in Figure 4.21 is 10 mL. The volume in **Figure 4.22** is 18 mL.

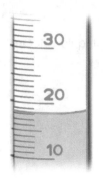

Figure 4.22   The markings on this graduated cylinder are in milliliter increments.

Recall Activity

1. A(n) _____ will form when liquid climbs up the side of a graduated cylinder.

2. Read the cylinder at the _____ of the meniscus.

3. Liquid volume is measured with a graduated _____.

4. If the bottom of the meniscus were halfway between 20 mL and 30 mL, the reading would be _____ mL.

5. View the graduated cylinder and record the measurement. Include units in your answer.

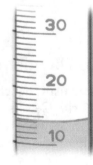

Liquid volume: _____

6. View the graduated cylinder and record the measurement. Include units in your answer.

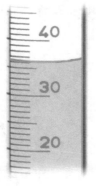

Liquid volume: _____

Concept 3: Celsius Scale

The metric unit for temperature is the *degree Celsius* (°C). In the metric system, temperature is *not* measured using degrees Fahrenheit (°F). Degrees Celsius is abbreviated °C. The scale for degrees Celsius is based on temperature variations of water. Water freezes at 0°C, and water boils at 100°C.

Recall Activity

1. Water freezes at _____ °C.

2. The abbreviation °C stands for _____.

3. Water boils at _____ °C.

Concept 4: The Celsius Thermometer

Degrees Celsius are measured using a Celsius thermometer. **Figure 4.23** shows a Celsius thermometer. On the Celsius thermometer, the numbers represent degrees Celsius. The marks in between the labeled numbers indicate individual degrees. Any markings below zero are considered negative degrees Celsius. The measurement in Figure 4.23 reads 18°C.

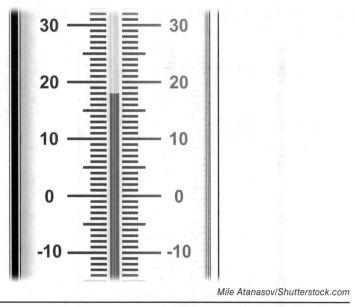

Mile Atanasov/Shutterstock.com

Figure 4.23 The level of mercury in this thermometer indicates temperature.

Recall Activity

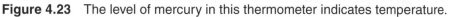

1. The numbers on a Celsius thermometer represent _____.

2. How many marks are found between 10 and 20 on a Celsius thermometer? _____

3. Each mark on a Celsius thermometer represents _____ degree.

4. View the Celsius thermometer below and record the temperature. Include units in your answer.

_____

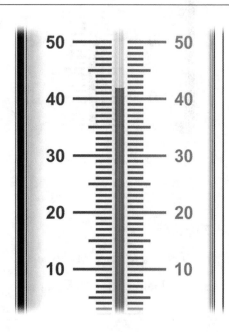

Mile Atanasov/Shutterstock.com

5. View the Celsius thermometer and record the temperature. Include units in your answer. _____

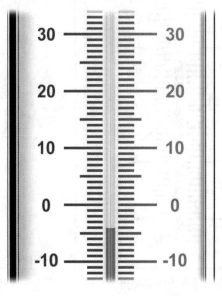

Mile Atanasov/Shutterstock.com

6. View the Celsius thermometer and record the temperature. Include units in your answer. _____

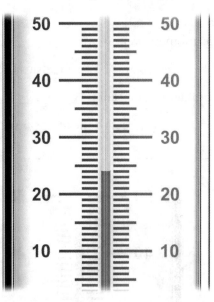

Mile Atanasov/Shutterstock.com

Section 4.6 Reinforcement

Answer the following questions using what you learned in this section.

1. Write the letters backward: sucsinem. Define the word that is formed. _____

_____

2. *True or False.* A volume of 1 mL is the same as 1 cc. _____

3. Water boils at _____ degrees Celsius.

4. There are _____ mL in 1 L.

5. °C is the abbreviation for _____.

6. Which of the following is the largest volume?
   A. 2.2 L   C. 16 mL
   B. 180 mL   D. 0.4 L

7. The scale for degrees _____ is based on temperature variations of water.

8. Unscramble the letters: cnessumi. Define the word that is formed. _____
   _____

9. The volume measurement of 100 mL is the same as _____ cc.

10. Water freezes at _____ °C.

11. *True or False.* A volume measurement in a graduated cylinder can be read by looking at the top of the meniscus. _____

12. Which of the following temperatures are below freezing?
    A. -1°C   C. 10°C
    B. 1°C   D. -15°C

13. The volume measurement of 100 mL is the same as _____ cc.

14. Which of the following measure volume?
    A. cc   C. L   E. cm²
    B. mL   D. cm   F. cm³

15. *True or False.* Liquid volume is measured with a graduated cylinder._____

16. Which of the following temperatures are above water's boiling point?
    A. 90°C   C. 101°C   E. 85°C
    B. 99°C   D. 120°C   F. 105°C

17. *True or False.* Ice forms at 0°C. _____

18. The volume measurement of 10 cc is the same as _____ mL.

19. The scale for degrees Celsius is based on temperature variations of _____.

20. Unscramble the letters: tirelmilli. Define the word that is formed. _____
    _____

21. _____ is the amount of liquid inside a three-dimensional space.

22. The semicircular surface of a liquid is known as a(n) _____.

Section 4.7 Mass

The metric unit for mass is the gram, which can also be expressed in milligrams or kilograms. In this section, you will learn about the difference between mass and weight, how to measure using grams, and how to read a platform balance and electronic balance.

The terms below are some of those that will be introduced in Section 4.7. To become familiar with these terms, reproduce each word on the line beside it. Pronounce each term as you write it. You will learn the definitions of these words as you complete this section.

1. mass _____

2. weight _____

3. platform balance _____

4. electronic balance _____

Concept 1: Mass Versus Weight

mass the amount of matter in an object

weight the force of gravity on the mass of an object

Mass and weight, while often used synonymously, refer to different measurements. *Mass* is the amount of matter in an object. *Weight* is the force of gravity on the mass of an object. On the earth, the mass and weight of an object are the same. If you were to take an object to the moon, however, the mass of the object would not change, but the object's weight would be smaller. This is because the force of gravity on the moon is less than the force of gravity on the earth.

Recall Activity

1. _____ is the amount of matter in an object.

2. Weight is the force of _____ on the mass of an object.

3. An object on the moon would weigh _____ than the same object on the earth.

Concept 2: Grams

The metric unit for mass is the gram. For example, the mass of one nickel is 5 grams (g). Mass can also be measured in milligrams (mg) and kilograms (kg). A *milligram* is ¹⁄₁₀₀₀ of a gram, and a *kilogram* is 1000 grams. The metric system is designed for simplicity and easy conversion. A mass of 1 mL of water equals 1 gram. The mass of 1 L (1000 mL) of water is 1 kg (1000 g).

Recall Activity

1. The metric unit for mass is the _____.

2. The mass of a(n) _____ is 5 g.

3. The mass of 1 mL of water is _____ g.

4. There are _____ mL of water in 1 L, and the mass of each mL of water is 1 g. Therefore, the mass of 1 L of water is _____ g or _____ kg.

Concept 3: The Platform Balance

A *platform balance* is used to measure the mass of an object in grams. A platform balance has three beams with markings that indicate the number of grams. Each beam measures grams in different increments. In the platform balance in **Figure 4.24**, the first beam measures individual grams, the second beam measures hundreds of grams, and the third beam measures tens of grams.

platform balance an instrument that measures the mass of an object in grams; has three beams with markings that indicate the number of grams

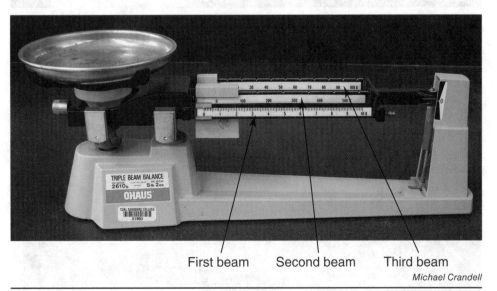

First beam   Second beam   Third beam

Michael Crandell

Figure 4.24   This platform balance has three beams.

Recall Activity

1. How many beams does the platform balance have? _____

2. In Figure 4.24, the first beam measures _____ grams, the second

   beam measures _____ grams, and the third beam measures

   _____ grams.

Concept 4: Using the Platform Balance

To use a platform balance, set an object on the platform with the balance pointer and weights set at zero (**Figure 4.25**). When the object is placed on the platform, the pointer will move up. To determine the object's mass, slide the weights along the beams to bring the pointer back down to zero (**Figure 4.26**). Each weight will be positioned above a number. Read the numbers at each weight to determine the mass of the object. Begin reading at the largest weight, followed by the middle weight, and finish with the smallest weight. The mass shown in Figure 4.26 is 4 g.

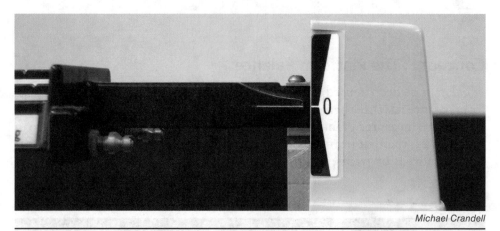

Michael Crandell

Figure 4.25 The pointer on the platform balance should be set at zero.

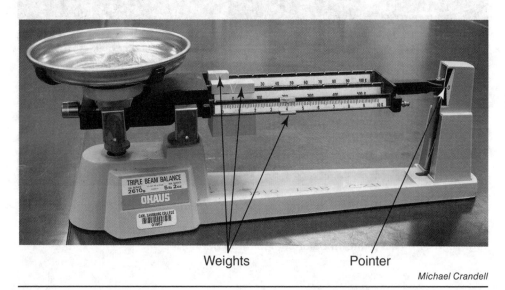

Weights   Pointer

Michael Crandell

Figure 4.26 Move the weights until the pointer is aligned to the zero. This balance reads 0 g, 0 g, and 4 g.

Recall Activity

1. Before placing the object on the platform, the pointer should be set at _____.

2. The object to be weighed should be placed on the _____.

3. Slide the weights along the _____ to bring the pointer back down to zero.

4. Mass is read from the positions of the _____.

5. Read the mass when the pointer is pointing at _____.

Concept 5: Reading a Platform Balance

When reading mass from a platform balance, read the largest weight (hundreds of grams) first. In **Figure 4.27**, this is 0 g. Then read the intermediate weight (tens of grams); it is 20 g. Finally, read the smallest weight (individual grams); it is 4.7 g. To figure mass, add the readings from the three weights together. The mass of this object is 24.7 g (0 g + 20 g + 4.7 g).

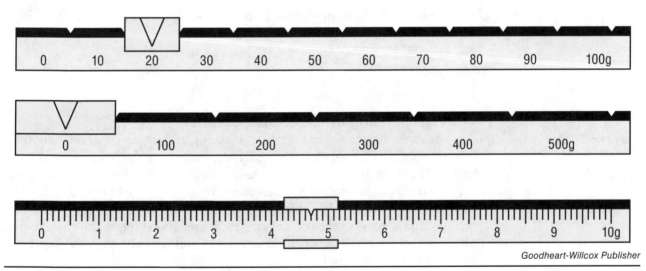

Figure 4.27   The mass of the object is 24.7 g.

Recall Activity

1. Read the platform balance below. What is the mass of the object? _____

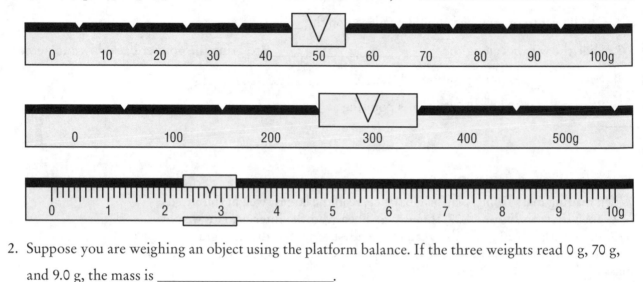

2. Suppose you are weighing an object using the platform balance. If the three weights read 0 g, 70 g, and 9.0 g, the mass is _____.

3. Suppose you are weighing an object using the platform balance. If the three weights read 100 g, 30 g, and 5.9 g, the mass is _____.

Concept 6: Using an Electronic Balance

electronic balance an instrument that measures the mass of an object in grams digitally

An *electronic balance* measures the mass of an object in grams digitally (**Figure 4.28**). To use an electronic balance, make sure the balance is on a flat surface. Turn the balance on and, if using a container to measure mass, place the container on the platform. Then press the *zero* or *tare* button to bring the measurement back to zero. This prevents the mass of the container from being included in the mass of the object being measured. Next, place the object being measured on the platform or in the container and read the object's mass from the screen of the electronic balance.

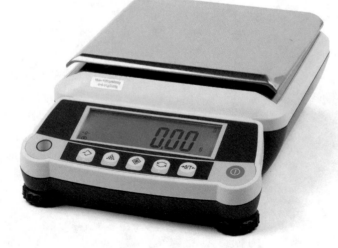

litchima/Shutterstock.com

Figure 4.28 An electronic balance records mass digitally.

Recall Activity

1. An electronic balance measures the mass of an object in _____ digitally.

2. What is the purpose of the *zero* or *tare* button?_____

_____

Section 4.7 Reinforcement

Answer the following questions using what you learned in this section.

1. *True or False.* An object has the same mass on the earth as it does on the moon._____

2. What is the mass of 500 mL of water in kg?_____

3. *True or False.* With the balance platform empty and the pointer set at zero, adding an object to the platform will cause the pointer to move. _____

4. The platform balance has _____ beam(s).

5. Unscramble the letters: nacable. Define the word that is formed. _____

_____

6. *True or False.* An object weighs more on the earth than it does on the moon._____

7. The weights of a platform balance read 100 g, 60 g, and 8.5 g. What is the mass of the object?

_____

8. The metric unit of mass is the _____.

9. Arrange these measurements from lightest to heaviest: 1.2 kg, 100 g, 1120 g, 710 g, and 0.75 kg.

_____

10. The weights of a platform balance read 0 g, 90 g, and 6.4 g. What is the mass of the object?

_____

11. *True or False.* An object has more mass on the earth than it does on the moon._____

12. Write the letters backward: ecnalab mroftalp. Define the term that is formed._____

_____

13. Does an object weigh more on the earth or on the moon? Explain._____

_____

14. Before placing an object on the platform, the pointer of the platform balance should point to

_____.

15. Unscramble the letters: higwet. Define the word that is formed. _____

_____

16. When weighing an object, move the weights of the platform balance until the pointer points to

_____.

17. If the mass of an object is 432.6 g, the reading in hundreds is _____,

the reading in tens is _____, and the reading in individual grams is

_____.

18. Can the three beams of a platform balance read 0 g, 50 g, and 66 g? Explain. _____

_____

_____

19. The metric unit for _____ is the gram.

20. The weights of a platform balance read 400 g, 10 g, and 2.3 g. What is the mass of the object?

_____

21. The amount of matter in an object is _____.

22. The force of gravity on the mass of an object is _____.

23. How is an electronic balance different from a platform balance? _____

_____

24. After placing a container on the platform of an electronic balance, press the

_____ or _____ button to bring the measurement

back to zero.

Comprehensive Review (Chapters 1–4)

Answer the following questions using what you have learned so far in this book.

25. The prefix _____ means "before."

26. There are _____ mm in 1 cm.

27. _____ is the deliberate effort to make long-term memories about subject
matter.

28. The two sources of facts in the diagnostic scientific method are _____ and

_____.

Section 4.8 Concentration, Pressure, and Rate

Concentration, pressure, and rate are measured using the metric system. These concepts are important in science. In this section, you will learn what concentration, pressure, and rate are and how they are measured.

The terms below are some of those that will be introduced in Section 4.8. To become familiar with these terms, reproduce each word on the line beside it. Pronounce each term as you write it. You will learn the definitions of these words as you complete this section.

1. concentration _____

2. solute _____

3. solvent _____

4. pressure _____

5. rate _____

Concept 1: Concentration

All matter—including solids, liquids, and gases—is made of particles called *atoms*. Atoms are so small they cannot be seen with a microscope. *Concentration* refers to the number of atoms or molecules per one unit of volume. An example is atoms dissolved in a volume of liquid. The liquid's concentration would refer to the number of atoms dissolved per one unit of volume (**Figure 4.29**).

concentration the number of atoms or molecules per one unit of volume; usually expressed in mg/L

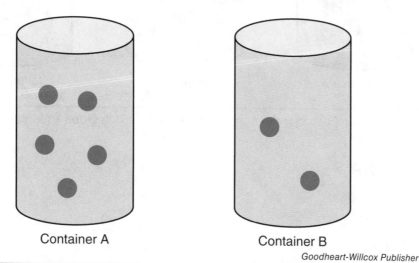

Container A   Container B

Goodheart-Willcox Publisher

Figure 4.29   The volume of water in container A is equal to the volume of water in container B. The purple dots represent atoms suspended in the same volume of water.

Recall Activity

View Figure 4.29 to answer the following questions.

1. Which container, A or B, has more purple dots? _____

2. Which container, A or B, has a higher concentration? _____

3. What is the difference in the concentration of purple dots between A and B? _____

4. The volume of water in A is _____ to the volume of water in B.

Concept 2: Concentration Units

solute the atoms dissolved in a solution

solvent the liquid in which atoms are dissolved in a solution

Concentration is often expressed in milligrams per liter or *mg/L*. For example, if you placed 5 mg of salt into 1 L of water, the salt concentration of the water would be 5 mg/L. When atoms are dissolved in a liquid, the liquid becomes known as a *solution*. A solution contains a solute and a solvent. The *solute* is the atoms dissolved, and the *solvent* is the liquid in which the atoms are dissolved. In the example of salt and water, salt is the solute, and water is the solvent. **Figure 4.30** shows three containers holding solutions. Each green square in the containers represents 1 mg of salt. Each container has 1 L of water. Therefore, each concentration will be expressed in mg of salt per 1 L.

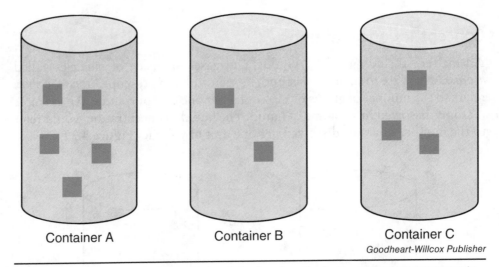

Container A   Container B   Container C

Goodheart-Willcox Publisher

Figure 4.30   Each cylinder contains 1 L of water. Each green square represents 1 mg of salt.

Recall Activity

View Figure 4.30 to answer the following questions.

1. What is the solute in the containers?_____

2. What is the solvent in the containers?_____

3. What is the concentration of salt (mg/L) in container A?_____

4. What is the concentration of salt (mg/L) in container B? _____

5. What is the concentration of salt (mg/L) in container C?_____

Concept 3: Pressure

pressure the collisions of atoms with other atoms and with the sides of a container

Atoms are constantly moving and colliding, and this ongoing motion produces pressure. *Pressure* refers to the collisions of atoms with other atoms and with the sides of a container (**Figure 4.31**).

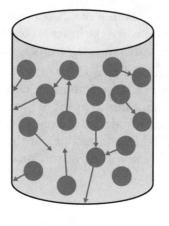

Figure 4.31   Pressure is caused by atoms colliding.

Pressure is dependent on the number of atoms in a container, regardless of the types of atoms. The more atoms there are in a container, the higher the pressure is. The pressure of a gas inside a container is also dependent on temperature. The higher the temperature, the more atoms move. Atoms moving more causes more collisions between the atoms and the sides of the container, thus increasing pressure. If the number of atoms in a container remains constant, then pressure also depends on the container's volume. If the volume of a container increases, a gas expands, and pressure inside the container decreases. If the volume of a container decreases, a gas is compressed, and pressure inside the container increases.

Recall Activity

1. If the container size stays the same, but more atoms are added to the container, pressure _____.

2. If the number of atoms in a container stays the same, but the container size is increased, pressure _____.

3. If the number of atoms in a container and container size stay the same, but the temperature inside the container increases, pressure _____.

4. If the container size is decreased, but the number of atoms stays the same, pressure _____.

Concept 4: Blood Pressure

A liquid does not expand and compress like a gas. One type of liquid pressure used often in healthcare is *blood pressure*. Blood pressure is measured in millimeters of mercury, abbreviated *mmHg*. A blood pressure reading has two components: pressure when the heart is contracting and pressure when the heart is relaxed. In a blood pressure reading of 120/90 mmHg, the number above the line (120) represents pressure when the heart is contracting. The number below the line (90) represents pressure when the heart is relaxed.

A normal blood pressure reading is 120/80 mmHg; a reading of 140/90 mmHg is high. If your diet includes a large amount of cholesterol, your blood vessels may accumulate *plaque*. Plaque builds inside of blood vessels, causing the diameters of the vessels to gradually decrease even as the amount of blood in the vessels remains the same. When contractions of the heart force blood through smaller-diameter vessels, this increases pressure on the walls of the blood vessels, thus increasing blood pressure.

Recall Activity

1. The unit of measurement for blood pressure is _____.

2. A normal blood pressure reading is _____.

3. A high blood pressure reading is _____.

4. Would blood pressure increase or decrease if a blood vessel became smaller in diameter? _____

5. What are the two parts of a blood pressure reading? _____

_____

Concept 5: Rate and Heart Rate

rate the number of events that occur during a specific unit of time

Rate refers to the number of events that occur during a specific unit of time. *Heart rate* is one example of rate. Heart rate measures the number of heartbeats per minute. A normal heart rate is 72 beats per minute (abbreviated as *bpm*).

To determine your own heart rate, begin by locating the pulse in your forearm or throat. Press lightly on your forearm or on the right side of your throat. Count the number of heartbeats for 20 seconds and then multiply the number of beats by 3 to calculate beats per minute.

Recall Activity

1. What is your heart rate in beats per minute? _____

2. If you multiplied your number of heartbeats for 20 seconds by 2 instead of by 3, you would express the number in beats per _____ second(s).

3. A rate measures the number of events that occur during a specific unit of

_____.

Section 4.8 Reinforcement

Answer the following questions using what you learned in this section.

1. Unscramble the letters: tisoluno. Define the word that is formed. _____
   _____

2. *True or False.* If the temperature inside a container increases, then the pressure inside the container increases. _____

3. A(n) _____ measures the number of events that occur during a specific unit of time.

4. In a solution of salt and water, salt is the _____.

5. Which of the following is the greatest concentration?
   A. 4.2 mg/L   C. 10.4 mg/L
   B. 0.85 mg/L   D. 9.8 mg/L

6. If the volume of a container increases, the pressure inside the container _____.

7. Which of the following are *not* rates?
   A. miles/hour   C. mg/L
   B. pounds/square inch   D. feet/second

8. *True or False.* If the temperature inside a container is decreased, the pressure inside the container increases. _____

9. Write the letters backward: erusserp. Define the word that is formed. _____
   _____

10. The unit of concentration is _____.

11. A(n) _____ is dissolved in a solvent.

12. Which of the following affect pressure?
    A. container size   C. number of atoms
    B. temperature   D. types of atoms

13. Atoms are constantly _____.

14. Suppose you have a salt water concentration of 10 mg/L. How many mg of salt do you have per 1 L of water? _____

15. Unscramble the letters: cationtrocnen. Define the word that is formed. _____
    _____

16. *True or False.* Atoms move faster at lower temperatures. _____

17. Concentration tells you how many atoms are in _____ of liquid.

18. In a solution of salt and water, water is the _____.

19. In the blood pressure reading of 135/95 mmHg, _____ is pressure when the heart is relaxed.

20. A solute is dissolved in a(n) _____.

Match the following terms with their definitions.

_____ 21. Events per unit of time

_____ 22. The liquid that dissolves the solute

_____ 23. Collisions between atoms

_____ 24. The atoms dissolved in a solvent

_____ 25. Atoms per unit of volume

A. concentration
B. solute
C. solvent
D. pressure
E. rate

Comprehensive Review (Chapters 1–4)

Answer the following questions using what you have learned so far in this book.

26. The combining forms in the term *osteoarthritis* mean "_____" and
   "_____."

27. Calculate the surface area of a 10 cm × 10 cm square. _____

28. Patient history is obtained by asking a patient to fill out a(n) _____ with yes-or-no answers.

29. An explanation is _____ if it is observable and testable.

Section 4.9 Converting Between Metric and English Units of Measurement

The metric system is the scientific standard of measurement, but you may be more familiar with the English system of measurement. In this section, you will learn how to convert between metric units and units in the English system of measurement.

The terms below are some of those that will be introduced in Section 4.9. To become familiar with these terms, reproduce each word on the line beside it. Pronounce each term as you write it. You will learn the definitions of these words as you complete this section.

1. English system of measurement _____

2. conversion factor_____

Concept 1: Metric and English Measuring Systems

The metric system is used in scientific measurement and is the standard measurement in most countries around the world. However, in the United States, the

English system of measurement is the standard. Although the English system is just as accurate as the metric system, the metric system is easier to use because it is based on powers of 10. Various *conversion factors* (values that can be multiplied to convert a unit) can help you change an English measurement into a metric measurement or change a metric measurement into an English measurement.

English system of measurement the measurement system used in the United States

conversion factor a value that is multiplied to convert a unit

Recall Activity

1. The United States uses the _____ system of measurement as the standard.

2. Scientific measurement uses the _____ system.

Concept 2: Length Conversions

To convert a measurement from the English system to the metric system or vice versa, multiply the measurement by the appropriate conversion factor. In the English system of measurement, inches, feet, yards, and miles measure length. The conversion factors for metric and English linear measurements are shown in **Figure 4.32**. You can review all of the conversion factors in this section in Appendix B.

English to Metric		Metric to English	
Conversion	**Multiply by**	**Conversion**	**Multiply by**
inches to centimeters	2.54 cm/inch	centimeters to inches	0.39 inches/cm
feet to meters	0.30 m/foot	meters to feet	3.28 feet/m
yards to meters	0.91 m/yard	meters to yards	1.09 yards/m
miles to kilometers	1.61 km/miles	kilometers to miles	0.62 miles/km

Figure 4.32 Conversion factors are values that can be multiplied by a measurement to convert that measurement into another unit.

For example, to convert a measurement of 3 inches into centimeters, multiply the inch measurement by 2.54 cm/inch. Because 3 inches × 2.54 cm/in = 7.62 cm, 3 inches is equivalent to 7.62 cm.

Recall Activity

1. Convert 5 inches into cm. _____

2. Convert 6 inches into cm. _____

3. Convert 1.5 feet into m. _____

4. Convert 6 m into yards. _____

5. Convert 10 km into miles. _____

6. Convert 2.25 inches into cm. _____

7. Convert 7.5 cm into inches._____

Concept 3: Volume Conversions

In the United States, both metric and English units measure volume. For example, food packaging labels list the volume of food contained in both metric and English units (**Figure 4.33**).

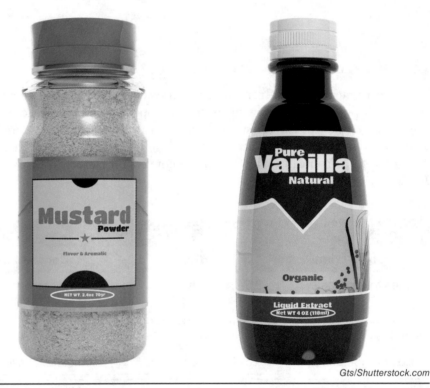

Gts/Shutterstock.com

Figure 4.33   These food package labels list volume in both English and metric units.

In the English system of measurement, gallons, quarts, and fluid ounces measure volume. As with length measurements, to convert volume measurements, multiply the measurement by the appropriate conversion factor. The conversion factors for metric and English volume measurements are shown in **Figure 4.34**.

English to Metric		Metric to English	
Conversion	**Multiply by**	**Conversion**	**Multiply by**
gallons to liters	3.79 L/gallon	liters to gallons	0.26 gallons/L
quarts to liters	0.95 L/quart	liters to quarts	1.06 quarts/L
fluid ounces to milliliters	29.57 mL/fluid ounce	milliliters to fluid ounces	0.03 fluid ounces/mL

Figure 4.34   Use these conversion factors to make volume conversions.

Recall Activity

1. Convert 2 gallons into L. _____

2. Convert 0.5 fluid ounces into mL. _____

3. Convert 10 quarts into L. _____

4. Convert 5 L into quarts. _____

5. Convert 4.5 mL into fluid ounces. _____

6. Convert 6 L into gallons. _____

Concept 4: Mass Conversions

In the English system of measurement, ounces and pounds measure mass. The conversion factors for metric and English mass measurements are shown in **Figure 4.35**.

English to Metric		Metric to English	
Conversion	**Multiply by**	**Conversion**	**Multiply by**
ounces to grams	28.35 g/ounce	grams to ounces	0.035 ounces/g
pounds to kilograms	0.45 kg/pound	kilograms to pounds	2.21 pounds/kg

Figure 4.35   Use these conversion factors to make mass conversions.

Recall Activity

1. Convert 100 g into ounces. _____

2. Convert 10 kg into pounds. _____

3. Convert 5 pounds into kg. _____

4. Convert 2 ounces into g. _____

Concept 5: Temperature Conversions

In the English system of measurement, degrees Fahrenheit (°F) measure temperature. In **Figure 4.36**, degrees Farenheit are shown on the left, and degrees Celsius are shown on the right. This figure shows some equivalencies between degrees Fahrenheit and degrees Celsius.

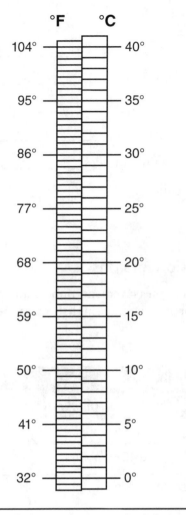

°F   °C

104° — 40°

95° — 35°

86° — 30°

77° — 25°

68° — 20°

59° — 15°

50° — 10°

41° — 5°

32° — 0°

Figure 4.36 Degrees Fahrenheit are shown on the left, and degrees Celsius are shown on the right.

To convert a measurement from degrees Fahrenheit into degrees Celsius, subtract 32 from the number of degrees Fahrenheit and then multiply that value by $\frac{5}{9}$. You would convert 34°F into degrees Celsius as follows: 34°F − 32 = 2, and $2 \times \frac{5}{9} = 1.1$°C.

To convert a measurement from degrees Celsius into degrees Fahrenheit, multiply the number of degrees Celsius by $\frac{9}{5}$ and then add 32 to that value. You would convert 27°C into degrees Fahrenheit as follows: 27°C $\times \frac{9}{5} = 48.6$, and 48.6 + 32 = 80.6°F.

Recall Activity

1. Convert 50°F into °C. _____

2. Convert 20°C into °F. _____

3. Convert 100°F into °C. _____

4. Convert 35°C into °F. _____

5. Convert 66°F into °C. _____

6. Convert 0°C into °F. _____

Section 4.9 Reinforcement

Answer the following questions using what you learned in this section.

1. Convert 4 L into gallons. _____

2. *True or False.* One inch is longer than 1 cm. _____

3. Convert 12 inches into cm. _____

4. How many liters are in 12 gallons? _____

5. Which of the following is the largest measurement?

   A. 10 cm   C. 55 mm

   B. 2 inches   D. 1.5 inches

6. *True or False.* One hundred degrees Fahrenheit is the same temperature as 32°C. _____

7. Which of the following are metric units of measurement?

   A. liters   C. ounces   E. inches   G. millimeters

   B. kilograms   D. pounds   F. centimeters   H. grams

8. The _____ system of measurement is used in the United States.

9. The conversion factor for meters to feet is _____.

10. Unscramble the letters: roonscievn. Define the word that is formed. _____

    _____

11. Convert 100 km into miles. _____

12. Convert 5 kg into pounds. _____

13. The metric unit of length is the _____.

14. Convert 10 feet into m. _____

15. *True or False.* Zero degrees Fahrenheit is the same temperature as 32°C. _____

16. Which of the following are English units of measurement?

    A. grams   C. liters   E. inches

    B. ounces   D. pounds   F. gallons

17. *True or False.* One inch is the same as 2.54 cm. _____

18. Convert 100 miles into km. _____

19. Convert 4 pounds into kg. _____

20. *True or False.* Metric measurements are more accurate than English measurements. _____

Section 4.10 Graphs

In science, graphs are used to record and organize data. In this section, you will learn about two types of graphs, how to read them, and how to construct them.

The terms below are some of those that will be introduced in Section 4.10. To become familiar with these terms, reproduce each word on the line beside it. Pronounce each term as you write it. You will learn the definitions of these words as you complete this section.

1. graph _____
2. line graph _____
3. y-axis _____

4. x-axis _____
5. coordinate pair _____
6. bar graph _____

Concept 1: Parts of a Line Graph

graph a visual representation of information

line graph a graph that shows changes in information or values over time

y-axis the vertical side of a graph

x-axis the horizontal side of a graph

A *graph* is a visual representation of information. A *line graph* shows changes in information or values over time. The parts of a line graph are the title, y-axis, x-axis, scale, and points connected by a line. The *title* of a line graph should explain the graph's meaning or purpose and what is measured in the graph. The two sides of a graph are called *axes*. The *y-axis* is the vertical side, and the *x-axis* is the horizontal side. If a graph contains a measurement per unit of time, time should be represented on the x-axis and measurement on the y-axis (**Figure 4.37**). A line graph's *scale* is the numbers or words on each axis. Points are positioned on a line graph by moving the specified number of lines *across* the x-axis (to the right) and moving the specified number of lines *up* the y-axis. A line connects the points on a line graph.

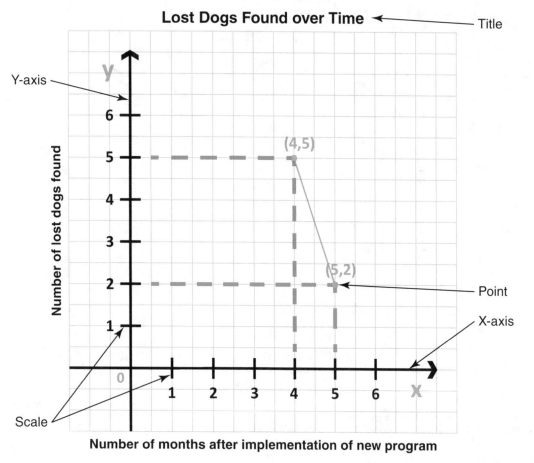

Figure 4.37 Five months after the implementation of the new program, two lost dogs were found. To place this point, you would move five lines across the x-axis and two lines up the y-axis.

Recall Activity

1. The _____ of a line graph explains what is measured in the graph.

2. The _____-axis is vertical.

3. The _____ is the numbers or words on each axis.

Concept 2: Reading a Line Graph

To read a line graph, first note the title of the graph and the labels on the x- and y-axes. These will help you understand what each point on the graph represents. Then view each point on the line to understand the general progression of the data.

To determine the value of a single point, count how many lines the point is across the x-axis. Record this number first. Then count how many lines the point is up the y-axis. Record this number. The value of a point can be written as *X, Y* (number of lines across the x-axis, number of lines up the y-axis). For example, in **Figure 4.38**, the point representing day 8 would be written as *8, 19.* This value (X,Y) is known as a *coordinate pair*.

coordinate pair the values representing where a data point is placed on a graph; X, Y

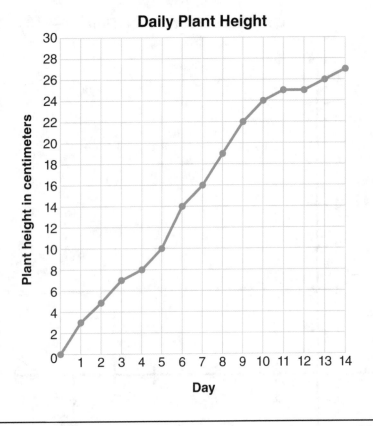

Daily Plant Height

Goodheart-Willcox Publisher

Figure 4.38 This line graph represents plant height in centimeters over the course of 14 days.

Recall Activity

View the line graph in Figure 4.38 to answer the following questions.

1. What is the title of the graph? _____

2. What is the unit of measurement on the y-axis? _____

3. What was the plant height on day 3? _____

4. On what day was the plant height 24 cm? _____

5. On what day was the plant height 22 cm? _____

6. How often were measurements taken in this study? _____

7. Does plant height increase the same amount each day? _____

8. Circle the period of time that had the greatest increase in height.

   days 3–4   days 7–8   days 12–13

9. How tall was the plant on day 6? _____

10. What is the range of the scale for the x-axis? _____

11. What was the maximum height of the plant? _____

12. Circle the period of time that had the greatest increase in height.

   days 0–1   days 2–3   days 5–6

Concept 3: Placing Points on a Line Graph

A point's coordinate pair (X, Y) determines where it is placed on a line graph. The point is placed by counting X lines across the x-axis and Y lines up the y-axis. For a coordinate pair of 2,3, you would count two lines across the x-axis and three lines up the y-axis. After all of the points from a set of data have been placed, draw a line connecting the points to show the data's progression.

Recall Activity

1. On the graph paper below, give the graph a title of your choosing. Also label the x- and y-axes.

2. Using the data shown, plot the coordinate pairs on the graph by moving across the x-axis and up the y-axis.

3. Connect the points by drawing a straight line from one point to the next.

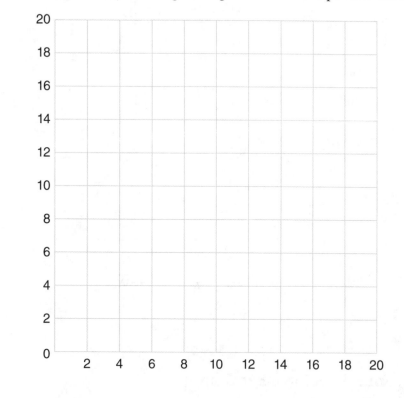

X	Y
2	2
4	5
6	4
8	3
10	9
12	17
14	7
16	5
18	10

Concept 4: Setting Up a Line Graph

When setting up a line graph, pay attention to the *range* (the smallest and largest values in the data). The graph should be able to include the entire range of the data. For example, for the data in **Figure 4.39**, the scale of the graph's y-axis could be 0 to 100.

Weeks	1	2	3	4	5	6	7	8
Weight (kg)	90.8 kg	93.1 kg	91.7 kg	92.6 kg	91.3 kg	89.9 kg	89.0 kg	87.2 kg

Figure 4.39 The data represents the weight of an adult male, recorded weekly.

Recall Activity

1. When setting up a line graph, pay attention to the _____ and _____ values in the data.

2. The graph should be able to include the entire _____ of the data.

3. On the graph paper, plot the data points from Figure 4.39. The data points represent the weight of an adult male, recorded each week. Remember to give the graph a title. Connect the points on the graph to create a line showing the progression of data.

4. The range of weight in Figure 4.39 is from _____ to _____.

Concept 5: Reading a Bar Graph

bar graph a graph that visually compares information

A *bar graph* is a graph that visually compares information. There are no connected points in a bar graph. Instead, the heights of the bars indicate number values on the y-axis. Each bar indicates a different piece of data on the x-axis. Bars may be color-coded to present even more varied sets of information. In **Figure 4.40**, for example, bars represent systolic or diastolic blood pressure on each day.

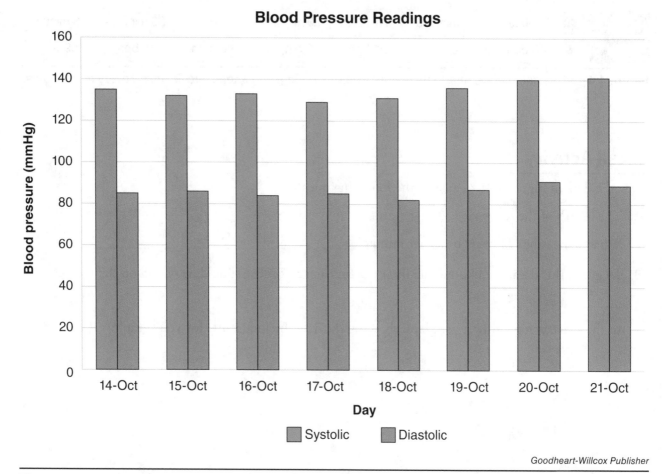

Blood Pressure Readings

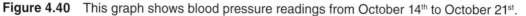

Figure 4.40 This graph shows blood pressure readings from October 14th to October 21st.

Recall Activity

View the bar graph in Figure 4.40 to answer the following questions.

1. On which day was the diastolic blood pressure reading highest? _____

2. What is the range of values for systolic blood pressure? _____

3. What is the range of values for diastolic blood pressure? _____

Concept 6: Drawing a Bar Graph

To create a bar graph, first use the data to construct the scale on the y-axis. Consider the highest and lowest values when labeling the y-axis. For example, the data in **Figure 4.41** might require a y-axis scale of 0 to 130. Because, in the data, the person's heart rate was recorded every five minutes, place five-minute increments on the x-axis. After constructing the axes, plot each coordinate pair on the bar graph and draw bars showing the data values.

Minutes	5 minutes	10 minutes	15 minutes	20 minutes	25 minutes	30 minutes	35 minutes
Heart Rate	68 bpm	110 bpm	121 bpm	118 bpm	98 bpm	70 bpm	69 bpm

Figure 4.41 This data shows heart rate readings before, during, and after exercise, taken every five minutes.

Recall Activity

View the data in Figure 4.41 to answer the following questions.

1. The length of the test was _____ minutes.

2. What is the range of heart beats per minute?_____

3. To graph this data, the five-minute intervals for each recording should be placed on the
    _____-axis.

4. In the space below, draw a bar graph showing the data. Include a title for your graph.

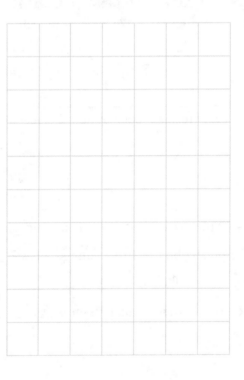

Section 4.10 Reinforcement

Answer the following questions using what you learned in this section.

1. The two sides of a graph are called _____.

2. Unscramble the letters: pragh. Define the word that is formed._____
    _____

3. What is the range for the following set of data: 14 mm, 27 mm, 5 mm, 15 mm, 8 mm, and 2 mm?

_____

4. *True or False.* The x-axis is vertical._____

5. In a graph of body weight by month, the month scale would be on the _____-axis.

6. Unscramble the letters: hagpr. Define the word that is formed._____

_____

7. The _____-axis is horizontal.

8. *True or False.* The y-axis is vertical. _____

9. Unscramble the letters: notlahiroz. Define the word that is formed._____

_____

10. In a graph of heart rate by minute, heart rate would be listed on the _____-axis.

11. The _____-axis is vertical.

12. What is the range for the following set of data: 0.6 g, 0.4 g, 1.5 g, 0.8 g, 1.1 g, and 0.3 g?

_____

13. *True or False.* The y-axis is horizontal. _____

14. A graph's _____ explains what is measured in the graph.

15. In a graph of heart rate by minute, the minute scale would be listed on the _____-axis.

16. What is the range for the following set of data: 3 g, 11 g, 2 g, 7 g, 6 g, and 10 g?_____

_____

17. Which of the following does *not* belong on a graph?
    A. y-axis   C. x-axis
    B. r-axis   D title

18. The scale of a graph is the _____ or words on the axes.

Comprehensive Review (Chapters 1–4)

Answer the following questions using what you have learned so far in this book.

19. If the diameter of a circle is 100 cm, the radius is _____.

20. *True or False.* The prefix *micro-* means "small."_____

21. *True or False.* Scientific laws tell you that the natural world is predictable. _____

22. Why is it helpful to see the natural and the supernatural as two sides of one coin?_____

_____

Chapter 4 Review

Answer the following questions using what you learned in this chapter.

1. Which of the following are linear units of measurements?

    A. grams   C. degrees Celsius   E. liters

    B. millimeters   D. meters   F. milliliters

2. Convert 34 mm into cm. _____

3. Which of the following is the heaviest measurement?

    A. 0.1 kg   C. 10 g

    B. 1 mg   D. 100 mg

4. To convert 0.01 to 1, move the decimal point to the _____.

5. *True or False.* The metric unit of volume is the liter. _____

6. Measure the length of this line in cm. Record the measurement here. _____

    ▬▬▬▬

7. Which is the smaller measurement: the diameter or the radius? _____

8. The _____ of a circle is the longest measurement across the circle.

9. *True or False.* Surface area is measured in cubic units. _____

10. Which of the following are surface area measurements?

    A. cm   C. cm²   E. mm²

    B. mm³   D. mm   F. cm³

11. Measure the length of this line in mm. Record the measurement here. _____

    ▬▬▬▬▬▬▬

12. The abbreviation for cubic centimeters is _____.

13. Calculate the surface area of a 4 cm × 4 cm × 4 cm cube. _____

14. _____ is measured in cubic units.

15. The unit of dry volume is _____.

16. A volume measurement of 150 mL is the same as _____ cc.

17. Water _____ at 100°C.

18. *True or False.* Ice forms at 10°C. _____

19. The metric unit of _____ is the gram.

20. Does an object weigh more on the earth or on the moon? Explain. _____

    _____

21. If the weights on a platform balance read 100 g, 20 g, and 7.5 g, what is the mass of the object being

    weighed? _____

22. What is the mass of 1500 mL of water in kg? _____

23. The mass of an object placed on a platform balance is 213.1 g. In this case, the largest weight would read _____, the middle weight would read _____, and the smallest weight would read _____.

24. Convert 2 L into gallons. _____

25. Which is the longer measurement: 1 inch or 1 cm? _____

26. Convert 100 feet into m. _____

27. *True or False.* One hundred degrees Celsius is the same as 32°F. _____

28. What is the range of the following data: 5, 2, 6, 10, 14, 1, and 8? _____

29. A graph's title explains what is _____ in the graph.

30. The _____-axis is horizontal.

31. To create a line graph, connect the data points with a straight _____ from one data point to the next.

32. A circle is ¼ red, and the rest is blue. What fraction of the circle is blue? _____

33. If a circle is divided into five equal parts, each part is _____% of the circle.

34. Convert ¹⁵⁄₃₅ into a percentage. _____

35. _____ measures how many atoms there are in a volume of liquid.

36. In a solution of salt and water, salt is the _____.

37. *True or False.* Atoms move slower at lower temperatures. _____

Comprehensive Review (Chapters 1–4)

Using what you have learned so far in this book, match the following terms with their definitions.

_____ 38. A combining form that means "red"

_____ 39. The study of inheritance

_____ 40. A combining form that means "skin"

_____ 41. The best explanation today of why a phenomenon occurs

_____ 42. A combining form that means "kidney"

_____ 43. The liquid in which atoms are dissolved in a solution

_____ 44. A combining form that means "bone"

_____ 45. A combining form that means "intestine"

_____ 46. A general statement of fact

_____ 47. The atoms dissolved in a solution

A. ren/o
B. scientific theory
C. scientific law
D. solvent
E. rubr/o
F. oste/o
G. solute
H. derm/o
I. enter/o
J. genetics

Chapter 5
Chemistry

Introduction

Knowledge of chemistry is essential for learning about anatomy and physiology. All of the human body's cells, tissues, and organs are composed of *atoms*, or extremely small particles that together make up the universe. Knowledge of how atoms interact will help you understand how the body functions. Learning about macromolecules, or combinations of atoms, will help you grasp cell function. Knowledge of pH will help you understand homeostasis.

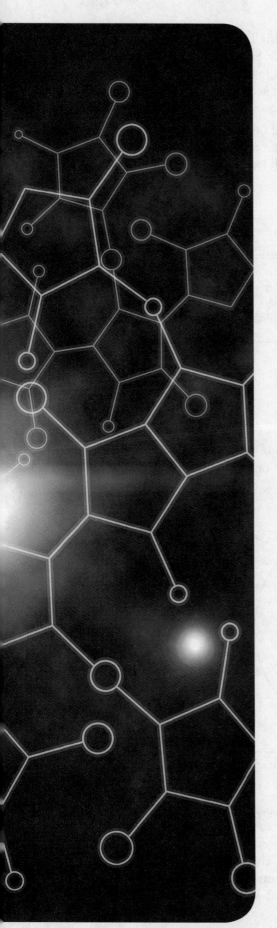

Objectives

After completing this chapter, you will be able to

- locate the protons, neutrons, and electrons in an atom
- determine the atomic symbol, atomic number, and atomic mass of an atom
- retrieve information from the periodic table of elements
- draw an atomic diagram for a given atomic number
- predict how atoms will bond
- describe ionic, covalent (single and double), and hydrogen bonding of atoms
- list the subunits of carbohydrates, lipids, proteins, and nucleic acids
- identify the types of carbohydrates
- describe the types of lipids
- explain protein structure
- understand enzyme action
- recognize types of nucleic acids
- explain the pH scale

Key Terms

The following terms and phrases will be introduced and explained in Chapter 5. Read through the list to become familiar with the words.

acid	electrolyte	nucleic acid
atom	electron	nucleotide
atomic diagram	electron capacity	partial charge
atomic mass	electron shell	periodic table of
atomic number	element	elements
atomic symbol	enzyme	pH
ATP	essential amino	polysaccharide
attraction	acid	polyunsaturated fat
base	fiber	primary structure
Bohr model	full outer shell	protein
bonding	hydrogen bond	proton
buffer	hydrogenation	relative atomic mass
calories	ion	RNA
carbohydrate	ionic bond	saturated fat
complementary	isotope	secondary structure
base	lipid	single bond
core	macromolecule	substrate
covalent bond	molecule	tertiary structure
disaccharide	monosaccharide	*trans* fat
DNA	neutral	turnover rate
double bond	neutron	unsaturated fat

Section 5.1 Atoms

Atoms, also known as *elements*, are extremely small particles that make up the universe. You might be familiar with some atoms. Some examples of atoms are hydrogen, carbon, and helium. Atoms contain subatomic particles and can be classified by symbol, number, and mass. In this section, you will learn about atoms and their properties.

The terms below are some of those that will be introduced in Section 5.1. To become familiar with these terms, reproduce each word on the line beside it. Pronounce each term as you write it. You will learn the definitions of these words as you complete this section.

1. atom _____

2. core _____

3. electron shell _____

4. proton _____

5. neutron _____

6. electron _____

7. bonding _____

8. element _____

9. atomic symbol _____

10. atomic number _____

11. atomic mass _____

Concept 1: Subatomic Particles

atom a core of protons and neutrons surrounded by orbiting electrons

core the center of an atom, which contains the atom's protons and neutrons

electron shell the outside part of an atom that contains the atom's orbiting electrons

The structure of an *atom* includes a *core* and one or more *electron shells*. **Figure 5.1** shows the structure of an atom.

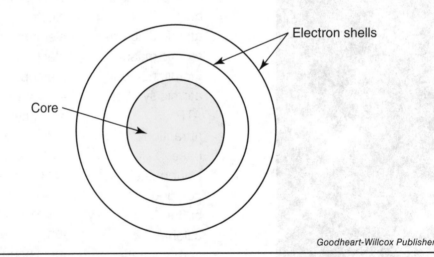

Figure 5.1   The core of an atom is surrounded by electron shells.

proton a subatomic particle found in the core of an atom; has a positive charge and a mass of 1 amu

neutron a subatomic particle found in the core of an atom; has no charge and a mass of 1 amu

electron a subatomic particle found in an atom's electron shells; has a negative charge and no mass

An atom is made of *subatomic particles*, or particles smaller than atoms. There are three types of subatomic particles: *protons*, *neutrons*, and *electrons*. Protons and neutrons are located in an atom's core, and electrons are found in an atom's electron shells. In the electron shells, the electrons *orbit*, or travel in a curved path around, the atom's core. The number of protons in an atom is equal to the number of electrons. **Figure 5.2** shows the arrangement of subatomic particles in an atom. Note that the atom in Figure 5.2 contains an equal number of protons and electrons. Atoms combine to make up all matter, including solids, liquids, and gases. The subatomic particles within an atom affect its properties.

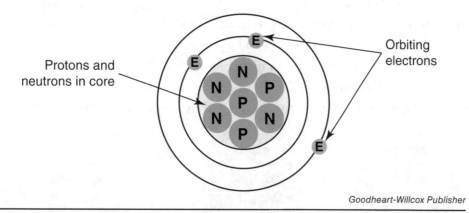

Figure 5.2 Protons and neutrons are in the core, and electrons orbit the core in electron shells.

Recall Activity

1. Draw a core and two electron shells in the space below. Label the *core* and the *electron shells*.

2. Write the names of the three subatomic particles. _____

3. The number of _____ in an atom must be equal to the number of

   _____.

4. Where are protons and neutrons found in an atom? Add protons and neutrons to the diagram of an atom you created in question 1._____

5. Where are electrons found in an atom? Add electrons to the diagram of an atom you created in question 1. _____

Concept 2: Mass and Charge

The subatomic particles—protons, neutrons, and electrons—vary in weight and attraction. When referring to atoms, *weight* is called *mass*, and *attraction* is called *charge*. Mass is expressed in *atomic mass units* or *amu*. Charge is expressed as either positive (+), negative (−), or no charge. The mass and charge of each subatomic particle is as follows:

- Protons have a mass of 1 amu and a positive charge (+).
- Neutrons have a mass of 1 amu and no charge.
- Electrons have no mass (0 amu) and a negative charge (−).

  See **Figure 5.3** to review the masses and charges of the subatomic particles.

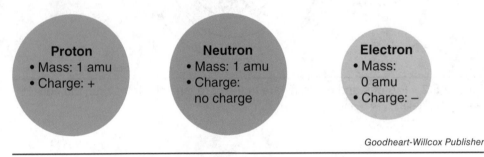

Figure 5.3 The subatomic particles have different masses and charges.

Recall Activity

1. A proton has a mass of _____ and _____ charge.

2. A neutron has a mass of _____ and _____ charge.

3. An electron has a mass of _____ and _____ charge.

4. What does the abbreviation *amu* represent?_____

5. In the diagram of an atom below, label the core and the electron shell. Add one more circle around the outer circle to represent two electron shells.

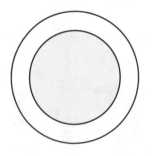

6. Where are electrons found? Add three electrons to the diagram of an atom in question 5.

7. Where are neutrons found? Add four neutrons to the diagram of an atom in question 5.

_____

8. Where are protons found? Add three protons to the diagram of an atom in question 5.

_____

Concept 3: Bonding

As you have learned, an atom consists of a core of protons and neutrons surrounded by orbiting electrons (**Figure 5.2**). In an atom, protons and neutrons do not leave the core. Electrons, however, can be exchanged or shared between atoms in an interaction called *bonding*. Bonding can take place in three ways:

bonding the exchange or sharing of electrons between atoms; holds atoms together

- One or more electrons can be donated to another atom.
- One or more electrons can be accepted from another atom.
- One or more electrons can be shared between atoms.

Bonding holds atoms together. Bonded atoms make up most matter—solids, liquids, and gases.

Recall Activity

1. An atom consists of a(n) _____ of protons and _____ surrounded by orbiting _____.

2. Which subatomic particles do not leave the core? _____

3. Which subatomic particle is involved in bonding? _____

4. List the three ways that electrons are involved in bonding._____

   _____

Concept 4: Atomic Symbol

You may have heard the names of some atoms, such as *chlorine*, *aluminum*, or *barium*. Remember that atoms are also referred to as *elements*. Abbreviations known as *atomic symbols* are used to refer to atoms. An atomic symbol may be a letter or a group of letters. Many atomic symbols are simply the first letter of the atom's name. Only the first letter of an atomic symbol is capitalized. **Figure 5.4** shows some atomic symbols and the atoms they represent.

element an atom

atomic symbol an abbreviation used to refer to an atom

Atomic Symbol	Name of Atom
N	Nitrogen
O	Oxygen
C	Carbon
H	Hydrogen

Figure 5.4 Atoms are represented by their atomic symbols.

Recall Activity

1. A letter or group of letters used to abbreviate the name of an atom is known as a(n)
   _____.

2. What is another name for atoms? _____

3. Many atomic symbols are simply the first _____ of the atom's name.

4. List the name of the atom indicated by each atomic symbol.

   N _____   C _____

   O _____   H _____

Concept 5: Atomic Number

atomic number the number of protons or electrons in an atom

Atoms and elements are also described by atomic number. The *atomic number* of an atom is equal to the number of protons in the atom's core. It is also equal to the number of electrons in the atom's electron shells. As you have learned, the number of protons in an atom's core is identical to the number of electrons in an atom's electron shells. For example, the atom boron, atomic number 5, would have five protons in its core and five electrons in its electron shells.

Recall Activity

1. The number of protons in an atom's core determines the atom's _____.

2. The number of electrons that should be in an atom's electron shells determines the atom's

   _____.

3. Which subatomic particle does *not* determine an atom's atomic number? _____

4. The atom helium has an atomic number of 2. Add the appropriate number of protons and electrons to the diagram of a helium atom below.

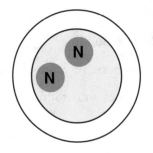

Concept 6: Atomic Mass

As you learned in Concept 2, in atoms, *weight* is referred to as *mass*. Each atom or element has an *atomic mass*. The atomic mass of an atom is equal to the number of protons plus the number of neutrons in the atom's core. Protons and neutrons each have a mass of 1 amu. Electrons have no mass, so they do not contribute to an atom's atomic mass.

atomic mass the number of protons plus the number of neutrons in an atom's core

Recall Activity

1. Which subatomic particles have mass?_____

2. Which subatomic particle has *no* mass?_____

3. Which subatomic particle is *not* used in calculating atomic mass? _____

4. The atomic mass of an atom is equal to the number of protons _____ the number of neutrons.

5. If an atom's core contains two neutrons and two protons, what is the atom's atomic mass? _____

6. View the diagram of an atom below. What is the atom's atomic mass?_____

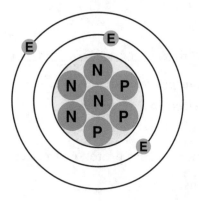

Section 5.1 Reinforcement

Answer the following questions using what you learned in this section.

1. Write the atomic symbol for carbon. _____

2. Which subatomic particle is involved in bonding? _____

3. *True or False.* Electrons can be shared between atoms. _____

4. Which of the following subatomic particles are found in an atom's core?

   A. proton   C. electron

   B. neutron

5. Which of the following subatomic particles are involved in determining atomic mass?

   A. proton   C. electron

   B. neutron

6. The _____ of an atom is equal to the number of protons plus the number of neutrons in the atom's core.

7. *True or False.* Neutrons are located in an atom's core. _____

8. Where in an atom are electrons found? _____

9. Write the atomic symbol for nitrogen. _____

10. In an atom, the number of protons is _____ the number of electrons.

11. *True or False.* In an atom, protons in the atom's core orbit the atom's electron shells. _____

12. How would you determine the atomic mass of an atom?_____

    _____

13. Write the following letters backward: nortcele. Define the word that is formed._____

    _____

14. *True or False.* C is the atomic symbol for nitrogen. _____

15. Which of the following subatomic particles is found in the atom's electron shells?

    A. proton   C. electron

    B. neutron

16. Write the atomic symbol for hydrogen._____

17. Which of the following subatomic particles are involved in determining atomic number?

    A. proton   C. electron

    B. neutron

18. Which subatomic particle has more mass: a proton or an electron?_____

19. *True or False.* Elements are atoms._____

Match the following terms with their definitions.

_____ 20. A subatomic particle that has no charge

_____ 21. The number of protons or electrons in an atom

_____ 22. A subatomic particle that has a positive charge

_____ 23. A subatomic particle that has a negative charge

_____ 24. A core of protons and neutrons surrounded by orbiting electrons

_____ 25. The number of protons plus the number of neutrons in an atom's core

A. atom

B. proton

C. neutron

D. electron

E. atomic number

F. atomic mass

Comprehensive Review (Chapters 1–5)

Answer the following questions using what you have learned so far in this book.

26. The letters *amu* stand for _____.

27. Which of the following prefixes means "below"?

    A. hyper-   C. iso-

    B. hypo-

28. How many milliliters are in 1 liter?_____

29. A(n) _____ is a general statement of fact.

30. *True or False.* Facts are independent of people and opinions. _____

Section 5.2 The Periodic Table of Elements

Atoms are organized on the periodic table of elements. As you have learned, an *element* is another word used to describe an *atom*. In this section, you will learn about the periodic table of elements and the atoms it contains.

The terms below are some of those that will be introduced in Section 5.2. To become familiar with these terms, reproduce each word on the line beside it. Pronounce each term as you write it. You will learn the definitions of these words as you complete this section.

1. periodic table of elements _____

2. isotope_____

3. relative atomic mass _____

Concept 1: Reading the Periodic Table of Elements

periodic table of elements
a grid that arranges elements by their atomic numbers and properties

The *periodic table of elements* is a grid that arranges elements (or atoms) by their atomic numbers and properties. If you can read the periodic table of elements, you can obtain many facts about an atom just by looking at it.

Information on the periodic table of elements is arranged in a consistent manner. Each square represents an atom. For each atom, the atomic number is listed on top; the atomic symbol is represented in the middle, followed by the atom's full name; and the relative atomic mass is recorded on the bottom. In most cases, the relative atomic mass of an atom is not a whole number. This is due to isotopes, which you will learn about in Concept 5 of this section. To determine atomic mass from relative atomic mass, round relative atomic mass to the nearest whole number. **Figure 5.5** shows the arrangement of information for each atom.

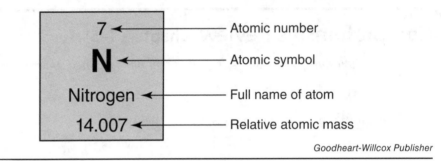

Goodheart-Willcox Publisher

Figure 5.5 The periodic table of elements shows an atom's atomic number, atomic symbol, full name, and relative atomic mass.

Recall Activity

1. In the diagram below, label each piece of information about the atom.

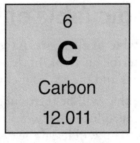

2. What is represented by the number 6 at the top of the diagram?_____

3. What is represented by the letter *C* in the middle of the diagram?_____

4. What is represented by the number 12.011 at the bottom of the diagram? _____

5. To determine atomic mass from relative atomic mass, round relative atomic mass to the nearest

    _____.

6. What is the atomic mass of carbon? _____

Periodic Table of Elements

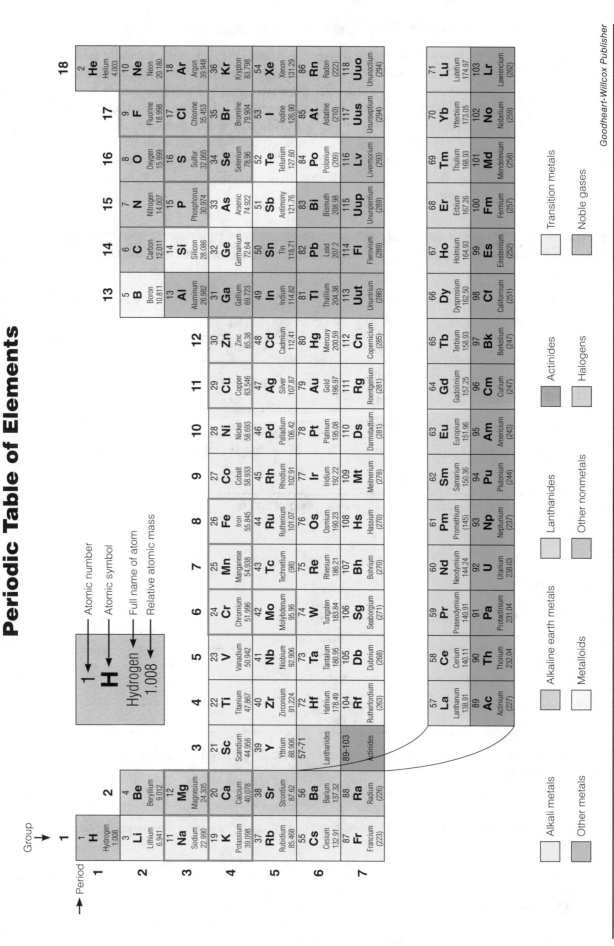

Figure 5.6 The periodic table lists elements.

Concept 2: Atoms of the Periodic Table

The periodic table organizes atoms. View the full periodic table of elements in **Figure 5.6** on the previous page. You may notice that some atomic symbols are one letter, while others are two letters. For some atoms, the atomic symbol is the first two letters of the atom's full name. For other atoms, the atomic symbol has no visible relationship to the full name of the atom (for example, the atomic symbol *Fe* for iron). **Figure 5.7** shows a selection of atomic symbols and the atoms they represent. The periodic table of elements can also be found in Appendix C. Remember that only the first letter of an atomic symbol is capitalized.

Atomic Symbol	Full Name of Atom	Atomic Symbol	Full Name of Atom
He	Helium	Be	Beryllium
Li	Lithium	F	Fluorine
Cl	Chlorine	Ne	Neon
K	Potassium	Mg	Magnesium
Ca	Calcium	Al	Aluminum
B	Boron	Si	Silicon
Ar	Argon	Fe	Iron
Na	Sodium	P	Phosphorus
S	Sulfur		

Figure 5.7 An atomic symbol may be one letter or a group of letters.

Recall Activity

1. List the full name of the atom after each atomic symbol. Say each atom's name as you write it.

   Fe_____   Ca _____

   H_____   Mg_____

   Si _____   Na_____

   B _____   S_____

2. List nine atomic symbols that are only one letter. Say the full name of each atom as you write its atomic symbol.

   _____

3. List 12 atomic symbols that are two letters. Say the full name of each atom as you write its atomic symbol.

   _____

   _____

4. Using what you have learned about the periodic table and atoms, complete the information in the following chart.

Name	Atomic Symbol	Atomic Number	Relative Atomic Mass
Hydrogen			
Carbon			
Nitrogen			
Oxygen			
Sodium			
Sulfur			
Chlorine			
Potassium			
Calcium			

Concept 3: Number of Neutrons

In an atom, protons and neutrons are located in the core, and electrons are located in the electron shells. You can determine the number of protons, electrons, and neutrons in an atom using information in the periodic table.

   You learned in the previous section that atomic mass is calculated by adding the masses of protons and neutrons in the atom's core. To determine the number of neutrons in an atom, subtract an atom's atomic number (the number of protons in the atom's core) from its atomic mass (the number of protons plus the number of neutrons in the atom's core). As an example, the atom lithium has the atomic number 3 and an atomic mass of 7 amu (relative atomic mass rounded to the nearest whole number). Using this information, you can calculate that $7 - 3 = 4$. There are four neutrons in a lithium atom's core.

Recall Activity

1. How many neutrons are in a helium atom's core? _____

2. How many neutrons are in a fluorine atom's core? _____

3. How many neutrons are in a sulfur atom's core? _____

4. How many neutrons are in a sodium atom's core? _____

5. How many neutrons are in a calcium atom's core? _____

Concept 4: Construct a Brief Periodic Table

In the periodic table, atoms are arranged by atomic number. Atomic numbers increase as you read the table from left to right and from top to bottom.

Recall Activity

1. In the brief periodic table below, arrange the first 18 atoms by atomic number. Start in the upper left corner and follow the order in the periodic table, moving from left to right. Write the appropriate atomic symbol in each square. Place the correct atomic number above each atomic symbol and the correct relative atomic mass below each atomic symbol.

2. What determines the order in which atoms are arranged in the periodic table?

   _____

3. Which atom is between aluminum and phosphorus on the periodic table? _____

4. Which atom has an atomic number of 13? _____

5. Which atom has an atomic mass of 16 amu? Remember to round relative atomic mass to the nearest

   whole number. _____

6. Which atom has five electrons? _____

Concept 5: Isotopes

An atom's atomic number is determined by its number of protons or electrons. Atomic mass is equal to the number of protons plus the number of neutrons. Atomic masses on the periodic table, however, are usually not whole numbers. This is because some atoms, known as *isotopes*, have the same atomic numbers, but have different atomic masses.

isotope a form of an atom that has the same atomic number as, but a different atomic mass than, another form of that atom

For example, carbon (atomic number 6) can have an atomic mass of 12 or 14. The carbon atom with an atomic mass of 12 is known as *carbon 12*. The carbon atom with an atomic mass of 14 is known as *carbon 14*. Their atomic masses are different because carbon 12 has six neutrons, while carbon 14 has eight. Carbon 12 is the most common form of carbon, and carbon 14 is considered an isotope (**Figure 5.8**). Atoms may have up to 10 different isotopes. The *relative atomic mass* listed on the periodic table is an average mass for the atom and all of its isotopes. Atomic mass, then, is relative atomic mass rounded to the nearest whole number.

relative atomic mass the average mass for an atom and all of its isotopes

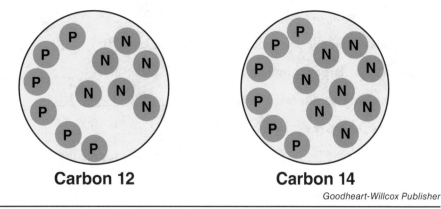

Carbon 12   **Carbon 14**

Figure 5.8 Isotopes have the same number of protons but different numbers of neutrons, resulting in different atomic masses.

Recall Activity

1. Atomic _____ is determined by the number of protons or electrons in an atom.

2. Atomic mass is equal to the number of _____ plus the number of

   _____.

3. A(n) _____ is an atom with the same atomic number as another atom but with a different atomic mass.

4. The most common form of carbon is carbon _____.

5. Among isotopes, atomic number remains the same, while atomic mass is _____.

6. To determine atomic mass, round relative atomic mass to the nearest _____ number.

Section 5.2 Reinforcement

Answer the following questions using what you learned in this section.

1. Which of the following atoms has the greatest atomic mass: B, Si, Mg, or Na? _____

2. What is the atomic mass of an atom with a relative atomic mass of 47.346 amu? _____

3. Which of the following is the atomic symbol for sodium: S, Si, Na, or N?_____

4. Write these atoms in order from the smallest to the greatest atomic mass: Mg, Li, N, and Cl._____

   _____

5. How many electrons are in the atom Li?_____

6. *True or False.* An aluminum atom contains 14 neutrons. _____

7. Unscramble the letters: tonrune. Define the word that is formed. _____

   _____

8. What is the atomic mass of an atom with a relative atomic mass of 3.49? _____

9. Which of the following atoms has the smallest atomic number: Al, O, Li, or Be?_____

10. Which of the following atoms has the largest atomic number: Al, C, Li, or Ne?_____

11. What is the full name of the atom with the atomic symbol B?_____

12. Which of the following atoms has the most electrons: O, Al, N, or Cl? _____

13. In the periodic table, an atom's atomic _____ can be found above its atomic symbol.

14. Which atom has 15 electrons? _____

15. Write the letters backward: epotosi. Define the word that is formed. _____

_____

16. *True or False.* The atomic number of He is 4. _____

17. How many electrons are in the atom Al? _____

18. The atomic mass of hydrogen is _____ amu.

19. *True or False.* The atomic number of Si is 28. _____

20. What atom has an atomic mass of 20 amu? _____

21. Two atoms that have the same atomic number, but have different atomic masses, are called

_____.

22. Which of the following atoms has the largest atomic number: Na, H, Si, or F? _____

23. How many electrons are in the atom argon? _____

24. Which of the following is *not* an atomic symbol: Na, D, Ne, or F? _____

25. *True or False.* The atom with atomic number 3 has an atomic mass of 7 amu._____

Comprehensive Review (Chapters 1–5)

Answer the following questions using what you have learned so far in this book.

26. Which atom has an atomic number of 7? _____

27. Explain the difference between natural and supernatural explanations. _____

_____

28. The two sources of facts in the diagnostic scientific method are _____ and

_____.

29. Which of the following is the largest mass?
    A. 1000 mg   C. 0.01 kg
    B. 0.5 g

30. What does the prefix *ab-* mean? _____

Section 5.3 Atomic Diagrams

Thus far in this chapter, you have drawn and interpreted several illustrations of atoms, including their cores and electron shells. These illustrations are known as *atomic diagrams*. They are also sometimes known as *Bohr models*, named for Niels Bohr, who introduced the diagrams in 1913. Atomic diagrams provide information about how an atom will interact with other atoms. An atomic diagram should represent both an atom's electrons and its protons.

The terms below are some of those that will be introduced in Section 5.3. To become familiar with these terms, reproduce each word on the line beside it. Pronounce each term as you write it. You will learn the definitions of these words as you complete this section.

atomic diagram an illustration of an atom that shows its protons, electrons, and electron shells

Bohr model another name for an atomic diagram; named for Niels Bohr

1. atomic diagram _____

2. Bohr model _____

3. electron capacity _____

Concept 1: Electron Shells

Electrons are subatomic particles found in the electron shell or shells surrounding an atom's core. In an atom, the *first electron shell* is closest to the core. The *second electron shell* surrounds the first shell, the *third electron shell* surrounds the second shell, and so on (**Figure 5.9**).

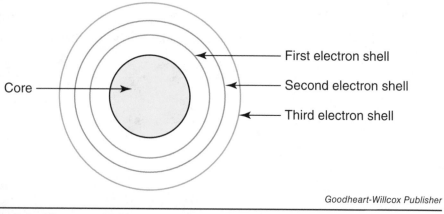

Goodheart-Willcox Publisher

Figure 5.9 Electron shells surround an atom's core.

Recall Activity

1. In Figure 5.9, which shell is closest to the core? _____

2. In Figure 5.9, which shell is farthest from the core? _____

3. In Figure 5.9, what color is the second electron shell? _____

Concept 2: Electron Shell Capacity

electron capacity the number of electrons an electron shell can hold

The position of an electron shell (for example, first, second, or third) determines *electron capacity*, or how many electrons a shell can hold. In an atom, the first electron shell can hold up to two electrons. The second shell can hold up to eight electrons, and the third shell can hold up to eight electrons. **Figure 5.10** shows the three electron shells and their electron capacities.

First shell: two electrons

Second shell: eight electrons

Third shell: eight electrons

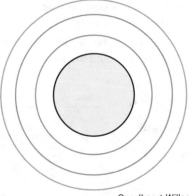

Figure 5.10   Electron shells can hold different numbers of electrons.

Recall Activity

1. Which electron shell holds up to two electrons? _____

2. Which electron shells hold up to eight electrons? _____

3. Draw an atom's core surrounded by three electron shells. Beside each shell, write the maximum number of electrons the shell can contain.

Concept 3: Core Diagram

Now that you understand electron capacity, you can begin creating an atomic diagram. Creating an atomic diagram involves two steps: diagramming the core and placing electrons in the electron shells. Diagramming the core is the first step in creating an atomic diagram. An atom's core contains its protons and neutrons. Neutrons are typically *not* included in an atomic diagram because they are not involved in bonding and do not influence an atom's charge. To diagram an atom's core, write the number of protons the atom contains, followed by a plus sign (+) to indicate the protons' positive charge. **Figure 5.11** represents nitrogen (N), which is atomic number 7. Seven protons exist in the atom's core.

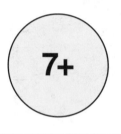

Figure 5.11 Nitrogen has seven protons in its core.

Recall Activity

1. What is the first step in creating an atomic diagram?_____
   _____

2. _____ are *not* included in an atomic diagram because they are not involved in bonding and do not influence an atom's charge.

Concept 4: Place Electrons

After diagramming an atom's core, the next step is to draw the electron shells and place the electrons. The number of electrons in an atom should equal the number of protons. For the atom nitrogen (N), atomic number 7, seven electrons will need to be placed.

Once you have determined the number of electrons to be placed, draw the first electron shell. The first electron shell can hold up to two electrons, so place two electrons in the first shell. For the atom nitrogen, this leaves five electrons that still need to be placed (7 – 2 = 5). Because the second electron shell can hold up to eight electrons, place the five remaining electrons in the second electron shell. If any electrons remained after the second electron shell reached its capacity, you would have to add a third electron shell, and so on. For the atom nitrogen, only two electron shells are needed (**Figure 5.12**).

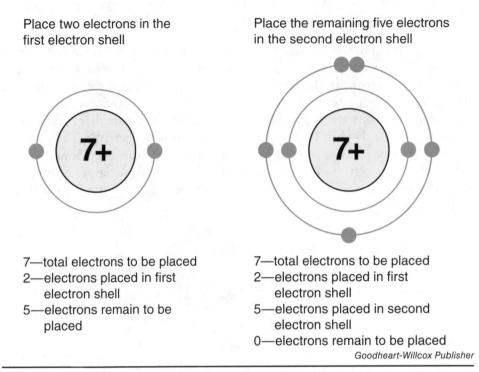

Place two electrons in the
first electron shell

Place the remaining five electrons
in the second electron shell

7—total electrons to be placed
2—electrons placed in first
electron shell
5—electrons remain to be
placed

7—total electrons to be placed
2—electrons placed in first
electron shell
5—electrons placed in second
electron shell
0—electrons remain to be placed

Goodheart-Willcox Publisher

Figure 5.12   Two electron shells are needed to place nitrogen's seven electrons.

Recall Activity

1. In an atomic diagram, how many electrons can the first electron shell hold? _____

2. In an atomic diagram, the second electron shell can hold up to _____
   electron(s).

3. If you needed to place five electrons, how many electrons would be placed in the first electron shell,
   and how many electrons would be placed in the second shell? _____

4. When placing electrons, which electron shell should you always start with?_____

5. If you were drawing a diagram of an atom with an atomic number of 4, how many electrons would
   you place?_____

6. How many electrons would you have to place before you drew a third electron shell?_____

7. How many electrons would you have to place before you drew a second electron shell? _____

Concept 5: Diagram Lithium and Fluorine

In the next few concepts, you will practice diagramming several atoms from
the periodic table. Using the following instructions, create an atomic diagram
for lithium, atomic number 3, in the space below. Then, for question 6, create
an atomic diagram for fluorine.

Recall Activity

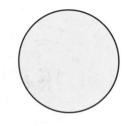

1. The circle to the right represents the core of a lithium atom. Write the number of protons in the core.

2. Draw a circle around the lithium atom's core to represent the first electron shell.

3. Place the appropriate number of electrons in the first electron shell.

4. Draw a circle around the first electron shell to represent the second electron shell.

5. Place the appropriate number of electrons in the second electron shell.

6. In the space below, draw an atomic diagram of the atom fluorine. Use the periodic table to determine fluorine's atomic number.

Concept 6: Diagram Phosphorus

Now that you have created atomic diagrams for atoms with two electron shells, apply the steps to diagramming an atom with three electron shells: phosphorus, atomic number 15. You should start by placing the protons. Phosphorus has an atomic number of 15, so write *15+* to represent 15 protons in the core (**Figure 5.13**).

Because phosphorus contains 15 protons, it also has 15 electrons. You should start with the electrons in the first electron shell. Follow Figure 5.13 to understand how electrons would be placed in the second and third electron shells.

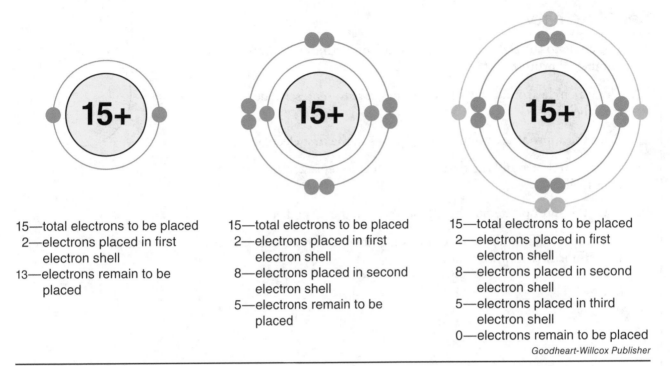

15—total electrons to be placed
2—electrons placed in first electron shell
13—electrons remain to be placed

15—total electrons to be placed
2—electrons placed in first electron shell
8—electrons placed in second electron shell
5—electrons remain to be placed

15—total electrons to be placed
2—electrons placed in first electron shell
8—electrons placed in second electron shell
5—electrons placed in third electron shell
0—electrons remain to be placed

Figure 5.13 Three shells are needed to place phosphorus' 15 electrons.

Recall Activity

1. How many protons are in the core of a phosphorus atom? _____

2. How many electrons are in a phosphorus atom's electron shells? _____

3. How many electron shells does a phosphorus atom contain? _____

Concept 7: Diagram Chlorine and Sodium

In this concept, you will practice diagramming chlorine and sodium. Using the following instructions, create an atomic diagram for chlorine, atomic number 17, in the space below. Then, for question 8, create an atomic diagram for sodium.

Recall Activity

1. The circle to the right represents the core of a chlorine atom. Write the number of protons in the core.

2. Draw a circle around the chlorine atom's core to represent the first electron shell.

3. Place the appropriate number of electrons in the first electron shell.

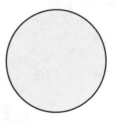

4. Draw a circle around the first electron shell to represent the second electron shell.

5. Place the appropriate number of electrons in the second electron shell.

6. Draw a circle around the second electron shell to represent the third electron shell.

7. Place the appropriate number of electrons in the third electron shell.

8. In the space below, draw an atomic diagram of the atom sodium. Use the periodic table to determine sodium's atomic number.

Concept 8: Electron Shells and the Periodic Table

Now that you understand atomic diagrams and electron shells, you can determine how many electron shells an atom has just by viewing the periodic table. In this concept, use your knowledge of electron shells and the periodic table to respond to the following statements.

Recall Activity

1. List the names, atomic symbols, and atomic numbers of two atoms containing only one electron shell.

2. List the names, atomic symbols, and atomic numbers of eight atoms containing only two electron shells.

3. List the names, atomic symbols, and atomic numbers of eight atoms containing only three electron shells.

_____

_____

Section 5.3 Reinforcement

Answer the following questions using what you learned in this section.

1. What is the first atomic number that contains a second electron shell? _____

2. *True or False.* The first electron shell holds up to three electrons. _____

3. How many electrons are in the outermost shell of a hydrogen atom?_____

4. How many electrons are in the outermost shell of a carbon atom? _____

5. Unscramble the letters: oreclent. Define the word that is formed. _____

_____

6. How many electrons are in the outermost shell of an oxygen atom?_____

7. *True or False.* Electrons are placed in an atom's core._____

8. Which of the following atoms has the greatest number of electrons in the outermost shell?
   A. carbon   C. magnesium
   B. oxygen   D. aluminum

9. Which of the following atoms has the greatest number of electron shells: He, B, Si, or Li?_____

10. *True or False.* An atom with an atomic number of 9 has three electron shells. _____

11. Among the atoms with atomic numbers 1–20, which atoms only have two electron shells? List the atoms' atomic symbols. _____

_____

12. Write the letters backward: elbat cidoirep. Define the word that is formed._____

_____

13. Which atom has a full second electron shell, but no third electron shell? _____

14. Which of the following atoms does *not* belong with the others: Ne, S, O, or Be? _____

15. *True or False.* The atom with atomic number 18 needs one more electron to fill its outermost shell.

_____

16. Which of the following atoms does *not* belong with the others: He, Ne, Si, or Ar? _____

17. Arrange the following atoms from the lowest atomic number to the highest atomic number: N, Be, Cl, and Mg. _____

Answer the following questions using what you have learned so far in this book.

18. Which of the following atoms has the most protons: S, Cl, O, or He? _____

19. How many centimeters is 124 mm? _____

20. Identify and define the prefix in the term *abiotic*. _____

21. The "then" portion of a hypothesis is the _____ variable.

22. _____ is the study of the parts of the body, and _____ explains the functions of these body parts.

Section 5.4 Ionic Bonding

Atoms bond to make up all the matter in the universe. *Bonding* is the process in which atoms donate, accept, or share electrons with other atoms. In this section, you will learn about one type of bonding: ionic bonding.

The terms below are some of those that will be introduced in Section 5.4. To become familiar with these terms, reproduce each word on the line beside it. Pronounce each term as you write it. You will learn the definitions of these words as you complete this section.

1. full outer shell _____

2. attraction _____

3. ion _____

4. ionic bond _____

5. molecule _____

Concept 1: How Atoms Bond

Bonding holds all the matter in the universe together. Bonding involves an atom's electrons. An important principle in bonding is that an atom will interact with other atoms to achieve a *full outer shell*, or an outermost electron shell that has the maximum number of electrons. For a first electron shell, this maximum would be two electrons. For a second or third electron shell, this maximum would be eight electrons.

In interacting, atoms can *donate electrons*, *accept electrons*, or *share electrons*. By looking at the number of electrons in an atom's outermost electron shell, you can predict how atoms will interact. The next few concepts will walk you through the process of two atoms interacting and then forming an ionic bond.

full outer shell an outermost electron shell that has the maximum number of electrons

Recall Activity

1. Atoms will interact with other atoms to achieve a(n) _____ outer shell.

2. By looking at the number of electrons in an atom's _____,
   you can predict how atoms will interact.

3. List the three ways that electrons can be involved in bonding.

   _____

Concept 2: Chlorine's Outer Shell

To understand how an atom's outer electron shell predicts how the atom will bond, look at the atomic diagram of chlorine. Chlorine is an example of an atom that must *accept* an electron in order to achieve a full outer shell. **Figure 5.14** shows a diagram of chlorine, atomic number 17. Notice that chlorine has seven electrons in its third and outermost shell. An atom's third electron shell has an electron capacity of eight. Chorine needs one more electron to have a full outer shell. As a result, when interacting with other atoms, chlorine must *accept* one more electron and achieve a full outer shell.

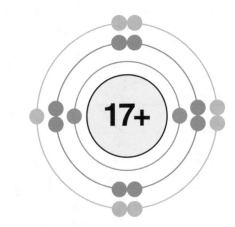

Figure 5.14   A chlorine atom has seven electrons in its outer shell.

Recall Activity

1. How many electrons are in the outermost electron shell of a chlorine atom? _____

2. How many electrons would chlorine have to accept to have a full outer shell? _____

3. By looking at the number of electrons in an atom's _____,
   you can predict how atoms will interact.

Concept 3: Sodium's Outer Shell

While chlorine must accept an electron to achieve a full outer shell, the atom sodium must *donate* an electron to achieve a full outer shell. **Figure 5.15** shows a diagram of a sodium atom, atomic number 11. Notice there is only one electron in sodium's outermost electron shell. If sodium were to donate the single electron in its outer shell, the third electron shell would disappear, and sodium's second electron shell would become its outer shell. Because sodium's second electron shell is full (containing eight electrons), this would achieve a full outer shell.

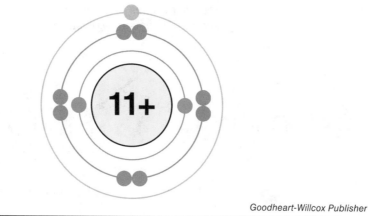

Figure 5.15   A sodium atom has one electron in its outer shell.

Recall Activity

1. How many electrons are in the outermost electron shell of a sodium atom? _____

2. How many electrons would sodium have to donate to have a full outer shell? _____

3. By looking at the number of electrons in an atom's _____, you can predict how atoms will interact.

4. If sodium donates its single electron in the third electron shell, which shell will become its outer shell? _____

5. With the donation of the single electron in the third electron shell, the outer shell of sodium is now its _____ electron shell.

Concept 4: Chlorine and Sodium Interact

attraction the tendency of an atom to keep, donate, or accept an electron

By diagramming chlorine and sodium, you can conclude that chlorine must *accept* one additional electron and sodium must *donate* one of its electrons. This is typically expressed in terms of *attraction*. Sodium does *not* have a very strong attraction for the single electron in its outer shell, while chlorine has a *very strong* attraction for that electron. As a result of their difference in attraction, sodium and chlorine are likely to interact. When they do interact, sodium will donate the electron in its outer shell, and chlorine will accept sodium's donated electron (**Figure 5.16**).

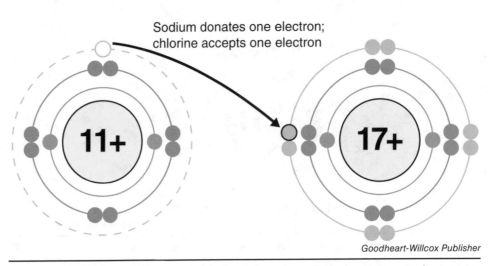

Sodium donates one electron; chlorine accepts one electron

Goodheart-Willcox Publisher

Figure 5.16 When sodium and chlorine interact, sodium donates one electron to chlorine.

Recall Activity

1. In the interaction shown above, sodium _____ an electron.

2. In the interaction shown above, chlorine _____ an electron.

3. In an interaction between sodium and chlorine, which atom has a stronger attraction for the other atom's outer shell electron? _____

4. Prior to interaction, how many electrons did chlorine need to accept to have a full outer shell?

   _____

5. Prior to interaction, how many electrons did sodium need to donate to have a full outer shell?

   _____

Concept 5: Full Outer Shells

After the interaction described in Concept 4, both chlorine and sodium have full outer shells. **Figure 5.17** shows atomic diagrams of chlorine and sodium after their interaction. Notice that both sodium and chlorine now have full outer shells.

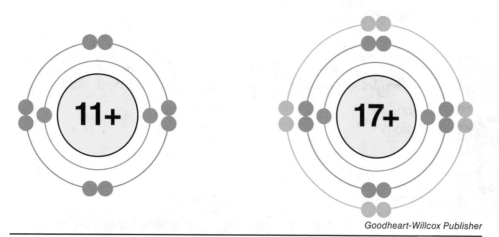

Figure 5.17   Chlorine and sodium now have full outer shells.

Recall Activity

1. How many protons are in sodium's core?_____

2. How many electrons are in sodium's electron shells? _____

3. How many protons are in chlorine's core?_____

4. How many electrons are in chlorine's electron shells?_____

Concept 6: Ions and Charges

You learned in Section 5.1 that, in an atom, the number of protons in the core equals the number of electrons in the electron shells. In ionic bonding, however, the number of protons and electrons in an atom becomes unequal. After donating one electron, for example, the number of protons and electrons is not equal in sodium. The same is true for chlorine, except that chlorine has accepted one electron. Once atoms have interacted and have donated or accepted electrons so that their numbers of protons and electrons are unequal, they are known as *ions*.

ion an atom that has donated or accepted an electron; has a charge

Ions formed from ionic bonding have a charge. As you have learned, protons have positive (+) charges, and electrons have negative (–) charges. When the numbers of protons and electrons are equal, these charges cancel out. When the numbers of protons and electrons are *not* equal, however, an atom that has donated or accepted an electron gains a charge. See **Figure 5.18** to understand how charge is determined. After the transfer of one electron from sodium to chlorine, both sodium and chlorine have a charge. Sodium has a positive charge (1+), and chlorine has a negative charge (1–).

	Sodium (Before Interaction)	Chlorine (Before Interaction)
Protons and Electrons	11 protons 11 electrons	17 protons 17 electrons
Sum of Charges	+ + + + + + + + + + + – – – – – – – – – – –	+++++++++++++++++ —————————————————
Charge	No charge	No charge
	Sodium Ion	**Chloride (Chlorine) Ion**
Protons and Electrons	11 protons 10 electrons (donated one electron)	17 protons 18 electrons (accepted one electron)
Sum of Charges	+ + + + + + + + + + + – – – – – – – – – –	+++++++++++++++++ —————————————————
Charge	1+	1–

Figure 5.18 Charge is determined by comparing the numbers of positive charges (protons) and negative charges (electrons) in an atom.

Recall Activity

1. In interacting with chlorine, sodium _____ one electron.

2. In interacting with sodium, chlorine _____ one electron.

3. Atoms that have donated or accepted electrons are called _____.

4. Atoms that have interacted through ionic bonding have a(n) _____.

5. After donating one electron, sodium has _____ positive charges (protons) and _____ negative charges (electrons).

6. After accepting one electron, chlorine has _____ positive charges (protons) and _____ negative charges (electrons).

Concept 7: Ionic Symbols

Ions that have charges are represented by their atomic symbols, followed by a + or – to indicate charge. Cl^- (chlorine's atomic symbol with one minus sign) is the symbol for the chloride (chlorine) ion. This represents that the chlorine atom has accepted one electron. Na^+ (sodium's atomic symbol with one plus sign) is the symbol for the sodium ion. This represents that the sodium atom has donated one electron.

You can tell what interaction an ion has undergone by analyzing its symbol. For example, the symbol Ca^{++} (calcium's atomic symbol with two plus signs) indicates that the calcium atom has donated two electrons, losing two negative charges. As a result, the calcium ion now has two more positive charges (protons) than negative charges (electrons).

Recall Activity

1. An atom that has donated one electron has a(n) _____ charge.

2. An atom that has accepted one electron has a(n) _____ charge.

3. How many electrons has the calcium ion C^{++} donated? _____

4. What is the symbol for a calcium ion that has donated two electrons? _____

Concept 8: Opposite Charges Attract

The ions created by sodium and chlorine interacting are Na^+ and Cl^-. These ions have opposite charges. These *opposite charges attract*, binding the ions together. The attraction between the Na^+ ion and the Cl^- ion is called an *ionic bond*. In an ionic bond, one atom has lost one or two electrons, and another atom has gained one or two electrons. Because the ions have opposite charges, they are attracted to each other and bind together. Ionic bonds hold atoms together. When a combination of atoms is held together by a bond or bonds, the resulting structure is known as a *molecule*.

ionic bond an atomic bond formed by the attraction between ions that have opposite charges

molecule a combination of atoms held together by bonds

Recall Activity

1. Two ions with opposite charges _____ each other.

2. Na^+ and Cl^- have _____ charges.

3. Na^+ has a(n) _____ charge.

4. Cl^- has a(n) _____ charge.

5. The bond that forms between a Na^+ ion and a Cl^- ion is called a(n) _____ bond.

6. A(n) _____ is a combination of atoms held together by a bond or bonds.

Section 5.4 Reinforcement

Answer the following questions using what you learned in this section.

1. If sodium were to donate the single electron in its outer shell, its third electron shell would

   _____, and the second shell would become the _____

   shell.

2. *True or False.* A positive ion is attracted to a negative ion._____

3. Because sodium has only one electron in its outer shell, sodium is likely to

   _____ the electron when interacting with other atoms.

4. Atoms will interact to achieve a(n) _____ outer shell.

5. If sodium donates the electron in its third electron shell, which shell will become its outer shell?

   _____

6. After interacting with sodium, the chloride ion will have a(n) _____ charge.

7. Atoms that have donated or accepted electrons are called _____.

8. In an interaction between sodium and chlorine, which atom has a stronger attraction for the other

   atom's outer shell electron? _____

9. Write the letters backward: cinoi. Define the word that is formed. _____

   _____

10. The ion Na^+ has a(n) _____ charge.

11. Na^+ and Cl^- have _____ charges.

12. Which subatomic particle is involved in bonding? _____

13. *True or False.* A positive ion is formed when an atom accepts electrons from another atom._____

14. Unscramble the letters: coemuell. Define the word that is formed. _____

    _____

15. *True or False.* An ion has a charge._____

16. A(n) _____ is a combination of atoms held together by a bond or bonds.

17. The bond that forms between a Na^+ ion and a Cl^- ion is called a(n) _____

    bond.

18. An atom with atomic number 16 needs to _____ two electrons to have a full

    outer shell.

19. Which atomic number would have a full outer shell: 2, 6, 5, or 12? _____

20. *True or False.* If an atom has seven electrons in its outer shell, it will accept two electrons when

    interacting with another atom. _____

21. Because chlorine needs only one electron to fill its outer shell, chlorine is likely to

    _____ an electron when interacting with other atoms.

Comprehensive Review (Chapters 1–5)

Answer the following questions using what you have learned so far in this book.

22. Arrange the following measurements from largest to smallest: 15 mm, 235 cm, 75 mm, and 0.09 m.

    _____

23. The atomic number of He is _____.

24. In the last step of the experimental scientific method, you decide to _____ or

    _____ the hypothesis.

25. Disassemble the word *physiology* by identifying its combining form and suffix._____

    _____

26. A fact is a(n) _____ observation.

Section 5.5 Covalent Bonding

When atoms bond, they donate, accept, or share electrons. In ionic bonding, atoms donate or accept electrons. In covalent bonding, the type of bonding discussed in this section, atoms share electrons.

The terms below are some of those that will be introduced in Section 5.5. To become familiar with these terms, reproduce each word on the line beside it. Pronounce each term as you write it. You will learn the definitions of these words as you complete this section.

1. covalent bond _____

2. single bond _____

3. double bond _____

Concept 1: Equal Attraction

As with ionic bonding, covalent bonding follows the principle that an atom will interact to achieve a full outer shell. In ionic bonding, one atom has a stronger attraction for an electron than another atom. In covalent bonding, two atoms have *equal* attraction for an electron. **Figure 5.19** shows atomic diagrams of hydrogen and carbon. Hydrogen has one electron in its outer shell. Carbon has four electrons in its outer shell. Because hydrogen and carbon have equal attraction for electrons, they neither donate nor accept electrons. Instead, they *share electrons* to achieve full outer shells.

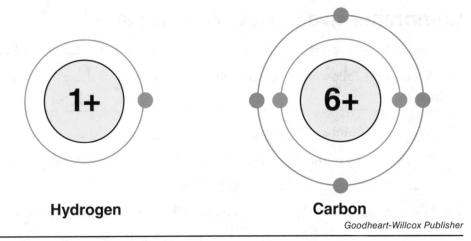

Hydrogen **Carbon**

Goodheart-Willcox Publisher

Figure 5.19 Hydrogen has one electron in its outer shell; carbon has four electrons in its outer shell.

Recall Activity

1. Hydrogen has _____ electron(s) in its outer shell.

2. Carbon has _____ electron(s) in its outer shell.

3. Because hydrogen and carbon need to accept electrons to achieve full outer shells, they _____ electrons.

4. Instead of donating or accepting electrons, atoms that form covalent bonds _____ electrons.

Concept 2: Forming a Covalent Bond

covalent bond an atomic bond in which electrons are shared

When atoms share electrons, they form *covalent bonds*. In covalent bonding, multiple atoms bond to one another to achieve full outer shells. In **Figure 5.20**, four hydrogen atoms bond to one carbon atom. In each pair of shared electrons, carbon shares one electron with hydrogen, and hydrogen shares one electron with carbon. Hydrogen's outer shell contains two electrons, and carbon's outer shell contains eight electrons. In forming these bonds, all five atoms achieve full outer shells. The five atoms bonded together are known as a *molecule*.

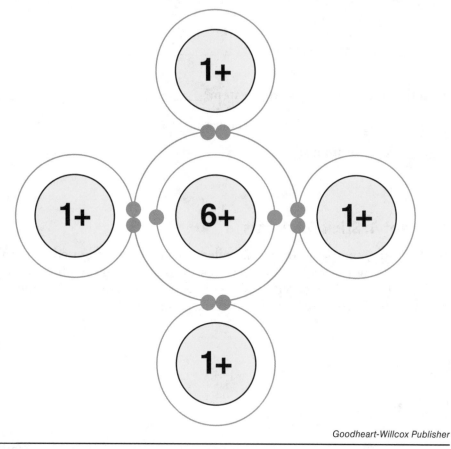

Goodheart-Willcox Publisher

Figure 5.20 Four atoms of hydrogen bond with one carbon atom.

Recall Activity

1. The molecule in Figure 5.20 contains _____ hydrogen atom(s) and _____ carbon atom(s).

2. A(n) _____ bond is formed when atoms share electrons.

3. In Figure 5.20, how many electrons are shared between the hydrogen and carbon atoms? _____

4. All atoms in Figure 5.20 have _____ outer shells.

5. In a covalent bond, electrons are _____ among atoms.

Concept 3: Molecular Symbols

Molecules are represented by chemical formulas that indicate the atoms bonded. The molecule discussed in Concept 2, one carbon atom and four hydrogen atoms, would be written CH_4 (one molecule of CH_4; *C* for carbon and *H* for hydrogen, with *4* indicating the number of hydrogen atoms). The name of that molecule is *methane*. Carbon will also interact with other atoms to achieve a full outer shell with eight electrons. For example, in CO_2, commonly called *carbon dioxide*, a carbon atom bonds with two oxygen atoms to achieve a full outer shell.

Recall Activity

1. CH₄ has _____ carbon atom(s) and _____ hydrogen atom(s).

2. How many electrons are in the outer shell of a hydrogen atom? _____

3. The molecule C_3H_8 has _____ carbon atom(s) and

    _____ hydrogen atom(s).

Concept 4: Stick Diagrams

In chemistry, shorthand diagrams called *stick diagrams* are used to simplify atomic drawings of molecules. In a stick diagram, atomic symbols represent individual atoms. If two electrons are shared between atoms, this is indicated by one stick. See **Figure 5.21** for a stick diagram of CH₄.

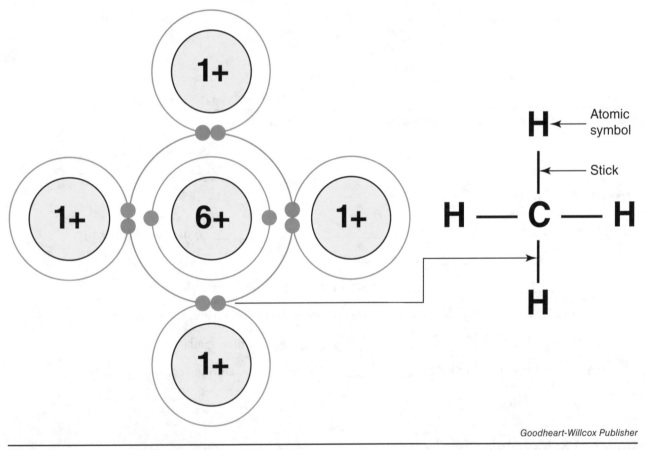

Figure 5.21   Each stick represents two shared electrons.

Recall Activity

1. In the stick diagram for CH_4, how many sticks are attached to the carbon atom?_____

2. Each stick represents _____ shared electron(s) in the outer shell.

3. When added together, all of the sticks attached to the carbon atom in CH_4 represent

   _____ shared electron(s).

4. How many sticks are attached to each hydrogen atom in CH_4? _____

5. When added together, all of the sticks attached to hydrogen atoms in CH_4 represent

   _____ shared electron(s).

6. In the stick diagram for CH_4, each hydrogen atom has _____ electron(s) in its
   outer shell.

Concept 5: Single and Double Covalent Bonds

Once you know how many sticks can be attached to each atom, you can diagram chains of atoms. See the stick diagram of C_4H_8 below. Each carbon atom has four sticks attached (sharing four electrons to achieve a full outer shell); each hydrogen atom has one stick attached (sharing one electron to achieve a full outer shell). One stick between atoms (–) represents a *single bond*. Two sticks between atoms (=) represents a *double bond*. In a single bond, two electrons are shared between the atoms. In a double bond, four electrons are shared (**Figure 5.22**).

single bond a covalent bond in which two electrons are shared

double bond a covalent bond in which four electrons are shared

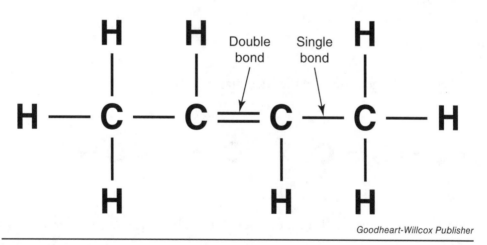

Goodheart-Willcox Publisher

Figure 5.22 Single bonds are represented by one stick. Double bonds are represented by two sticks.

Recall Activity

1. Each stick represents _____ shared electron(s).

2. Two sticks (=) represent _____ shared electron(s).

3. Each carbon atom has _____ stick(s) attached to it.

4. Each hydrogen atom has _____ stick(s) attached to it.

5. In a single bond, _____ electrons are shared.

6. In a double bond, _____ electrons are shared.

7. What is the symbol for a single bond? _____

8. What is the symbol for a double bond? _____

9. If a carbon atom has one double bond, how many additional sticks will be attached to it? _____

10. The molecule C_4H_{10} has _____ carbon atom(s) and
    _____ hydrogen atom(s).

Concept 6: Construct a Stick Diagram

In this concept, you will learn more about how to construct a stick diagram of a carbon-hydrogen molecule. When creating a stick diagram for a carbon-hydrogen molecule, first place the carbon atoms. Then add the hydrogen atoms using what you know about full outer shells.

Recall Activity

1. Add the appropriate number of hydrogen atoms to the stick diagrams below.

$$C - C - C - C - C \qquad C - C = C - C$$

2. Place sticks to represent single and double bonds in the stick diagrams below; some will require double bonds.

```
H H H H H              H H H H H                  H   H H
H C C C C H            H C C C C C H         H
H H H H H                  H    H H          H  C C C C C H
                                             H    H   H
```

Section 5.5 Reinforcement

Answer the following questions using what you learned in this section.

1. Describe what is wrong with the following stick diagram. _____

_____

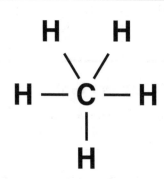

2. Which of the following terms does *not* belong with the others: donate, share, ion, or ionic bond?

_____

3. Unscramble the letters: latvocen. Define the word that is formed. _____

_____

4. In a stick diagram, each carbon atom should have _____ stick(s) attached to it.

5. In a double bond, _____ electrons are shared.

6. *True or False.* Three electrons are shared in a double bond. _____

7. The molecule C_6H_{14} has _____ carbon atom(s) and
_____ hydrogen atom(s).

8. In a stick diagram, each hydrogen atom should have _____ stick(s) attached
to it.

9. *True or False.* All ionic bonds are double bonds. _____

10. A(n) _____ bond results when atoms share electrons.

11. Unscramble the letters: rahse. Define the word that is formed. _____

_____

12. Which bond has more shared electrons: a single bond or a double bond? _____

13. In a single bond, _____ electrons are shared.

14. Describe why the following statement is incorrect: Protons are shared between atoms in a covalent
bond. _____

15. In a stick diagram, what is the symbol for a single bond? _____

16. *True or False.* Electrons are shared in a covalent bond. _____

17. List the names of the two types of covalent bonds discussed in this section. _____

_____

18. Two sticks (=) represents _____ shared electron(s).

19. *True or False*. In a stick diagram, one stick represents two shared electrons. _____

20. Which of the following words is misspelled?

A. covalant   C. hydrogen

B. stick   D. accept

Comprehensive Review (Chapters 1–5)

Answer the following questions using what you have learned so far in this book.

21. An atom's first electron shell can hold up to _____ electron(s).

22. How many millimeters are in 1.56 m? _____

23. Constants are _____ factors.

24. What is the prefix in the word *antibacterial*? _____

25. *True or False*. Science invokes supernatural explanations. _____

Section 5.6 Hydrogen Bonding

Thus far in this chapter, you have learned about two types of bonding between atoms: ionic bonding and covalent bonding. In this section, you will learn about a third type of bonding: hydrogen bonding.

The terms below are some of those that will be introduced in Section 5.6. To become familiar with these terms, reproduce each word on the line beside it. Pronounce each term as you write it. You will learn the definitions of these words as you complete this section.

1. partial charge _____

2. hydrogen bond _____

Concept 1: Water Molecule

To understand hydrogen bonding, first analyze a water molecule. The chemical formula for water is one atom of oxygen and two atoms of hydrogen, written as H_2O. The shape of a water molecule resembles a mouse head, as shown in **Figure 5.23**. Some atoms, including the oxygen atom in a water molecule, have an especially intense attraction for electrons. In a water molecule, covalent bonds bind the oxygen atom and the hydrogen atoms together. However, because oxygen's attraction for electrons is especially intense, electrons tend to spend more time in the "chin" (oxygen atom) of the water molecule than in the "ears" (hydrogen atoms). Because of this, the "chin" of the water molecule has a partial negative charge, and the "ears" have partial positive charges.

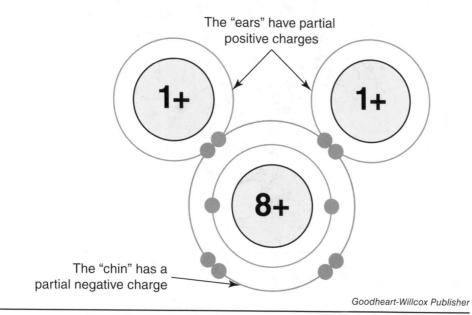

The "ears" have partial positive charges

1+

1+

8+

The "chin" has a partial negative charge

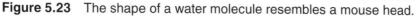

Goodheart-Willcox Publisher

Figure 5.23 The shape of a water molecule resembles a mouse head.

Recall Activity

1. A water molecule contains _____ oxygen atom(s) and _____ hydrogen atom(s).

2. What type of bond exists between the hydrogen and oxygen atoms in H_2O? _____

3. In a water molecule, electrons tend to spend more time in the _____ than in the _____ .

4. Electrons have a(n) _____ charge.

5. The presence of more electrons in the chin of a water molecule gives the chin a partial _____ charge.

6. The absence of electrons in the ears of a water molecule gives the ears a partial _____ charge.

Concept 2: Forming a Hydrogen Bond

Hydrogen bonds are formed based on *partial charges*. To represent a partial charge, use the symbol ~. A partial positive charge will be written as ~+, and a partial negative charge will be written as ~−. See the partial charges represented on the water molecule in **Figure 5.24**.

partial charge a slight negative or positive charge in a part of a molecule

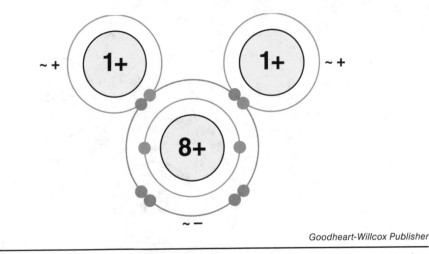

Goodheart-Willcox Publisher

Figure 5.24 The chin of the water molecule has a partial negative charge, and the ears have partial positive charges.

As you may recall, opposite charges attract. This includes even partial charges, like the partial negative charge of a water molecule's chin and the partial positive charges of its ears. Because of this, the ear (hydrogen atom) of one water molecule is attracted to the chin (oxygen atom) of another water molecule. This attraction is called a *hydrogen bond*. Hydrogen bonding can also occur when hydrogen atoms bond with other atoms that have especially intense attractions for electrons (for example, nitrogen and fluorine). Because they are based on partial charges, hydrogen bonds are weaker than ionic or covalent bonds. See **Figure 5.25** for an illustration of how hydrogen bonds are formed by partial charges.

hydrogen bond an atomic bond in which the partial charges of water molecules attract; the weakest type of atomic bond

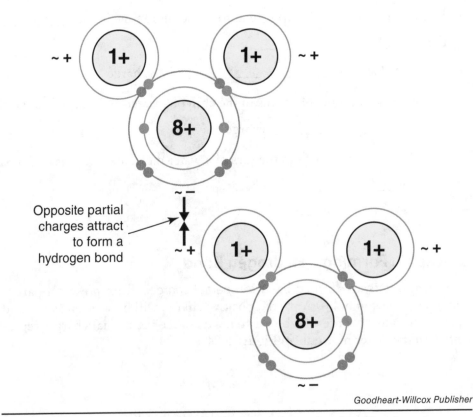

Opposite partial charges attract to form a hydrogen bond

Goodheart-Willcox Publisher

Figure 5.25 The opposite partial charges in water molecules attract.

Recall Activity

1. The ear of one water molecule is attracted to the _____ of another water molecule.

2. Opposite partial charges _____.

3. Because they are based on partial charges, hydrogen bonds are _____ than ionic or covalent bonds.

4. What is the symbol for a partial charge? _____

5. What is the partial charge of the chin of a water molecule?_____

6. In the space below, draw two water molecules with the ear of one molecule below the chin of the other. Draw in the partial charges to represent a hydrogen bond.

Concept 3: Hydrogen Bonds and Water Characteristics

The water molecule interacts with various ions. Water is a *solvent*, which means it is capable of dissolving *ionic molecules* (molecules formed from ions). It can do this because of its partial charges.

As you have learned, a water molecule has partial positive and negative charges. Because of these charges, ions (which also have charges) are attracted to water. If an ionic molecule such as NaCl is added to water, the Na^+ ion will be attracted to the partial negative charge of the water molecule's chin, and the Cl^- ion will be attracted to the partial positive charge of the water molecule's ear. This will cause the molecule NaCl to *dissolve*, or break apart.

The nature of the hydrogen bond also affects other characteristics of water. Hydrogen bonds cause water molecules to stick together or be cohesive. Water is less dense as a solid (ice) than as a liquid. As water freezes, water molecules spread out so that a volume of ice (for example, a cubic centimeter) contains fewer water molecules than the same volume of liquid water. Water also has a high heat capacity and resists changes in temperature. When heat is applied to an object, the activity of the molecules composing the object increases. This increase in molecular activity increases the temperature of the object. In water, heat energy is absorbed or released by hydrogen bonds before the activity of water molecules increases or decreases.

Recall Activity

1. Water is capable of dissolving _____ molecules.

2. A water molecule has partial positive and negative _____.

3. _____ are attracted to water.

4. If NaCl is added to water, the Na^+ ion will be attracted to the partial _____ of the water molecule's _____, and the Cl^- ion is attracted to the partial _____ of the water molecule's _____.

5. Hydrogen bonding causes water molecules to stick together, or be _____.

6. Water is _____ dense as a solid (ice) than as a liquid.

7. Water has a high heat capacity and _____ changes in temperature.

Concept 4: Types of Bonds

In this chapter, you have learned about three types of bonds between atoms:
- *ionic bonds*—the attraction between ions with opposite charges
- *covalent bonds*—the sharing of electrons between atoms
- *hydrogen bonds*—the attraction of partial charges between molecules made of hydrogen atoms and atoms with an especially intense attraction for electrons

Of these three types of bonds, hydrogen bonds are the weakest. This is because the charges in a hydrogen bond are only partial, not full.

Recall Activity

1. List and describe the three types of bonds.

_____

2. Of these bonds, the weakest is the _____ bond.

Concept 5: Chemical Formulas

As you learned in Section 5.5, molecules are represented by *chemical formulas*. In this last concept of Section 5.6, you will learn more about reading and writing chemical formulas. Chemical formulas indicate the numbers and names of atoms in a molecule. The chemical formula for glucose, $C_6H_{12}O_6$, means there are 6 carbon, 12 hydrogen, and 6 oxygen atoms in one glucose molecule.

When referring to more than one molecule, a number placed in front of the chemical formula indicates how many molecules exist. The formula $2C_6H_{12}O_6$ represents two molecules of glucose. In two molecules of glucose, there are 12 carbon, 24 hydrogen, and 12 oxygen atoms. To determine this, simply multiply the 2 preceding the formula by the number of carbon (6), hydrogen (12), and oxygen (6) atoms in one molecule. As another example, the formula $3H_2NO_3$ represents three molecules of nitric acid. In one molecule of nitric acid, there are 2 hydrogen, 1 nitrogen, and 3 oxygen atoms. In three molecules of nitric acid, there are 6 hydrogen, 3 nitrogen, and 9 oxygen atoms.

Recall Activity

1. How many molecules are in the formula $3NaHCO_3$? _____

2. How many molecules are in the formula H_2NO_3? _____

3. The formula H_2SO_4 has _____ hydrogen, _____ sulfur, and _____ oxygen atoms.

4. The formula $3NaCl$ has _____ sodium and _____ chlorine atoms.

5. The formula $2NaHCO_3$ has _____ sodium, _____ hydrogen, _____ carbon, and _____ oxygen atoms.

6. The formula $4H_2O$ has _____ hydrogen and _____ oxygen atoms.

Section 5.6 Reinforcement

Answer the following questions using what you learned in this section.

1. How many molecules are in the formula $5NaHCO_3$? _____

2. The formula $4H_2SO_4$ has _____ hydrogen, _____ sulfur, and _____ oxygen atoms.

3. What are the three types of bonds discussed in this chapter?_____

_____

4. Of the three types of atomic bonds, the weakest is the _____ bond.

5. Which of the following words are misspelled?

   A. molacule   C. covalent

   B. hydrgen

6. The chin of one water molecule is attracted to the _____ of another water molecule.

7. *True or False*. The ear of a water molecule has a full positive or negative charge. _____

8. The three types of atomic bonds are hydrogen bonds, ionic bonds, and _____.

9. Write the letters backward: negordyh. Define the word that is formed. _____
    _____

10. The formula 8H$_2$O has _____ hydrogen and _____ oxygen atoms.

11. *True or False*. One water molecule is held to another water molecule by a covalent bond. _____

12. Which of the following bonds is the weakest?
    A. hydrogen   B. covalent   C. ionic

13. *True or False*. The ear of a water molecule has a partial positive charge. _____

14. Unscramble the letters: ratpail. Define the word that is formed. _____
    _____

15. The hydrogen and oxygen atoms in a water molecule are held together by _____ bonds.

16. Which of the following statements are true?
    A. Water is a solvent.   C. Water molecules are cohesive.
    B. Ice is more dense than liquid water.

17. Opposite partial charges _____.

18. Which atom has a greater attraction for electrons: oxygen or hydrogen? _____

19. *True or False*. The water molecule consists of two hydrogen atoms and one oxygen atom. _____

20. Because the charges are partial, hydrogen bonds are _____ than other bonds.

21. Unscramble the letters: kawe. Define the word that is formed. _____
    _____

22. What is the total number of atoms in the formula 2H$_2$NO$_3$? _____

23. In your own words, describe a hydrogen bond. _____
    _____
    _____

Comprehensive Review (Chapters 1–5)

Answer the following questions using what you have learned so far in this book.

24. In a double bond, _____ electrons are shared.

25. Convert 1567 m into km. _____

26. Biology is the science that studies _____.

27. *True or False.* Both *ad-* and *ab-* mean "toward." _____

28. What is the difference between the experimental group and the control group? _____

_____

_____

Section 5.7 Carbohydrates

Now that you have learned about atoms and atomic bonding, you can understand various macromolecules in the human body, including carbohydrates, lipids, proteins, and nucleic acids. All of these macromolecules are important for body function. In this section, you will learn about carbohydrates.

The terms below are some of those that will be introduced in Section 5.7. To become familiar with these terms, reproduce each word on the line beside it. Pronounce each term as you write it. You will learn the definitions of these words as you complete this section.

1. macromolecule_____   5. polysaccharide_____

2. carbohydrate_____   6. fiber _____

3. monosaccharide_____   7. calories _____

4. disaccharide_____

Concept 1: Macromolecules

As you have learned, a *molecule* is a combination of atoms. When many atoms combine, they form a *macromolecule*. Macromolecules are big because they contain so many atoms. A macromolecule made of repeating subunits is called a *polymer*. In this section and in the sections that follow, you will learn about four main types of macromolecules: carbohydrates, lipids, proteins, and nucleic acids.

macromolecule a combination of many atoms held together by bonds

Recall Activity

1. List the four main types of macromolecules._____

_____

2. A(n) _____ is a combination of many atoms.

Concept 2: Sugars

carbohydrate a macromolecule that is a sugar; types include monosaccharides, disaccharides, and polysaccharides

The first type of macromolecule is the carbohydrate. *Carbohydrates* are sugars, which are also known as *saccharides*. There are three main categories of carbohydrates: monosaccharides, disaccharides, and polysaccharides. Carbohydrates are polymers, meaning they are made of repeating subunits. The repeating subunit in disaccharides and polysaccharides is a six-carbon or five-carbon sugar. The six-carbon sugar is commonly diagrammed as a hexagon, while the five-carbon sugar is drawn as a pentagon.

Recall Activity

1. What are saccharides? _____

2. List the three main types of carbohydrates._____

_____

3. What are carbohydrates? _____

Concept 3: Monosaccharides

monosaccharide a type of carbohydrate containing one sugar

A *monosaccharide* is one sugar. This word is formed from the prefix *mono-*, which means "one," and the combining form *sacchar/o*, which means "sugar." Monosaccharides are the simplest type of sugar. Glucose is one example of a monosaccharide. When you eat carbohydrates, your digestive system breaks down the carbohydrates into glucose. Glucose is then shipped by your blood to the cells in your body. Inside your cells, the energy contained in glucose is converted into a form of energy your cells can use. Your life is dependent on this process. A glucose molecule looks like a hexagon, as shown in **Figure 5.26**. The basic structure of glucose contains 6 carbon atoms, 12 hydrogen atoms, and 6 oxygen atoms.

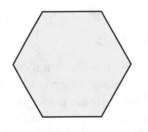

Figure 5.26 A glucose molecule is represented as a hexagon.

Recall Activity

1. The prefix _____ means "one."

2. The combining form _____ means "sugar."

3. The simplest sugars are _____.

4. One example of a monosaccharide is _____.

5. When you eat _____, your digestive system breaks them down into

   _____.

6. Glucose is shipped by your blood to the _____ in your body.

7. The glucose molecule looks like a(n) _____.

8. Write the chemical formula of glucose. _____

Concept 4: Disaccharides

A *disaccharide* consists of two monosaccharides bonded together. One example of a disaccharide is *maltose*, commonly known as *malt sugar*. Two other examples are *sucrose* (table sugar) and *lactose* (milk sugar). A disaccharide is drawn as two hexagons to represent the two bonded monosaccharides (**Figure 5.27**).

disaccharide a type of carbohydrate containing two sugars bonded together

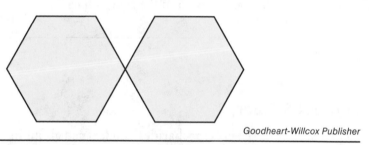

Goodheart-Willcox Publisher

Figure 5.27 This diagram represents the disaccharide maltose.

Recall Activity

1. Two monosaccharides bonded together make a(n) _____.

2. One example of a disaccharide is _____.

3. Sucrose is also called _____ sugar.

4. A disaccharide is made of two _____.

Concept 5: Polysaccharides

A *polysaccharide* consists of many monosaccharides linked together. The prefix *poly-* in polysaccharide means "many." One example of a polysaccharide is *glycogen*. Glycogen is stored in your liver. When your body needs blood sugar, stored glycogen is broken down into many glucose molecules. Other examples of polysaccharides are *cellulose* and *starch*. A polysaccharide is drawn as many hexagons linked together (**Figure 5.28**).

polysaccharide a type of carbohydrate containing more than two sugars bonded together

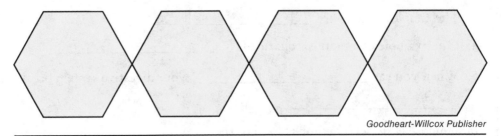

Goodheart-Willcox Publisher

Figure 5.28 Polysaccharides are drawn as many hexagons.

Recall Activity

1. The basic shape of a monosaccharide is a(n) _____.

2. A polysaccharide is many _____ linked together.

3. The prefix _____ means "many."

4. List three examples of polysaccharides._____

5. What is the name of the polysaccharide that is stored in the body's liver? _____

6. What is glycogen broken down into? _____

Concept 6: Fiber

Cellulose, one of the polysaccharides you learned about in Concept 5, is found in many plant cells. When you eat plants such as vegetables, your digestive system cannot break down cellulose into monosaccharides. Plant material that you eat and that is indigestible is called *fiber*. Although you cannot obtain energy from cellulose, fiber should be a part of your diet.

fiber plant material that is eaten, but is indigestible

Recall Activity

1. Plant cells contain _____.

2. Your digestive system cannot break down cellulose into _____.

3. Indigestible cellulose is called _____ in your diet.

Concept 7: Complex Carbohydrates

Carbohydrates can be classified as *simple* or *complex*. Complex carbohydrates are polysaccharides, and simple carbohydrates are monosaccharides. As you might imagine, one molecule of a complex carbohydrate contains more energy than one molecule of a simple carbohydrate. A monosaccharide or disaccharide, such as sugar or a candy bar, is quickly digested and rapidly increases your blood sugar or energy level. A polysaccharide, however, takes longer to digest and provides energy over a longer period of time. Examples of complex carbohydrates include bread and pasta.

Recall Activity

1. Bread and pasta are _____ carbohydrates.

2. Which type of carbohydrate provides quick energy?_____

3. Which type of carbohydrate provides energy over a longer period of time? _____

   _____

4. A candy bar contains _____ carbohydrates.

5. Which type of carbohydrate is digested quickly? _____

Concept 8: Calories in Carbohydrates

Carbohydrates are a major source of energy in a person's diet. The energy provided by macromolecules is measured in *calories* or in *kilocalories* (one thousand calories). One gram of carbohydrates contains 4 kilocalories of energy.

calories a measurement of the energy provided by macromolecules

Recall Activity

1. The amount of energy provided by carbohydrates is measured in _____ or

   _____ .

2. One gram of carbohydrates contains _____ kilocalories of energy.

Section 5.7 Reinforcement

Answer the following questions using what you learned in this section.

1. Which of the following words is misspelled?
   A. saccaride   C. macromolecule
   B. hydrogen

2. Which of the following are polysaccharides?
   A. starch   C. glycogen
   B. sucrose

3. Bread and pasta are _____ carbohydrates.

4. Unscramble the letters: rusag. Define the word that is formed. _____

_____

5. What is the name of the polysaccharide stored in the liver? _____

6. Name the three types of carbohydrates in alphabetical order. _____

_____

7. Your digestive system cannot break down cellulose into _____.

8. Which of the following are macromolecules?

   A. amino acids   B. nucleotides   C. proteins   D. lipids

9. _____ is the polysaccharide that is stored in the liver.

10. Write the letters backward: etardyhobrac. Define the word that is formed. _____

_____

11. *True or False.* A polysaccharide is represented by many hexagons linked together. _____

12. Which type of molecule is bigger: a monosaccharide, disaccharide, or polysaccharide? _____

_____

13. What is glycogen broken down into? _____

14. Which of the following are polysaccharides?

   A. glucose   C. starch

   B. sucrose   D. glycogen

15. The simplest sugars are _____.

16. Unscramble the letters: negohax. Define the word that is formed. _____

_____

17. Does a candy bar contain simple or complex carbohydrates? _____

18. Indigestible cellulose is called _____ in your diet.

19. Write the letters backward: edirahccas. Define the word that is formed. _____

_____

Match the following terms with their definitions.

_____ 20. Two sugars   A. carbohydrate

_____ 21. One sugar   B. monosaccharide

_____ 22. Three sugars   C. disaccharide

_____ 23. Sugar   D. polysaccharide

Comprehensive Review (Chapters 1–5)

Answer the following questions using what you have learned so far in this book.

24. How many molecules are in the formula $2NaHCO_3$? _____

25. Which of the following is the lowest temperature?

    A. 76°F   C. 34°C

    B. 14°C   D. 42°F

26. The two variables in a hypothesis are the _____ and the

    _____.

27. *True or False.* A polygon has one side. _____

28. Studying is the deliberate effort to make _____ memories about subject matter.

Section 5.8 Lipids

The second category of macromolecules is lipids. Lipids are made of glycerol molecules and fatty acids (or fats). In this section, you will learn about the properties and types of lipids.

The terms below are some of those that will be introduced in Section 5.8. To become familiar with these terms, reproduce each word on the line beside it. Pronounce each term as you write it. You will learn the definitions of these words as you complete this section.

1. lipid _____

2. saturated fat_____

3. unsaturated fat_____

4. polyunsaturated fat _____

5. *trans* fat_____

6. hydrogenation _____

Concept 1: Types of Lipids

Lipids include the macromolecules that make up fats, waxes, and oils. A *lipid* is one glycerol molecule ($C_3H_8O_3$) bonded to three fatty acids. Fatty acids are called *fats*. There are four types of fats: saturated fat, unsaturated fat, polyunsaturated fat, and *trans* fat.

> **lipid** a macromolecule that is a fat; one glycerol molecule bonded to three fatty acids

Recall Activity

1. Lipids make up _____, _____, and
    _____.

2. A lipid is one _____ molecule bonded to three _____.

3. Fatty acids are called _____.

4. List the four types of fats. _____
    _____

Concept 2: Saturated Fat

saturated fat a lipid in which all bonds between carbon atoms are single bonds and each carbon atom has the maximum number of hydrogen atoms bonded to it; is solid at room temperature

A fat is a *saturated fat* if all of the bonds between carbon atoms are single bonds and if each carbon atom has the maximum number of hydrogen atoms bonded to it (**Figure 5.29**). Saturated fats are solids at room temperature. The fat on meat is an example of saturated fat. Saturated fat makes many foods taste good. Fat is high in calories, and many people crave high-fat foods.

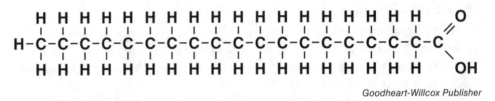

Goodheart-Willcox Publisher

Figure 5.29 In a saturated fat, all of the bonds between carbon atoms are single bonds. The stick diagram in this figure represents stearic acid, a saturated fat. The tasty fat on meat is saturated fat.

Recall Activity

1. In a saturated fat, all of the bonds between carbon atoms are _____ bonds.

2. In a saturated fat, each carbon atom has the _____ number of hydrogen atoms bonded to it.

3. At room temperature, a saturated fat is a(n) _____.

4. Name an example of a saturated fat. _____

Concept 3: Unsaturated Fat

unsaturated fat a lipid in which there is one double bond between carbon atoms and fewer than the maximum number of hydrogen atoms bonded to each carbon atom; is liquid at room temperature

A fat is an *unsaturated fat* if there is one double bond between the carbon atoms and if there are fewer than the maximum number of hydrogen atoms attached to each carbon atom (**Figure 5.30**). Unsaturated fats (for example, olive oil) are liquids at room temperature.

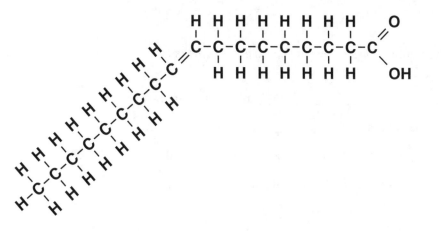

Goodheart-Willcox Publisher

Figure 5.30 In an unsaturated fat, there is one double bond between carbon atoms. The stick diagram in this figure represents oleic acid, an unsaturated fat. Unsaturated fat is liquid at room temperature, like olive oil.

Recall Activity

1. An unsaturated fat has one _____ bond between carbon atoms.

2. An unsaturated fat has _____ than the maximum number of hydrogen atoms bonded to each carbon atom.

3. At room temperature, unsaturated fats are _____.

4. An example of an unsaturated fat is _____ oil.

Concept 4: Polyunsaturated Fat

A fat is a *polyunsaturated fat* if there is more than one double bond between the carbon atoms and if there are far fewer than the maximum number of hydrogen atoms bonded to each carbon (**Figure 5.31**). Polyunsaturated fats (for example, corn oil) are liquids at room temperature.

polyunsaturated fat a lipid in which there is more than one double bond between carbon atoms and far fewer than the maximum number of hydrogen atoms bonded to each carbon atom; is liquid at room temperature

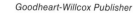

Goodheart-Willcox Publisher

Figure 5.31 In a polyunsaturated fat, there is more than one double bond between carbon atoms. The stick diagram in this figure represents linoleic acid, a polyunsaturated fat. Polyunsaturated fat is liquid at room temperature, like corn oil.

Recall Activity

1. A fat with more than one double bond between the carbon atoms is a(n) _____ fat.

2. Polyunsaturated fats are _____ at room temperature.

3. An example of a polyunsaturated fat is _____ oil.

4. In a polyunsaturated fat, there are far fewer than the maximum number of _____ atoms bonded to each carbon atom.

Concept 5: *Trans* Fat

trans *fat* an unsaturated or polyunsaturated fat that has had hydrogen atoms added to it

hydrogenation the process of adding hydrogen atoms to an unsaturated or polyunsaturated fat; creates *trans* fat

A trans *fat* is an unsaturated or polyunsaturated fat that has had hydrogen atoms added to the molecule. This process of adding hydrogen atoms is called *hydrogenation*. Foods that have had hydrogen atoms added are called *hydrogenated*. When shopping, you may see the phrases *partially hydrogenated* or *trans fat* on food labels. Hydrogenated and partially hydrogenated fats are used in making many processed foods because hydrogenation makes the fat easier to work with.

Recall Activity

1. A(n) _____ fat is a hydrogenated unsaturated fat.

2. Adding hydrogen atoms to fats is called _____.

3. Fats are hydrogenated to make the fat _____ to work with when making foods.

4. A *trans* fat is made by adding _____ atoms to an unsaturated fat.

Concept 6: Calories in Lipids

Fats are a concentrated source of energy. One gram of fat contains 9 kilocalories of energy. Compared to carbohydrates, fats have more than twice the energy per gram. Fats are long-term energy storage in the body.

Recall Activity

1. _____ are long-term energy storage in the body.

2. One gram of fat contains _____ kilocalories.

Section 5.8 Reinforcement

Answer the following questions using what you learned in this section.

1. Is C_6H_{12} a saturated, unsaturated, or polyunsaturated fat? _____

2. A fat with more than one double bond between the carbon atoms is a(n)

   _____ fat.

3. In a saturated fat, each carbon atom has the _____ number of hydrogen atoms bonded to it.

4. A(n) _____ fat is a hydrogenated unsaturated fat.

5. Unscramble the letters: lopy. Define the word that is formed. _____

   _____

6. At room temperature, a saturated fat is a(n) _____.

7. Fats are hydrogenated to make the fat _____ to work with when making foods.

8. Write the letters backward: detarutasnuylop. Define the word that is formed. _____

   _____

9. A *trans* fat is made by adding _____ atoms to an unsaturated fat.

10. In a saturated fat, all of the bonds between carbon atoms are _____ bonds.

11. Unscramble the letters: detatrasu. Define the word that is formed. _____

    _____

12. Adding hydrogen atoms to fats is called _____.

13. List the four types of fats. _____

    _____

Match the following terms with their definitions.

_____ 14. Hydrogenation

_____ 15. Two double bonds between carbon atoms

_____ 16. One double bond between carbon atoms

_____ 17. Single bonds between carbon atoms

A. saturated fat
B. unsaturated fat
C. polyunsaturated fat
D. *trans* fat

Section 5.9 Proteins

Another category of macromolecules includes proteins. Proteins are chains of amino acids. In this section, you will learn about amino acids and protein structures.

The terms below are some of those that will be introduced in Section 5.9. To become familiar with these terms, reproduce each word on the line beside it. Pronounce each term as you write it. You will learn the definitions of these words as you complete this section.

1. protein _____

2. essential amino acid _____

3. primary structure _____

4. secondary structure _____

5. tertiary structure _____

Concept 1: What Is a Protein?

protein a macromolecule that is a chain of amino acids

Proteins are another class of macromolecules important for body functions. A *protein* is a chain of amino acids. A protein is also a polymer. The repeating subunit of a protein is an amino acid. There are 20 different amino acids. Ten are represented by the different-colored circles in **Figure 5.32**. The green lines represent *peptide bonds*, or bonds that hold the amino acids together.

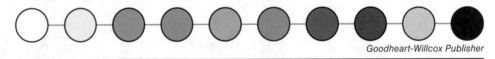

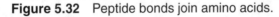

Goodheart-Willcox Publisher

Figure 5.32 Peptide bonds join amino acids.

Recall Activity

1. A protein is a chain of _____.

2. How many different amino acids are there? _____

3. What type of bond holds amino acids together? _____

Concept 2: Amino Acids

Each of the 20 amino acids has a similar structure. This structure includes a central carbon atom, a hydrogen atom, a carboxyl group of atoms, an amino group of atoms, and a remainder (**Figure 5.33**). The central carbon atom is one carbon atom in the middle of the molecule. Similarly, the hydrogen atom is one hydrogen bonded to the central carbon atom. The *carboxyl group* can be written as COOH, containing one carbon atom, two oxygen atoms, and one hydrogen atom. The *amino group* contains one nitrogen atom and several hydrogen atoms. In the diagram below, the amino group is written as NH_2. The final part of the amino acid is the *remainder (R) group*. The R group is different among the 20 amino acids.

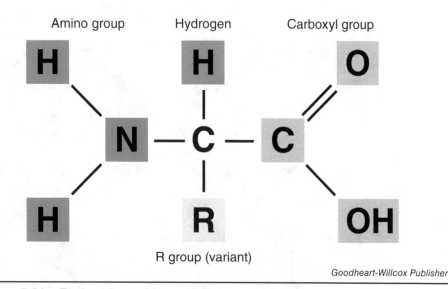

Amino group   Hydrogen   Carboxyl group

R group (variant)

Figure 5.33 Each amino acid consists of a central carbon, an amino group, a carboxyl group, a hydrogen, and an R group.

Recall Activity

1. List the five parts of an amino acid. _____

2. In the space below, draw the symbols that represent the five different parts of the amino acid.

Concept 3: Types of Amino Acids

There are 20 different types of amino acids. **Figure 5.34** shows these types. The amino acids' R groups are shown in yellow. Amino acids are building blocks that make up proteins. The diversity in life is due to different combinations of these building blocks.

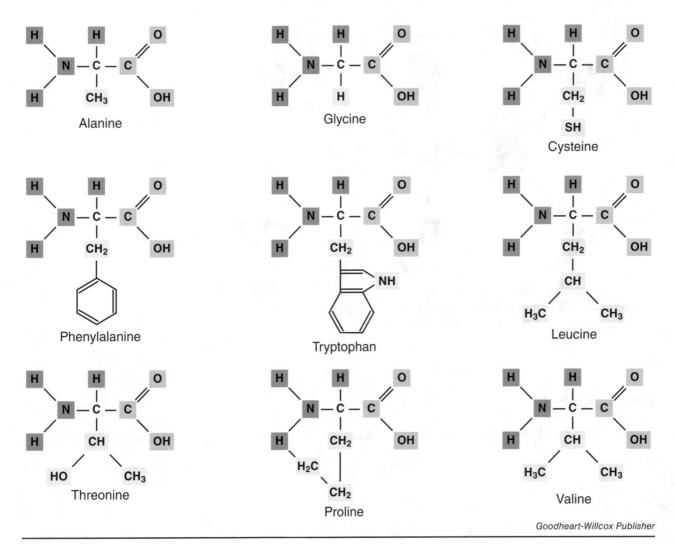

Goodheart-Willcox Publisher

Figure 5.34 The R groups of these amino acids are shown in yellow.

246 Chapter 5 *Chemistry*

Copyright Goodheart-Willcox Co., Inc.

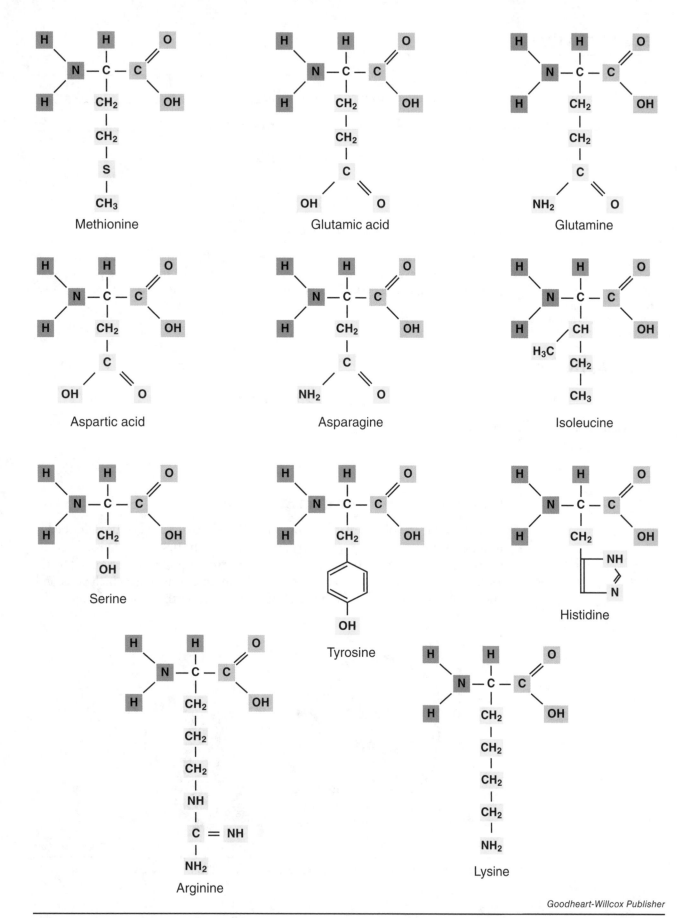

Methionine

Glutamic acid

Glutamine

Aspartic acid

Asparagine

Isoleucine

Serine

Tyrosine

Histidine

Arginine

Lysine

Goodheart-Willcox Publisher

Figure 5.34 *Continued.*

Recall Activity

1. How many different types of amino acids are there?_____

2. Which amino acid has a single hydrogen atom as the R group?_____

3. List three amino acids that have the molecule CH₃ in the R group._____

_____

Concept 4: Essential Amino Acids

essential amino acid an amino acid that the body cannot make and that must be included in a person's diet

While there are 20 different types of amino acids, the human body can only make some of these. Amino acids that the body *cannot* make need to be part of your diet. Amino acids that the body cannot make are called *essential amino acids*.

Recall Activity

1. Your body *cannot* make _____ amino acids.

2. Essential amino acids must be part of your _____.

Concept 5: Primary Protein Structure

primary structure the sequence of amino acids in a protein

Proteins are made of chains of amino acids. Protein structure can be described in terms of primary, secondary, and tertiary structure. The first type of protein structure is the *primary structure*. The primary structure of a protein is determined by the sequence of amino acids. A sequence—which amino acid is first, which is second, and so on—is illustrated in **Figure 5.35**. Circles represent the amino acids.

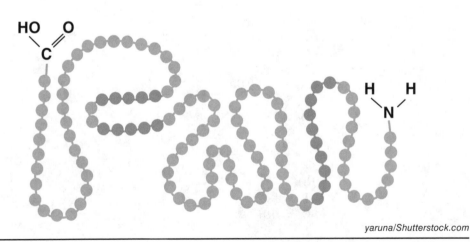

yaruna/Shutterstock.com

Figure 5.35 The primary structure of a protein is the amino acid sequence.

Recall Activity

1. List the three classifications of protein structure. _____

_____

2. The primary structure of a protein is determined by the _____ of amino acids.

Concept 6: Secondary Protein Structure

The second classification for protein structure is *secondary structure*. The secondary structure of a protein results from the attraction between amino acids that are close together. This attraction determines the shape of the molecule. Protein shape can be a pleated sheet, as shown in **Figure 5.36**, or a helix (twisted).

secondary structure the attraction between amino acids that are close together in a protein; determines the shape of the molecule (pleated sheet or helix)

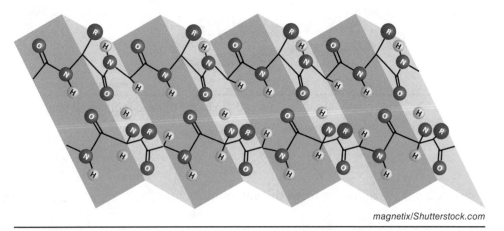

magnetix/Shutterstock.com

Figure 5.36 One shape the secondary structure of a protein can take is a pleated sheet.

Recall Activity

1. Secondary structure results from the _____ between amino acids that are close together.

2. List the two shapes that attraction between close-together amino acids can cause. _____

_____

Concept 7: Tertiary Protein Structure

The *tertiary structure* of a protein results from the attraction between *distant* amino acids. This attraction results in a hydrogen or a covalent bond. The tertiary structure forms the three-dimensional shape of the protein. This is because the hydrogen or covalent bonding of distant amino acids makes the chain of amino acids fold back on itself, creating a three-dimensional shape (**Figure 5.37**).

tertiary structure the attraction between distant amino acids in a protein; determines the three-dimensional shape of the molecule

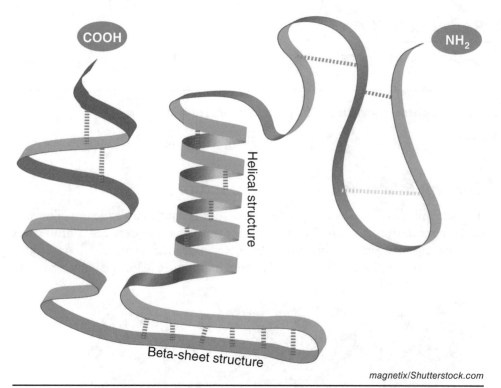

magnetix/Shutterstock.com

Figure 5.37 The tertiary structure of a protein is the three-dimensional shape.

Recall Activity

1. What protein structure results from attraction between distant amino acids? _____

_____

2. List the two types of bonds that affect a protein's tertiary structure. _____

_____

3. The tertiary structure forms the _____-dimensional shape of the protein.

4. The bonding of _____ amino acids makes the chain of amino acids

_____ back on itself.

Concept 8: Denaturing

The tertiary structure of a protein is required for protein function. High heat or low pH levels can *denature* a protein by causing its three-dimensional shape to unravel. Sometimes this unraveling can be reversed, but in extreme cases, it cannot. For example, the white of an egg contains protein. The heat in cooking the egg denatures the proteins, permanently changing the egg's clear liquid into a white solid.

Recall Activity

1. The tertiary structure of a protein is required for _____ function.

2. List two factors that can denature a protein. _____

3. The white of an egg contains _____.

4. Cooking an egg _____ the proteins.

Concept 9: Calories in Proteins

Proteins and their component amino acids can be broken down for energy. One gram of protein contains 4 kilocalories of energy. When an amino acid is broken down for energy, its amino group is removed. The amino group becomes waste, will form urea, and will then be expelled in urine.

Recall Activity

1. One gram of protein contains _____ kilocalories of energy.

2. When an amino acid is broken down for energy, the _____ group is removed.

Section 5.9 Reinforcement

Answer the following questions using what you learned in this section.

1. Which of the following can denature a protein?
   A. dryness   C. low pH
   B. high heat

2. One gram of protein contains _____ kilocalories of energy.

3. Which of the following is *not* part of the basic structure of an amino acid?
   A. carboxyl group   C. sulfur
   B. hydrogen   D. R group

4. Different _____ groups are what distinguish the 20 amino acids from one another.

5. Write the letters backward: yraitret. Define the word that is formed. _____

   _____

6. The three types of protein structure are _____, secondary, and tertiary.

7. Unscramble the letters: teppedi. Define the word that is formed. _____

   _____

8. List two factors that can denature a protein. _____

9. Which of the following terms does *not* belong with the rest: cysteine, tyrosine, lipid, or leucine?

   _____

10. List the three classifications of protein structure. _____

    _____

11. Write the letters backward: lyxobrac. Define the word that is formed. _____

_____

12. Which of the following words are misspelled?
    A. carboxil   C. tertiary
    B. protien

13. *True or False.* The sequence of amino acids is the primary structure of a protein._____

14. _____ bonds hold amino acids together.

15. Urea is produced when an amino acid's _____ group is broken down.

16. In denaturing, the _____ protein structure is unraveled.

17. *True or False.* Amino acids are carbohydrates. _____

18. List the three levels of protein structure in alphabetical order. _____

_____

19. Which of the following amino acids has the biggest R group?
    A. alanine   C. serine
    B. proline   D. glycine

20. *True or False.* Bonding between distant amino acids makes the primary structure of a protein. _____

21. Unscramble the letters: ropetin. Define the word that is formed. _____

_____

22. Which of the following is *not* part of an amino acid?
    A. amino group   C. hydrogen
    B. carboxyl group   D. sulfur

23. A(n) _____ is a chain of amino acids.

Comprehensive Review (Chapters 1–5)

Answer the following questions using what you have learned so far in this book.

24. In a single bond, _____ electrons are shared.

25. Which of the following is the highest temperature?
    A. 64°C   C. 73°C
    B. 85°F   D. 98°F

26. *True or False.* The prefix *anti-* means "toward."_____

27. If a fact contradicts a proposal, the proposal must be _____ and

_____ to test again.

28. *True or False.* Science builds upon itself. _____

Section 5.10 Enzymes

One class of proteins is enzymes, which perform a number of important functions in the body. In this section, you will learn about enzymes and their vital functions.

The terms below are some of those that will be introduced in Section 5.10. To become familiar with these terms, reproduce each word on the line beside it. Pronounce each term as you write it. You will learn the definitions of these words as you complete this section.

1. enzyme _____

2. substrate _____

3. turnover rate _____

Concept 1: Structural Proteins

Proteins in the body can be classified as *structural* or *functional*. *Structural proteins* compose body tissues. Two examples of structural proteins in the body are keratin and collagen. Keratin is the protein that makes up hair and fingernails. Keratin is also found in cells forming the outermost layer of the skin. Collagen is the most abundant protein in the body. Collagen fibers in the skin make skin tough.

Recall Activity

1. List the two classifications of proteins in the body. _____

2. What protein makes up hair and fingernails? _____

3. What is the most abundant protein in the body? _____

4. Collagen fibers make skin _____.

Concept 2: Functional Proteins

While structural proteins compose body tissues, *functional proteins* perform various tasks within the body. These tasks include

- carrying oxygen in the blood
- regulating the movement of materials through the cell membrane
- speeding up reactions in the body

For example, red blood cells contain the protein hemoglobin. Hemoglobin binds with oxygen, enabling red blood cells to carry oxygen throughout the body.

Recall Activity

1. List three tasks that functional proteins perform in the body._____

_____

2. What protein binds with oxygen in red blood cells? _____

Concept 3: What Are Enzymes?

enzyme a protein catalyst

substrate the atoms involved in an enzymatic reaction

Enzymes are a class of functional proteins. Enzymes are catalysts in that they speed up the rates of reactions in the body. The atoms involved in these reactions are called the *substrate* or substrates. Enzymatic reactions take place at the part of the enzyme known as the *active site* (**Figure 5.38**).

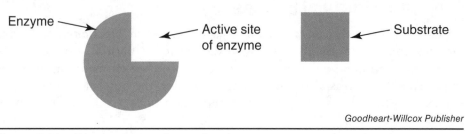

Goodheart-Willcox Publisher

Figure 5.38 Enzymatic reactions take place at an enzyme's active site.

Recall Activity

1. An enzyme is a class of _____ proteins.

2. _____ are catalysts.

3. A catalyst _____ up the rate of a reaction.

4. What are the atoms involved in an enzymatic reaction called?_____

5. An enzymatic reaction takes place at the _____ site of the enzyme.

Concept 4: Active Site

In an enzymatic reaction, notice that the substrate fits *exactly* into the enzyme's active site. Other molecules with different shapes would *not* fit into the enzyme's active site (**Figure 5.39**). All enzymes have specific molecules they will catalyze. They will not catalyze other types of molecules that do not have the correct shape.

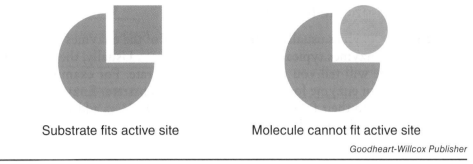

Substrate fits active site   Molecule cannot fit active site

Goodheart-Willcox Publisher

Figure 5.39   Only specific molecules will fit an enzyme's active site.

Recall Activity

1. If a molecule has the right _____, it will fit into the enzyme's active site.

2. All enzymes have specific molecules they will _____.

Concept 5: Enzyme-Substrate Complex

When a substrate fits into an enzyme's active site, this will form an *enzyme-substrate complex*. Once the enzyme-substrate complex is formed, an enzymatic reaction can occur. If a molecule is not the correct shape, it will not fit into the enzyme's active site, and no reaction will take place (**Figure 5.40**).

 Substrate fits into active site, and enzyme substrate-complex is formed

An enzymatic reaction will take place

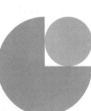 The shape of the molecule is wrong

The molecule cannot fit the active site, and no reaction can take place

Goodheart-Willcox Publisher

Figure 5.40   If a molecule will not fit an enzyme's active site, no reaction will take place.

Recall Activity

1. If the substrate fits into the active site, then a(n) _____ complex is formed.

2. If an enzyme-substrate complex is formed, a(n) _____ will take place.

3. If the shape of a molecule is wrong, a molecule cannot fit the _____.

4. If a molecule cannot fit the active site, no _____ can take place.

Section 5.10 Reinforcement

Answer the following questions using what you learned in this section.

1. The name of the enzyme that breaks down sucrose is _____.

2. Unscramble the letters: statcaly. Define the word that is formed. _____

   _____

3. The speed of an enzymatic reaction is called the _____.

4. Which of the following is *not* an enzyme?

   A. sucrase
   B. lactose
   C. maltase
   D. lipase

5. If the shape of a molecule is wrong, the molecule will not be able to fit an enzyme's

   _____.

6. Which of the following is an enzyme: lactase, sucrose, lipid, or fructose? _____

   _____

7. If a molecule has the right _____, it will fit into an enzyme's active site.

8. Write the two types of enzymatic reactions in alphabetical order. _____

   _____

9. What protein makes up the hair and fingernails? _____

10. If the molecule cannot fit the active site of an enzyme, no _____ can take place.

11. _____ add water during a reaction.

12. Write the letters backward: sisehtnys. Define the word that is formed. _____

    _____

13. Enzymes' names end in the letters _____.

14. Which of the following terms is misspelled?

    A. substraight
    B. catalyst
    C. enzyme

15. *True or False.* An enzyme is a functional protein. _____

16. Which of the following speeds up an enzymatic reaction?

    A. heat
    B. cold
    C. water

17. Which of the following terms does *not* belong with the others?

    A. enzyme
    B. catalyst
    C. structural
    D. substrate

18. *True or False.* All structural proteins are enzymes. _____

19. Unscramble the letters: nymeez. Define the word that is formed. _____

_____

20. The opposite of a degradative reaction is a(n) _____ reaction.

21. A(n) _____ is a protein catalyst.

Comprehensive Review (Chapters 1–5)

Answer the following questions using what you have learned so far in this book.

22. A(n) _____ is an atom with the same atomic number as another atom but with a different atomic mass.

23. *True or False.* The prefix *hyper-* means "front." _____

24. Which temperature is higher: 73°F or 73°C? _____

25. Facts are _____ of people and opinions.

26. A scientific _____ is the best explanation today of why a phenomenon occurs.

Section 5.11 Nucleic Acids

Nucleic acids link generations together and are involved in passing traits through DNA. In this section, you will learn about the structure and types of nucleic acids.

The terms below are some of those that will be introduced in Section 5.11. To become familiar with these terms, reproduce each word on the line beside it. Pronounce each term as you write it. You will learn the definitions of these words as you complete this section.

1. nucleic acid _____
2. nucleotide _____
3. complementary base _____

4. DNA _____
5. RNA _____
6. ATP _____

Concept 1: Nucleotides

Nucleic acids are the code for the genetic information in your cells. Some examples of nucleic acids include DNA and RNA, which you will learn about later in this section. A nucleic acid is a polymer. The basic unit of a nucleic acid is a *nucleotide*. There are three parts to a nucleotide: a phosphate, a sugar, and a base. Say the words *phosphate*, *sugar*, and *base* out loud three times. These are the three parts of a nucleotide. In diagramming a nucleotide, the phosphate is represented as a circle. The five-carbon sugar is drawn as a pentagon that looks like a house. The base is represented as either a hexagon or a hexagon combined with a pentagon (**Figure 5.43**).

nucleic acid a macromolecule that is a chain of nucleotides

nucleotide the basic unit of a nucleic acid; contains a phosphate, a sugar, and a base

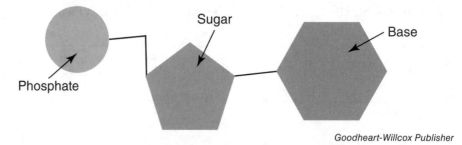

Figure 5.43 A nucleotide consists of a phosphate, a sugar, and a base.

Recall Activity

1. The basic unit of a nucleic acid is a(n) _____.

2. List the three parts of a nucleotide. _____

Concept 2: Bases

As you have learned, a nucleotide consists of a phosphate, a sugar, and a base. Bases can be drawn as either a hexagon or a hexagon combined with a pentagon. Bases represented as one hexagon are called *pyrimidines*. Bases represented as a hexagon-pentagon combination are called *purines* (**Figure 5.44**).

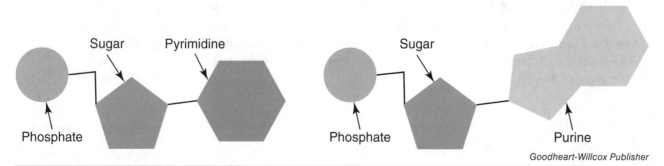

Figure 5.44 Nucleotide bases can be either one hexagon (pyrimidine) or a pentagon and a hexagon (purine).

Recall Activity

1. List the parts of a nucleotide. _____

2. List the two types of bases. _____

3. A base consisting of one hexagon is a(n) _____.

4. A base consisting of a hexagon and a pentagon is a(n) _____.

5. In the space below, draw a nucleotide with a purine base and a nucleotide with a pyrimidine base. Label the phosphate, sugar, and base of each.

Concept 3: Purines and Pyrimidines

Nucleotides can be formed from pyrimidine or purine bases. There are two purine bases: adenine (A) and guanine (G). There are three pyrimidine bases: cytosine (C), thymine (T), and uracil (U). **Figure 5.45** shows the pyrimidine and purine bases in DNA. The base uracil is found in RNA, but not in DNA.

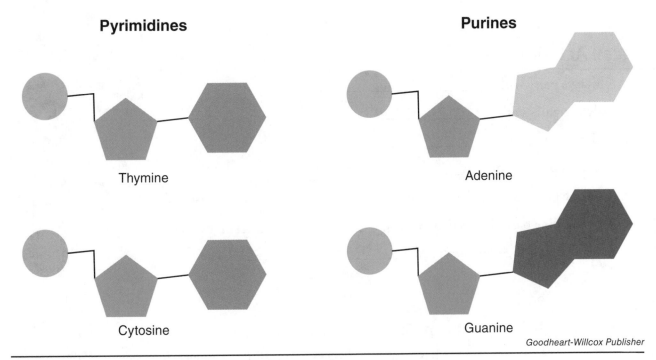

Pyrimidines

Thymine

Cytosine

Purines

Adenine

Guanine

Figure 5.45   T and C are pyrimidines. A and G are purines.

Recall Activity

1. List the two purine bases. _____

2. List the three pyrimidine bases. _____

3. What base does the abbreviation C represent? _____

4. What base does the abbreviation A represent? _____

5. What base does the abbreviation T represent? _____

6. What base does the abbreviation G represent? _____

Concept 4: Base Pairing

Nucleotides that have purine bases pair with nucleotides that have pyrimidine bases. A nucleotide containing an adenine (A) base is always paired with a nucleotide containing a thymine (T) base. A nucleotide containing a cytosine (C) base is always paired with a nucleotide containing a guanine (G) base. Bases that pair together are called *complementary bases* (**Figure 5.46**).

complementary base a nucleotide base that pairs with another base; purine and pyrimidine bases are complementary bases

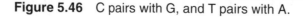

Pyrimidines ←——————→ Purines

Cytosine ←——————→ Guanine

Thymine ←——————→ Adenine

Goodheart-Willcox Publisher

Figure 5.46 C pairs with G, and T pairs with A.

Recall Activity

1. A always pairs with _____.

2. T always pairs with _____.

3. C always pairs with _____.

4. G always pairs with _____.

5. A purine base always pairs with a(n) _____ base.

6. A pyrimidine base always pairs with a(n) _____ base.

7. Bases that pair together are called _____ bases.

Concept 5: Base Bonding

Paired bases form hydrogen bonds, linking nucleotides together. Two hydrogen bonds bind adenine with thymine. Three hydrogen bonds bind cytosine with guanine (**Figure 5.47**).

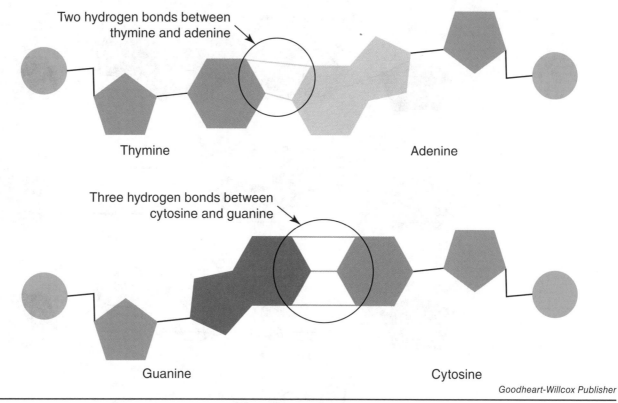

Figure 5.47   Hydrogen bonds join nucleotides.

Recall Activity

1. Paired bases are held together by _____ bonds.

2. There are _____ hydrogen bonds between C and G.

3. There are _____ hydrogen bonds between A and T.

Concept 6: DNA

A nucleic acid is a chain of nucleotides. One type of nucleic acid is *DNA*. DNA stands for *deoxyribonucleic acid*. This name is derived from the name of the sugar in DNA's nucleotides—deoxyribose—and the type of macromolecule that DNA is (nucleic acid). **Figure 5.48** is an illustration of DNA's arrangement. In DNA, the complementary bases of nucleotides are paired. Notice that the sugars on one side of DNA point up and that the sugars on the other side point down.

DNA deoxyribonucleic acid; a nucleic acid that makes up chromosomes

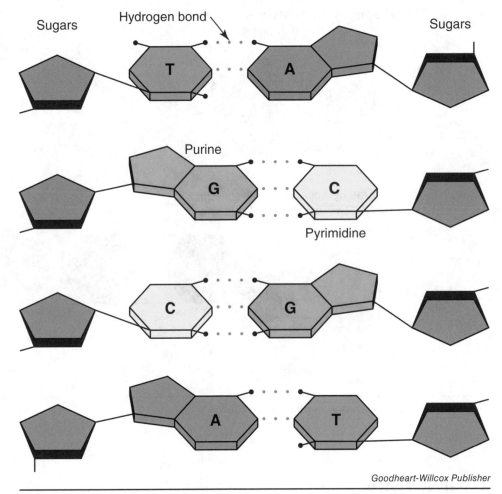

Figure 5.48 On one side of DNA, sugars point up. On the opposite side, sugars point down.

Goodheart-Willcox Publisher

Recall Activity

1. What is the name of the sugar in DNA? _____

2. What type of macromolecule is DNA? _____

3. What do the letters *DNA* stand for? _____

4. If the sugar of one nucleotide points up, the sugar of the paired nucleotide will point

   _____ .

Concept 7: Two Strands

A stack of nucleotides is called a *strand*. Nucleotides in a strand are held together by a covalent bond between the phosphate of one nucleotide and the sugar of the next nucleotide. The left and right strands are held together by hydrogen bonds between complementary bases.

Recall Activity

1. Adenine and cytosine would be considered _____ bases.

2. Bases are held together by _____ bonds.

3. A nucleotide consists of a(n) _____, _____, and

   _____.

Concept 8: Double Helix

DNA is described as a *double helix*. The *double* refers to the two strands of nucleotides. The two strands are coiled around each other. The *helix* refers to the coiled shape of the DNA molecule (**Figure 5.49**).

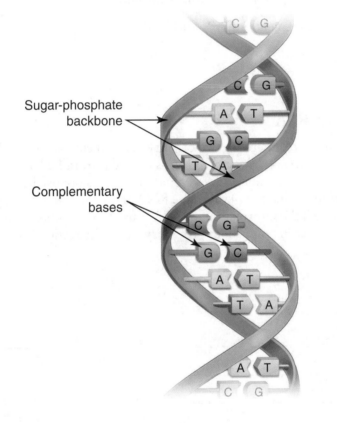

Sugar-phosphate backbone

Complementary bases

DNA molecule

Figure 5.49 Nucleotide strands are twisted around each other, forming a helix.

Recall Activity

1. DNA is described as a(n) _____.

2. In the double helix, there are two _____, or strings of nucleotides.

3. DNA's strands are a helix because they are _____ around each other.

Concept 9: Genes

Chromosomes are made of DNA. Each cell in your body that contains a nucleus has a full set of chromosomes. A gene is a segment of DNA within a chromosome that codes for a particular trait. A *trait* is an observable physical characteristic. Each color on the chromosome represents a gene. Each gene is responsible for making a particular protein. This protein, in turn, causes a certain trait to manifest.

Recall Activity

1. Genes are responsible for making particular _____.

2. _____ are made of DNA.

3. A gene is a(n) _____ of DNA within a chromosome.

4. A(n) _____ is a segment of DNA within a(n) _____ that codes for a particular trait.

Concept 10: RNA

RNA ribonucleic acid; a nucleic acid involved in protein synthesis

In addition to DNA, there are two other types of nucleic acids: RNA and ATP. *RNA* stands for *ribonucleic acid*. RNA is different from DNA in that RNA is only one strand. RNA nucleotides contain ribose (as opposed to deoxyribose) and the base uracil instead of thymine. RNA is used in *protein synthesis*, or the process in which the information in DNA is used to assemble a chain of amino acids. You will learn more about protein synthesis in Section 7.8.

Recall Activity

1. List the three types of nucleic acids. _____

2. What do the letters *RNA* stand for? _____

3. For what process is RNA used? _____

4. In protein synthesis, the information in _____ is used to assemble a chain of amino acids.

5. RNA nucleotides contain the base _____ instead of _____.

6. _____ is only one strand.

7. Instead of deoxyribose, RNA nucleotides contain _____.

Concept 11: ATP

The third type of nucleic acid is ATP. *ATP*, which stands for *adenosine triphosphate*, is the energy storage molecule inside a cell. The energy that is transformed from carbohydrates, lipids, and amino acids is stored in the bonds of ATP and is used to make reactions happen inside a cell.

ATP adenosine triphosphate; the energy storage molecule inside a cell

Recall Activity

1. What type of macromolecule is ATP? _____

2. What do the letters *ATP* stand for? _____

3. What is the function of ATP? _____

4. List the three sources of energy for a cell. _____

Section 5.11 Reinforcement

Answer the following questions using what you learned in this section.

1. In a string of nucleotides, pyrimidine bases tend to pair with _____ bases.

2. What is cytosine's complementary base? _____

3. What is thymine's complementary base? _____

4. List the three parts of a nucleotide. _____

5. Genes are responsible for making particular _____.

6. Which of the following terms does *not* belong with the others?

   A. base   C. purine

   B. helix   D. pyrimidine

7. Cytosine and guanine would be considered _____ bases.

8. Unscramble the letters: pnurie. Define the word that is formed. _____

   _____

9. What is the name of the sugar in DNA? _____

10. Write the letters backward: dica cielcunobir. Define the word that is formed. _____

    _____

11. A purine base always pairs with a(n) _____ base.

12. What type of macromolecule is DNA? _____

13. *True or False.* DNA is a protein. _____

14. What do the letters *DNA* stand for? _____

15. A chain of nucleotides is known as a(n) _____.

Match the following terms with their definitions.

_____ 16. Purine base

_____ 17. Pyrimidine base

_____ 18. Nucleotide

_____ 19. Nucleic acid

A. a phosphate, a sugar, and a base

B. DNA

C. adenine

D. thymine

Comprehensive Review (Chapters 1–5)

Answer the following questions using what you have learned so far in this book.

20. An ion that has donated an electron has a(n) _____ charge.

21. Science seeks natural _____ to phenomena.

22. *True or False.* The prefix *sub-* means "above." _____

23. The metric unit for linear measurements is the _____.

24. An abstract is a brief _____ of a scientific article.

Section 5.12 pH

In this chapter, you have learned about the term *pH* in relation to its ability to denature proteins. The pH scale is an important concept for understanding cell function. In this section, you will learn about pH and the effects of buffers and electrolytes.

The terms below are some of those that will be introduced in Section 5.12. To become familiar with these terms, reproduce each word on the line beside it. Pronounce each term as you write it. You will learn the definitions of these words as you complete this section.

1. pH_____

2. acid_____

3. base_____

4. neutral_____

5. buffer_____

6. electrolyte _____

pH the measurement of acid or base in a liquid

acid a liquid that contains more H^+ ions than OH^- ions

base a liquid that contains more OH^- ions than H^+ ions

neutral a liquid that contains equal amounts of OH^- ions and H^+ ions; is neither an acid nor a base

Concept 1: What Is pH?

pH is the measurement of acid or base in a liquid. Determining pH is simple. It involves comparing the number of hydrogen ions (H^+) in a liquid to the number of hydroxide ions (OH^-). If there are more H^+ ions than OH^- ions, the liquid is an *acid*. If there are fewer H^+ ions than OH^- ions, the liquid is a *base*. If the numbers of H^+ ions and OH^- ions are equal, the liquid is *neutral*, neither an acid nor a base.

Recall Activity

1. What is the abbreviation for the hydroxide ion? _____

2. What is the abbreviation for the hydrogen ion? _____

3. The measurement of acid or base in a liquid is known as _____.

4. Determining pH involves comparing the number of _____ ions to the number of _____ ions.

5. If there are more H^+ ions than OH^- ions, the liquid is a(n) _____.

6. If there are more OH^- ions than H^+ ions, the liquid is a(n) _____.

7. If the number of H^+ ions is equal to the number of OH^- ions, then the liquid is

   _____.

8. A neutral liquid is neither _____ nor _____.

Concept 2: pH Values

pH is expressed as a *value*, or a number that indicates whether a liquid is an acid or a base. pH values range from 0 to 14. On this scale, pH values from 0–6.9 indicate a liquid is an acid. pH values from 7.1–14 indicate a liquid is a base. The pH value of 7.0 indicates a neutral liquid.

Recall Activity

1. The range of pH values is _____ to _____.

2. Liquids with pH values from 0–6.9 are _____.

3. Liquids with pH values from 7.1–14 are _____.

4. A liquid with a pH value of 7.0 is a(n) _____.

Concept 3: Strong and Weak Acids and Bases

Acids and bases can be described as either *strong* or *weak*. To determine a liquid's pH value, compare the amounts of H^+ and OH^- ions in the liquid. If there are only a *few* more H^+ ions than OH^- ions, the liquid is a weak acid. If there are *many* more H^+ ions than OH^- ions, then the liquid is a strong acid. Similarly, if there are only a few more OH^- ions than H^+ ions, the liquid is a weak base. If there are many more OH^- ions than H^+ ions, then the liquid is a strong base.

On the pH scale, pH values of 0–1 are strong acids; values of 5–6 are weak acids; values of 8–9 are weak bases; and values of 13–14 are strong bases. Values of 2–4 are acids that are neither strong nor weak. Values of 10–12 are bases that are neither strong nor weak.

Recall Activity

1. If a liquid contains many more OH⁻ ions than H⁺ ions, then the liquid is a(n)

   _____.

2. If a liquid contains many more H⁺ ions than OH⁻ ions, then the liquid is a(n)

   _____.

3. If a liquid has a few more OH⁻ ions than H⁺ ions, then the liquid is a(n) _____.

4. If a liquid has a few more H⁺ ions than OH⁻ ions, then the liquid is a(n) _____.

5. A liquid with a pH value of 6 is a(n) _____.

Concept 4: pH Scale

Figure 5.50 illustrates the pH scale. On the pH scale, the concentration of H⁺ ions is shown in red. The concentration of OH⁻ ions is shown in blue. A liquid with more red than blue is an acid. A liquid with more blue than red is a base.

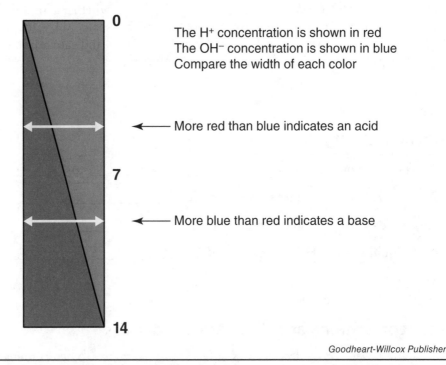

The H⁺ concentration is shown in red
The OH⁻ concentration is shown in blue
Compare the width of each color

← More red than blue indicates an acid

← More blue than red indicates a base

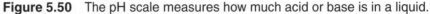

Figure 5.50   The pH scale measures how much acid or base is in a liquid.

Recall Activity

1. On the pH scale, what does blue indicate? _____

2. On the pH scale, what does red indicate? _____

Concept 5: pH Values of Liquids

Many liquids are classified on the pH scale. **Figure 5.51** shows some common liquids and their pHs. The strongest acid in the illustration is hydrochloric acid. The strongest base in the illustration is sodium hydroxide. With a pH of 7.0, pure water is a neutral liquid.

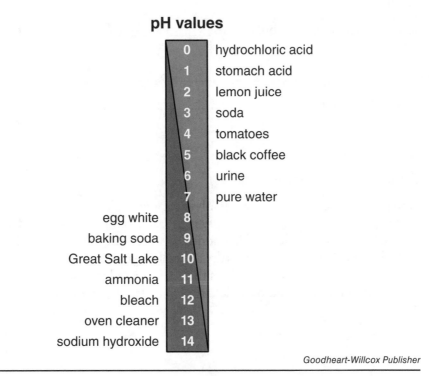

Figure 5.51 The pHs of some common liquids are shown on this scale.

Recall Activity

1. Are liquids with pH values from 0–6.9 acids or bases? _____

2. Are liquids with pH values from 7.1–14 acids or bases? _____

3. A liquid with a pH value of 7.0 is _____.

4. What is the pH value of stomach acid? _____

5. What liquid has a pH value of 14? _____

Concept 6: Buffers

Molecules that are added to a liquid can affect the liquid's pH. Molecules that help maintain the pH of a liquid when other ions are added are known as *buffers*. A *buffer* is a molecule that can accept or donate H^+ ions. A buffer in a liquid resists changes in pH. This is because buffers absorb H^+ ions, minimizing the change in pH if an acid is added. If a base is added to a liquid, a buffer can release H^+ ions to bond with the base's OH^- ions. When the H^+ and OH^- ions bond, they make water, which has a neutral pH.

buffer a molecule that can accept or donate H^+ ions to resist changes in pH

Recall Activity

1. A(n) _____ is a molecule that can accept or donate H^+ ions.

2. A buffer in a liquid resists _____ in pH.

3. If an acid is added to a liquid with a buffer, the buffer can absorb _____ ions and minimize the change in pH.

4. If a base is added to a liquid with a buffer, the buffer can _____ H^+ ions to bond with the base's OH^- ions.

5. When H^+ and OH^- ions bond, they make _____, which has a neutral pH.

6. What is the chemical formula for water? _____

Concept 7: Electrolytes

electrolyte an acid, base, or salt that releases ions when added to water

Water is a solvent capable of dissolving ionic molecules. If acid is added to water, the acid will release H^+ ions. If a base is added to water, the base will release OH^- ions. If salt, NaCl, is added to water, the salt will dissolve into Na^+ and Cl^- ions. Acids, bases, and salts are called *electrolytes* because they release ions when added to water. The ions that are released into water (H^+, OH^-, Na^+, Cl^-, or any other charged particle) are also called electrolytes.

Recall Activity

1. What does an acid release into water? _____

2. What does a base release into water? _____

3. What does salt release into water? _____

4. A substance that releases ions into water is called a(n) _____.

5. List three electrolytes. _____

Section 5.12 Reinforcement

Answer the following questions using what you learned in this section.

1. What does the abbreviation H^+ stand for? _____

2. If there are more H^+ than OH^- ions in a liquid, the liquid is a(n) _____.

3. Identify the most acidic and the most basic of these pH values: 4.0, 2.5, 10.1, and 7.8. _____

4. If a liquid has many more OH^- than H^+ ions, then the liquid is a(n) _____.

5. If a liquid has a few more H^+ than OH^- ions, then the liquid is a(n) _____.

6. Arrange the following terms from the lowest pH value to the highest: neutral, weak base, weak acid, strong base, and strong acid.

_____

7. What does the abbreviation OH⁻ stand for? _____

8. Which of the following is the strongest acidic pH value?
   A. 2   C. 6
   B. 4   D. 8

9. *True or False.* A buffer resists changes in pH. _____

10. If a liquid has a few more OH⁻ than H⁺ ions, then the liquid is a(n) _____.

11. A liquid with a pH value of 7.0 is a(n) _____.

12. Which of the following is the strongest basic pH value?
    A. 2   C. 6
    B. 4   D. 8

13. Which of the following pH values does *not* belong with the others?
    A. 6   C. 1
    B. 10   D. 4

14. *True or False.* A base has a high pH value. _____

15. The measurement of acid or base in a liquid is known as _____.

16. A(n) _____ resists pH changes in a liquid.

Match the following terms with their definitions.

_____ 17. Acid   A. many hydrogen ions and few hydroxide ions
_____ 18. Base   B. equal numbers of hydrogen ions and hydroxide ions
_____ 19. Neutral   C. few hydrogen ions and many hydroxide ions

Comprehensive Review (Chapters 1–5)

Answer the following questions using what you have learned so far in this book.

20. Compared to ionic bonds, hydrogen bonds are _____.

21. The meter stick is _____ meter(s) in length.

22. *True or False.* The prefix *hemi-* means "half." _____

23. A natural explanation can be _____ or _____ and proven to be false.

24. *True or False.* There is only one scientific method. _____

Chapter 5 Review

Answer the following questions using what you learned in this chapter.

1. Write these pH values in order from the most acidic to the least acidic: 5.6, 2.1, 3.4, and 4.9.

_____

2. *True or False.* The chin of a water molecule has a partial positive charge. _____

3. Molecules are brought together in a(n) _____ reaction.

4. Your body cannot make _____ amino acids.

5. A liquid with a pH value of 10 is a(n) _____.

6. Which of the following atoms have an atomic mass of 12: Al, C, N, or Ne? _____

7. *True or False.* Electrons have a negative charge and a mass of 1 amu. _____

8. In a double bond, _____ electrons are shared.

9. The substrate for the enzyme lactase is _____.

10. Which of the following has the largest atomic number: He, H, Al, or Ne? _____

11. Nucleotide bases are held together by _____ bonds.

12. In a water molecule, the "ears" are the _____ atoms.

13. The number of _____ or electrons determines an atom's atomic number.

14. Which of the following atoms has three electrons in its outer shell: C, N, O, or B? _____

15. In a covalent bond, electrons are _____.

16. Which subatomic particles do not leave the atom's core? _____

17. List the three types of atomic bonds in alphabetical order. _____

18. If a liquid has many H^+ ions and few OH^- ions, then the liquid is a(n) _____.

19. Which of the following has an atomic number of 12: Mg, Na, Si, or Al? _____

20. *True or False.* The atom with atomic number 10 has a full second shell.

21. The atomic number of magnesium is _____.

22. Arrange the following atoms from the fewest electrons to the most electrons: Al, S, O, and He.

_____

23. Which of the following has the smallest atomic number: Mg, S, F, or B? _____

24. How many electrons are in the outer shell of a sodium atom? _____

25. *True or False.* Nucleotides are made of nucleic acid. _____

26. Atomic mass is the number of _____ plus the number of

_____ in an atom.

27. The atomic symbol for boron is _____.

28. A lipid is one _____ molecule bonded to three _____.

29. *True or False.* Amino acids make up lipids. _____

30. The tertiary structure forms the _____-dimensional shape of the protein.

31. The third electron shell can hold _____ electron(s).

32. Which atom has a full first shell, but no electrons in its second shell? _____

33. Because hydrogen and carbon have equal attraction for electrons, they _____ electrons.

34. *True or False.* A substrate is broken down in a synthesis reaction. _____

35. Which of the following is solid at room temperature?
   A. saturated fat   C. polyunsaturated fat
   B. unsaturated fat

36. How many protons are in Ca? _____

37. In a water molecule, the "chin" is the _____ atom.

38. Which subatomic particle has no mass? _____

39. Which subatomic particle is *not* involved in determining atomic number? _____

Comprehensive Review (Chapters 1–5)

Using what you have learned so far in this book, match the following terms with their definitions.

_____ 40. A subatomic particle with no charge

_____ 41. A substance that dissolves a solute

_____ 42. The science that studies life

_____ 43. A protein catalyst

_____ 44. A prefix that means "two"

_____ 45. A subatomic particle with a negative charge

_____ 46. A prediction about the outcome of an experiment

_____ 47. Half the distance across a circle

_____ 48. A general statement of fact

_____ 49. The number of protons plus the number of neutrons in an atom's core

_____ 50. The number of atoms per one unit of volume

_____ 51. A subatomic particle with a positive charge

_____ 52. The study of cells

_____ 53. A prefix that means "one"

A. solvent
B. atomic mass
C. scientific law
D. neutron
E. biology
F. concentration
G. radius
H. proton
I. hypothesis
J. electron
K. di-
L. cytology
M. mono-
N. enzyme

Chapter 6
Cell Morphology

Introduction

This chapter is an introduction to the parts of a cell. All life consists of at least one cell. Humans have trillions of cells. Because all body parts are made of cells, understanding the cell is the essential first step in understanding the body. In this chapter, you will learn the three basic parts of the cell and will study all the parts of a typical cell.

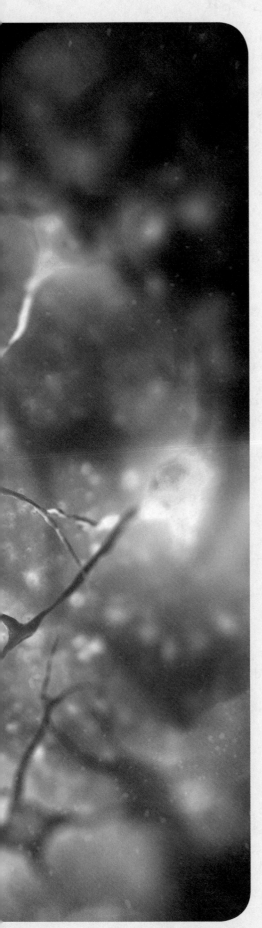

Objectives

After completing this chapter, you will be able to

- name the three basic parts of the cell
- list the components of the plasma membrane
- name the components of the nucleus
- explain how materials move inside the cell
- list the components of cytoplasm
- name the extensions and junctions of the plasma membrane

Key Terms

The following terms and phrases will be introduced and explained in Chapter 6. Read through the list to become familiar with the words.

anucleate
cholesterol
chromatin
chromosome
cilia
cytoplasm
cytoskeleton
desmosome
endoplasmic reticulum (ER)
flagella
fluid mosaic
gap junction
gene
globular protein
glycolipid
glycoprotein
Golgi
hydrophilic
hydrophobic
intermediate filament
lysosome
membrane junction
microfilament

microtubule
microvilli
mitochondrion
morphology
multinucleate
nuclear envelope
nucleolus
nucleus
permeable
peroxisome
phospholipid
phospholipid bilayer
plasma membrane
ribosome
rough endoplasmic reticulum (RER)
secretory vesicle
selective
smooth endoplasmic reticulum (SER)
specialized
tight junction
transport vesicle

Section 6.1 Overview of the Cell

The cell is the basic unit of life. Trillions of cells make up your body, and cells are responsible for numerous body functions. In this section, you will learn about the basic structure of the cell.

The terms below are some of those that will be introduced in Section 6.1. To become familiar with these terms, reproduce each word on the line beside it. Pronounce each term as you write it. You will learn the definitions of these words as you complete this section.

1. morphology _____

2. specialized _____

3. plasma membrane _____

4. nucleus _____

5. cytoplasm _____

Concept 1: What Are Cells?

The human body is a community made up of trillions of cells. In essence, your cells are *you*. You are alive because of the activities that occur inside your cells. Basic life processes, such as breathing and eating, serve the vital purpose of supplying nutrients to your cells. Without the activities that occur inside and the processes that sustain cells, life would not be possible.

Recall Activity

1. Your body is a(n) _____ of trillions of cells.

2. You are alive because of the activities that occur inside your _____.

Concept 2: The Morphology of Cells

morphology the study of structure or form

Morphology is the study of structure or form. To study cell morphology is to study cell structure. Think of a cell as a fluid-filled bag floating in more fluid. Inside the bag are smaller bags. In cell morphology, you will study the structure of a cell by identifying the parts of the fluid-filled bag, the two fluids, and the smaller bags.

Recall Activity

1. _____ is the study of structure or form.

2. You can think of a cell as a fluid-filled _____ containing smaller

_____ and floating in _____.

Concept 3: Cell Size

Although the sizes of cells vary, all cells are small. You can only see cells using magnification (for example, a microscope). Activities and chemical reactions inside a cell require that raw materials enter the cell and that waste and products exit the cell. During this entering and exiting, materials and products pass through the fluid-filled bag, or the surface area, of the cell. As a result, the number of chemical reactions that can take place inside the cell (also described as *cell volume*) is limited by the surface area of the cell. As you learned in Section 4.5, cells must be small to have a sufficient surface-area-to-volume ratio (**Figure 6.1**).

Volume of cell

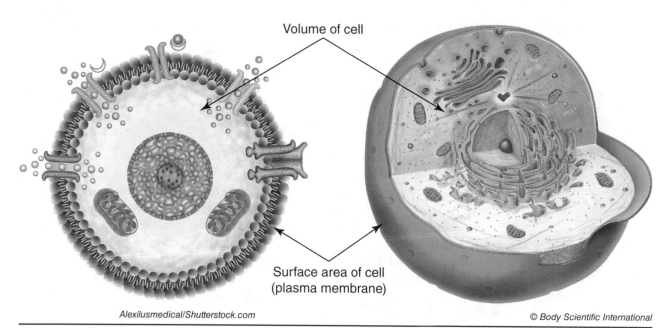

Surface area of cell
(plasma membrane)

Alexilusmedical/Shutterstock.com

© Body Scientific International

Figure 6.1   Cells are small because smaller volumes (small cells) have a large enough surface-area-to-volume ratio to allow the sufficient exchange of raw materials, products, and waste.

Recall Activity

1. During entering and exiting, materials and products pass through the fluid-filled bag, or the
   _____, of the cell.

2. The number of chemical reactions that can take place inside the cell is limited by the
   _____ of the cell.

3. You can only see cells using _____.

Concept 4: Cell Diversity

The human body is composed of many different types of cells. Cells in the human body are *specialized*, meaning that different types of cells have unique structures, components, or shapes that enable them to perform a specific

specialized a quality of cells that causes them to have unique structures, components, or shapes that enable them to perform a specific function

function. For example, the structure of muscle cells allows them to shorten or contract. The components in nerve cells allow them to conduct an electrical charge. The shape of skin cells allows them to form a barrier that protects underlying tissues. There are hundreds of different types of cells in your body. Each type of cell has a specific function.

Recall Activity

1. Cells in the human body are _____.

2. Different types of cells have unique structures, components, or shapes that enable them to perform a specific _____.

Concept 5: Cell Activities

Everything produced by your body is made in one of your cells. Think of the activities your body is engaged in right now. The cells of your stomach, small intestine, liver, and pancreas are producing enzymes to digest your food. The cells of your pituitary gland are producing hormones that regulate the functions of other endocrine glands. The cells in your brain are producing endorphins that give you a sense of pleasure as you study, and the cells of your blood are supplying vital oxygen to the cells of your organs. Your life is maintained by the activities of your cells.

Recall Activity

1. Everything produced by your body is made in one of your _____.
2. Your life is maintained by the _____ of your cells.

Concept 6: Basic Parts of a Cell

plasma membrane the barrier of a cell that acts as a gatekeeper and keeps molecules inside or outside of the cell

nucleus the control center of a cell; contains genetic information

cytoplasm all the material found inside a cell except for the nucleus; includes cytosol and organelles

The structure of a cell includes three basic parts: a plasma membrane, a nucleus, and cytoplasm (**Figure 6.2**). The *plasma membrane* is the bag part of the fluid-filled bag. It acts as a *gatekeeper* and keeps molecules inside or outside of a cell. The *nucleus* (one of the small bags) is the *control center* of the cell. It contains genetic information, or DNA, which directs the activities inside the cell. The *cytoplasm* is all the material found inside the bag except for the nucleus. Cytoplasm has two parts: cytosol and organelles (small bags). *Cytosol* is the fluid found inside the cell. *Organelles* are specialized structures that perform specific functions inside the cell. The fluid surrounding a cell is called *interstitial fluid*. Both cytosol and interstitial fluid are primarily water.

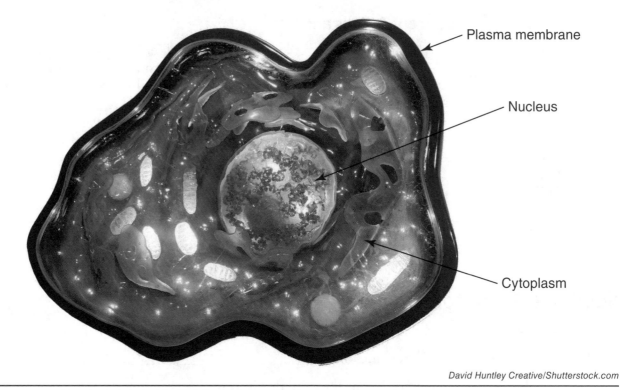

Plasma membrane

Nucleus

Cytoplasm

Figure 6.2 The three basic parts of the cell are the plasma membrane, nucleus, and cytoplasm.

Recall Activity

1. Circle the structure that is not a basic part of the cell.

   cytoplasm   plasma membrane
   cytosol   nucleus

2. The _____ is the barrier that keeps molecules inside or outside of a cell.

3. Both _____ and _____ fluid are primarily water.

4. Cytoplasm has two parts: _____ and _____.

5. Genetic information, or _____, controls the activities inside the cell.

6. Circle the liquid that is inside the cell.

   interstitial fluid   cytosol

7. List the three basic parts of the cell. _____

   _____

8. Specialized structures that perform specific functions inside the cell are known as

   _____.

9. The _____ contains genetic information.

Concept 7: Cells and Life

As you have learned, the cell is the basic unit of life. The individual parts of the cell—the plasma membrane, nucleus, and cytoplasm—are not, by themselves, alive. Together, however, they form a cell that is alive. All organisms, from bacteria to whales, consist of at least one cell.

Recall Activity

1. The _____ is the basic unit of life.

2. The individual parts of a cell are not, by themselves, _____.

Section 6.1 Reinforcement

Answer the following questions using what you learned in this section.

1. Your life is maintained by the activities of your _____.

2. Unscramble the letters: rongleela. Define the word that is formed. _____

_____

3. Which of the following is *not* a basic part of the cell?
   A. nucleus
   B. cytoplasm
   C. interstitial fluid
   D. plasma membrane

4. What structures are the smaller bags inside the fluid-filled bag of the cell? _____

_____

5. You can only see cells using _____.

6. What does it mean that cells in the human body are specialized? _____

_____

7. *True or False.* The nucleus of a cell is alive. _____

8. Which of the following words are misspelled?
   A. cytosolo
   B. cytoplasn
   C. organelle
   D. nucleus
   E. memebrane

9. Unscramble the letters: tocosly. Define the word that is formed. _____

_____

10. *True or False.* Organelles are primarily water. _____

11. The _____ is the fluid inside the cell, and the _____ is the fluid outside the cell.

12. The number of _____ that can take place inside the cell is limited by the surface area of the cell.

13. The _____ keeps molecules inside or outside of a cell.

14. Activities inside a cell require that raw materials _____ the cell and waste and products _____ the cell.

15. Both cytosol and interstitial fluid are primarily _____.

16. Which of the following structures are fluids?
    A. nucleus   C. interstitial fluid
    B. cytosol   D. plasma membrane

17. *True or False.* Human body cells are specialized. _____

18. What are the three basic parts of the cell?_____

19. Cells must be small to have a sufficient _____ ratio.

20. *True or False.* The nucleus contains cytoplasm. _____

21. Morphology is the study of _____ or _____.

Match the following terms with their definitions.

_____ 22. A specialized structure in the cytoplasm that performs a specific function inside the cell

_____ 23. All the material found inside the cell except for the nucleus

_____ 24. The gatekeeper of the cell that keeps molecules inside or outside of the cell

_____ 25. The control center of the cell that contains genetic information

_____ 26. The fluid found inside a cell

_____ 27. The basic unit of life

A. cell
B. organelle
C. cytosol
D. nucleus
E. cytoplasm
F. plasma membrane

Comprehensive Review (Chapters 1–6)

Answer the following questions using what you have learned so far in this book.

28. Isotopes have the same atomic number, but different atomic _____.

29. *True or False.* A scientific theory is an educated guess._____

30. The unit mg/L is a measurement of _____.

31. Which of the following word parts mean "toward"?
    A. ab-   C. af-   E. di-
    B. ad-   D. ef-

32. The fluid outside of a cell is known as _____.

33. Name and define the areas of biology. _____

_____

Section 6.2 Plasma Membrane

One of the three basic parts of the cell is the plasma membrane. As you have learned, the plasma membrane keeps molecules inside or outside of a cell. In this section, you will learn about the function and structure of the plasma membrane.

The terms below are some of those that will be introduced in Section 6.2. To become familiar with these terms, reproduce each word on the line beside it. Pronounce each term as you write it. You will learn the definitions of these words as you complete this section.

1. permeable_____
2. selective_____
3. phospholipid_____
4. hydrophilic_____
5. hydrophobic_____
6. phospholipid bilayer_____

7. globular protein_____
8. cholesterol_____
9. glycoprotein_____
10. glycolipid_____
11. fluid mosaic_____

Concept 1: Gatekeeper

The plasma membrane forms the border around a cell, keeping molecules inside or outside of the cell. The plasma membrane also acts as the *gatekeeper* of the cell border. This is because the plasma membrane allows some molecules to travel in or out of the cell and prevents other molecules from leaving or entering the cell.

The plasma membrane determines what molecules pass in or out of the cell; for this reason, it is sometimes called *selectively permeable*. The plasma membrane is *permeable* because atoms and molecules can move through it. It is *selective* because not *all* atoms and molecules can move through it.

permeable the quality of the plasma membrane that enables molecules to move through it

selective the quality of the plasma membrane that not *all* atoms and molecules can move through it

Recall Activity

1. The plasma membrane acts as the _____ of the cell border.

2. The plasma membrane allows some molecules to travel _____ or _____ of the cell and prevents other molecules from _____ or _____ the cell.

3. The plasma membrane is _____ because atoms and molecules can move through it.

4. The plasma membrane is _____ because not *all* atoms and molecules can move through it.

Concept 2: Components of the Plasma Membrane

The plasma membrane is composed of the following parts:
- phospholipid bilayer
- globular proteins
- cholesterol
- glycoproteins
- glycolipids

Figure 6.3 illustrates these parts. All of these parts are important for the function of the plasma membrane. In the concepts that follow, you will learn about each plasma membrane component.

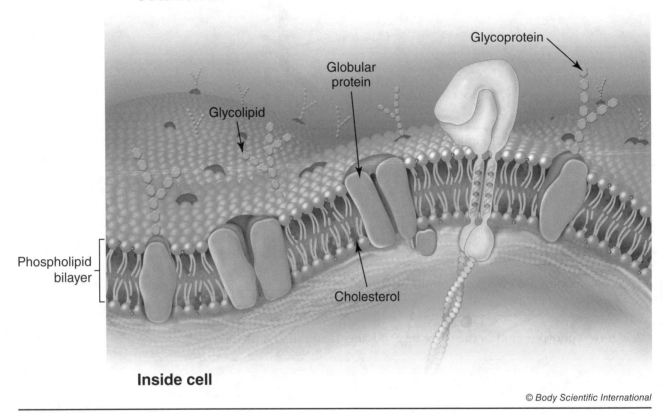

Outside cell

Glycoprotein

Globular protein

Glycolipid

Phospholipid bilayer

Cholesterol

Inside cell

© Body Scientific International

Figure 6.3   Illustrated here are the components of the plasma membrane.

Recall Activity

1. List the parts of the plasma membrane. _____

   _____

2. Write the parts of the plasma membrane in alphabetical order. _____

   _____

Concept 3: Phospholipids

phospholipid a molecule composed of one phosphate head and two lipid tails

hydrophilic attracted to water

hydrophobic not attracted to water

A *phospholipid* is a molecule composed of one phosphate head and two lipid tails (**Figure 6.4**). The phosphate head has a negative charge and therefore is *hydrophilic*, or attracted to water. The lipid tails do *not* have a charge and therefore are *hydrophobic*, or not attracted to water. For this reason, in a phospholipid layer, the phosphate heads will face toward a cell's cytosol or interstitial fluid, which are primarily water. The lipid tails will face away from the cytosol or interstitial fluid.

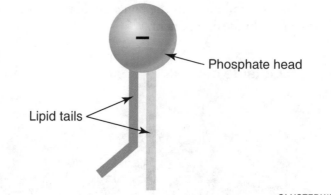

Phosphate head

Lipid tails

CLUSTERX/Shutterstock.com

Figure 6.4 A phospholipid has one head and two tails. The phosphate head has a negative charge and thus is attracted to the water-based cytosol and interstitial fluid inside and around a cell. The lipid tails have no charge.

Recall Activity

1. A phospholipid is composed of one phosphate _____ and two lipid _____.

2. Draw a phospholipid in the space below. Label the head and the tails.

3. The phosphate head has _____ charge and therefore

_____ attracted to water.

4. The lipid _____ do not have a charge and therefore

_____ attracted to water.

5. A(n) _____ molecule is not attracted to water; a(n)

_____ molecule is attracted to water.

Concept 4: Phospholipid Bilayer

In the plasma membrane, phospholipids are arranged in two layers. Because there are two layers of phospholipids, this component of the plasma membrane is referred to as the *phospholipid bilayer*. Notice how the lipid tails in the phospholipid bilayer point *away* from the cytosol or interstitial fluid and how the phosphate heads point *toward* the cytosol or interstitial fluid (**Figure 6.5**). This is due to the negative charges of the phosphate heads, which are attracted to water. The phospholipid bilayer forms the three-dimensional border around the cell.

phospholipid bilayer two layers of phospholipids that compose the plasma membrane; forms the three-dimensional border around the cell

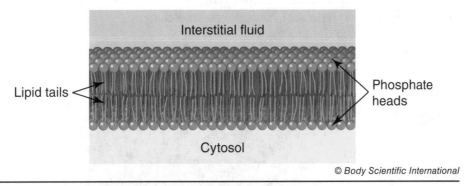

© Body Scientific International

Figure 6.5 In the phospholipid bilayer, the lipid tails face each other, and the phosphate heads face the water-based cytosol or interstitial fluid.

Recall Activity

1. There are _____ layers of phospholipids in the plasma membrane.

2. In the phospholipid bilayer, the _____ point away from the cytosol or interstitial fluid, and the _____ point toward the cytosol or interstitial fluid.

3. The phospholipid bilayer forms the _____ border around the cell.

Concept 5: Globular Proteins and Cholesterol

Wedged into the phospholipid bilayer are two types of structures: globular proteins and cholesterol. *Globular proteins* form channels that allow select

globular protein a protein that forms a channel to allow select molecules to pass through the plasma membrane

cholesterol a substance that separates individual phospholipids in the bilayer and helps them shift location

molecules to pass through the plasma membrane. *Cholesterol* separates the individual phospholipids in the bilayer, allowing flexibility so the components can change location. Phospholipids and proteins are constantly moving around the surface of the cell. Figure 6.3 shows how globular proteins and cholesterol are wedged into the phospholipid bilayer.

Recall Activity

1. Globular proteins form _____ that allow select molecules to pass through the plasma membrane.

2. _____ separates the individual phospholipids and helps them shift location.

Concept 6: Glycoproteins and Glycolipids

The final components of the plasma membrane are glycoproteins and glycolipids. A *glycoprotein* is a carbohydrate chain attached to a globular protein. A *glycolipid* is a carbohydrate chain attached to a lipid. In **Figure 6.6**, the glycoprotein and glycolipid carbohydrate chains are represented as strands of hexagons. Each hexagon represents one glucose molecule.

glycoprotein a carbohydrate chain attached to a globular protein

glycolipid a carbohydrate chain attached to a lipid

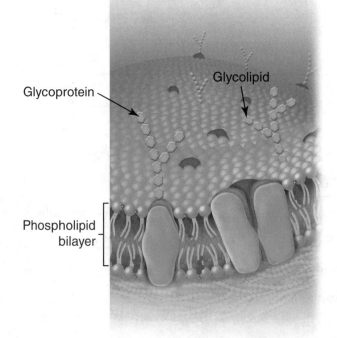

Figure 6.6 The terms *glycoprotein* and *glycolipid* contain the combining form *glyc/o*, which means "glucose" (or "sugar"). In this illustration, each hexagon represents one glucose molecule.

Glycoproteins and glycolipids form the "fingerprint" of a cell. This fingerprint is the same for all native cells in an organism. Cells in an organism that have a different fingerprint, such as invading bacteria, are recognized and attacked by the immune system.

Recall Activity

1. A(n) _____ is a chain of glucose molecules attached to a protein.

2. A(n) _____ is a chain of glucose molecules attached to a lipid.

3. Glycoproteins and glycolipids form the _____ of a cell.

Concept 7: Fluid Mosaic Model

The composition of the plasma membrane is described as a *fluid mosaic*. It is described as a *mosaic* because the plasma membrane is made of many distinct parts: the phospholipid bilayer, globular proteins, cholesterol, glycoproteins, and glycolipids. The plasma membrane is described as a *fluid* because the parts are not fixed in place. Rather, the parts constantly move around the surface of the cell. Do not think of the plasma membrane as a hard shell. On the contrary, the plasma membrane more resembles oil.

fluid mosaic a model used to describe how the plasma membrane has many distinct parts that are not fixed in place

Recall Activity

1. List the parts of the plasma membrane. _____

_____

_____

_____

_____

2. Are the parts of the plasma membrane fixed in place? Explain. _____

_____

3. The plasma membrane is not a hard shell. Instead, it resembles _____.

Section 6.2 Reinforcement

Answer the following questions using what you learned in this section.

1. The combining form *glyc/o* means "_____."

2. _____ form channels that allow select molecules to pass through the plasma membrane.

3. Which of the following is *not* a part of the plasma membrane?
   A. phospholipid bilayer
   B. cholesterol
   C. nucleus
   D. glycolipid

4. Unscramble the letters: sicamo. Define the word that is formed. _____
   _____

5. Cholesterol separates individual _____ and helps them shift location.

6. Write the letters backward: dipilocylg. Define the word that is formed. _____
   _____

7. *True or False*. Because the phosphate head is attracted to water, it is hydrophobic. _____

8. The fingerprint of a cell is formed from _____ and
   _____.

9. The plasma membrane is described as a(n) _____ because its parts are not fixed in place.

10. *True or False*. The composition of the plasma membrane is described as a fluid mosaic. _____

11. In the phospholipid bilayer, the _____ face *toward* the interstitial fluid or cytosol, and the _____ face *away* from the interstitial fluid or cytosol.

12. Unscramble the letters: slopophiphid. Define the word that is formed. _____
    _____

13. The phospholipid bilayer is made of two layers of _____.

14. The _____ of a phospholipid is hydrophilic.

15. Which of the following structures forms a channel that allows select molecules to pass through the plasma membrane?
    A. glycolipid
    B. globular protein
    C. cholesterol
    D. phospholipid

16. A glycolipid is a carbohydrate chain attached to a(n) _____.

17. *True or False*. The parts of the plasma membrane constantly move around the surface of the cell. _____

18. List the components of the plasma membrane that end in the word *lipid*._____
    _____

19. The parts of the plasma membrane are the phospholipid bilayer, cholesterol, glycolipids, glycoproteins, and _____.

20. *True or False*. The plasma membrane is selectively permeable._____

21. Which of the following words are misspelled?
    A. bilayer
    B. phopholipid
    C. glycolipid
    D. cloesterol

Match the following terms with their definitions.

_____ 22. The quality of being attracted to water

_____ 23. The quality of allowing materials to pass through

_____ 24. A structure composed of many different movable parts

_____ 25. The quality of not allowing all materials to pass through

_____ 26. The quality of not being attracted to water

A. permeable
B. selective
C. hydrophilic
D. hydrophobic
E. fluid mosaic

Comprehensive Review (Chapters 1–6)

Answer the following questions using what you have learned so far in this book.

27. The complementary base of adenine is _____.

28. The control group in an experiment is not given the _____ variable.

29. Which of the following word parts means "skin"?

    A. oste/o   C. derm/o   E. enter/o

    B. hepat/o   D. gastr/o   F. neur/o

30. Calculate the surface area of a cube that measures 10 cm by 10 cm by 10 cm. _____

31. What is morphology? _____

32. Studying is the deliberate effort to make _____ memories about subject matter.

Section 6.3 Nucleus

Inside the cell is a nucleus. The nucleus contains genetic information that directs cell activities. In this section, you will learn about the structure of the nucleus and its functions.

    The terms below are some of those that will be introduced in Section 6.3. To become familiar with these terms, reproduce each word on the line beside it. Pronounce each term as you write it. You will learn the definitions of these words as you complete this section.

1. chromosome _____

2. chromatin _____

3. gene _____

4. multinucleate _____

5. anucleate _____

6. nuclear envelope _____

7. nucleolus _____

Concept 1: Control Center

The nucleus (plural *nuclei*) is the control center of the cell. It houses the operating instructions for the many processes that take place inside the cell. These operating instructions are encoded in *DNA*. You learned about the structure and function of DNA in Section 5.11.

The DNA in the nuclei of your cells is 6 feet long. Within the cell nucleus, DNA packages itself by wrapping around proteins called *histones*. This enables the long length of DNA to fit inside the microscopic nucleus.

Recall Activity

1. The _____ is the control center of the cell.

2. DNA is wrapped around _____, allowing it to be packed inside the nucleus.

3. DNA controls many _____ that take place inside the cell.

Concept 2: Chromosomes and Chromatin

chromosome a structure inside the nucleus that contains packaged DNA during cell division

chromatin a structure inside the nucleus that contains packaged DNA most of the time

A cell's operating instructions, encoded in DNA, are located on chromosomes (**Figure 6.7**). A *chromosome* is a structure inside the nucleus that contains packaged DNA. However, DNA is only packaged in chromosomes during cell division. When a cell is *not* dividing—which is most of the time—DNA is packaged as *chromatin*.

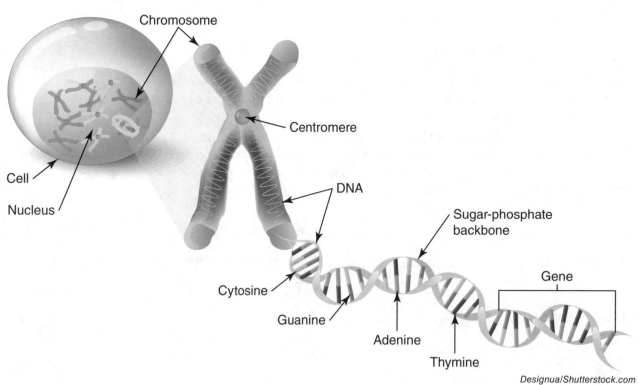

Designnua/Shutterstock.com

Figure 6.7 DNA is packaged on chromosomes.

The relationship between chromosomes and chromatin is similar to the relationship between ice and liquid water. Ice and liquid water are composed of the same H_2O molecules, but they are different forms of H_2O. Chromosomes and chromatin are the same strands of DNA, just different forms. For the purposes of this section, packages of DNA will be called *chromosomes*.

Recall Activity

1. DNA is located on _____.

2. Most of the time, DNA is packaged in a form called _____.

3. *True or False.* Chromatin is made of DNA. _____

4. *True or False.* Chromatin and chromosomes are the same strands of DNA. _____

Concept 3: Genes on Chromosomes

Humans possess 23 pairs of chromosomes (**Figure 6.8**). Each chromosome has hundreds to thousands of DNA segments called *genes*. The information encoded into genes is used to make proteins. Some of these proteins become

gene a segment of DNA within a chromosome that codes for a particular trait

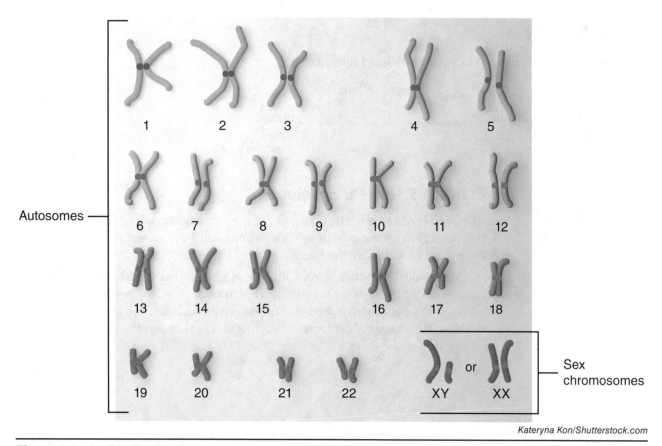

Autosomes

1   2   3   4   5

6   7   8   9   10   11   12

13   14   15   16   17   18

19   20   21   22   XY or XX

Sex chromosomes

Kateryna Kon/Shutterstock.com

Figure 6.8 Notice that humans have 22 pairs of autosomes plus one pair of sex chromosomes. This amounts to 23 pairs of chromosomes or 46 total chromosomes.

structures inside or outside of the cell. Other proteins, such as enzymes, control the processes involved in cell function. As you learned in Chapter 5, genes make proteins that cause certain traits to manifest.

Recall Activity

1. Humans possess _____ of chromosomes.

2. Genes are located on _____.

3. The information encoded into genes is used to make _____.

Concept 4: Multinucleate and Anucleate Cells

multinucleate having more than one nucleus

anucleate having no nucleus

Most of the trillions of cells in your body have one nucleus. Each nucleus contains a full set of your chromosomes. Some cells, however, are multinucleate. *Multinucleate* cells have many nuclei. One example of a multinucleate cell is the skeletal muscle cell. Other cells, such as red blood cells, lose their nuclei during development and thus do not have nuclei. A cell that has no nucleus is called *anucleate*.

Recall Activity

1. *True or False.* Every cell in your body has a nucleus. _____

2. _____ cells have no nuclei.

3. Multinucleate cells have _____ nuclei.

Concept 5: Nuclear Envelope

nuclear envelope the border of the nucleus

The border of the nucleus is called the *nuclear envelope*. The nuclear envelope separates the contents of the nucleus from a cell's cytoplasm. The liquid inside the nucleus is called *nucleoplasm*.

Much like the phospholipid bilayer of the plasma membrane, the nuclear envelope is a double-layer membrane (**Figure 6.9**). *Nuclear pores* form channels through the nuclear envelope and allow select molecules to enter or leave the nucleus. Raw materials enter and products leave through the nuclear pores.

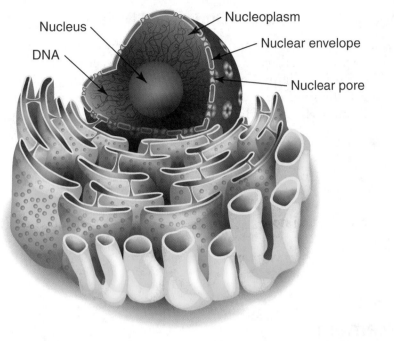

Nucleus

Nucleoplasm

Nuclear envelope

DNA

Nuclear pore

Tefi/Shutterstock.com

Figure 6.9   The nucleus has a double membrane.

Recall Activity

1. The liquid inside the nucleus is called _____.

2. Nuclear _____ form channels through the nuclear envelope.

3. The nuclear _____ separates the contents of the nucleus from a cell's

   _____.

Concept 6: Nucleoli

In addition to DNA and nucleoplasm, a nucleus may contain one or several areas called *nucleoli* (singular *nucleolus*). A *nucleolus* assembles the components needed to make organelles and to make ribosomes. *Ribosomes* are structures found in the cytoplasm that use operating instructions from the nucleus to assemble amino acids into specified proteins. This process of assembly is known as *protein synthesis* and will be discussed in more detail in Section 7.8. Nucleoli may not be present in a cell at all times. See Figure 6.9 to understand the placement of the nucleolus in a cell's nucleus.

nucleolus an area of the nucleus that assembles the components needed to make organelles and to make ribosomes

Recall Activity

1. A(n) _____ assembles the components needed to make organelles and

   _____.

2. Nucleoli _____ be present in a cell at all times.

Concept 7: The Nucleus During Cell Division

In your body, old cells die and are replaced by new cells. New cells are formed through a process called *cell division*, in which one cell divides into two daughter cells. During cell division, the nuclear envelope of a cell dissolves. At the end of cell division, the nuclear envelope reforms in each daughter cell. You will learn more about cell division in Section 7.9.

Recall Activity

1. _____ cell divides into _____ daughter cell(s).

2. During cell division, the nuclear envelope _____.

Section 6.3 Reinforcement

Answer the following questions using what you learned in this section.

1. The border of the nucleus is called the nuclear _____.

2. During cell division, DNA is packaged in the form of _____.

3. Which of the following structures is *not* found inside the nucleus?
   A. chromosome   C. nuclear pore
   B. chromatin   D. nucleoli

4. The liquid inside the nucleus is called _____.

5. *True or False.* A multinucleate cell has more than one nucleus. _____

6. The _____ dissolves during cell division.

7. *True or False.* The plural of nucleoli is nucleolus. _____

8. Unscramble the letters: ouscellun. Define the word that is formed. _____
   _____

9. Give an example of an anucleate cell. _____

10. *True or False.* Chromosomes and chromatin are different forms of DNA. _____

11. Give an example of a multinucleate cell. _____

12. Unscramble the letters: rathinmoc. Define the word that is formed. _____
    _____

13. Within the cell nucleus, DNA packages itself by wrapping around proteins called
    _____.

14. When a cell is not dividing, DNA is packaged in the form of _____.

15. Write the letters backward: emosomorhc. Define the word that is formed. _____

_____

16. Which of the following words are misspelled?

   A. chomosome   C. histone

   B. newcleoli   D. evelope

17. *True or False.* The singular form of nuclei is nucleus._____

18. Nuclear pores form _____ through the nuclear envelope.

19. The instructions to operate a cell are encoded in _____.

20. Humans possess 23 pairs of _____.

21. Which of the following are made in the nucleolus?

   A. histones   C. proteins

   B. ribosomes   D. nuclei

Match the following terms with their definitions.

_____ 22. A cell with no nucleus

_____ 23. The form in which DNA is packaged during cell division

_____ 24. A structure inside the nucleus that assembles ribosomes

_____ 25. A location on a chromosome

_____ 26. The border of the nucleus

_____ 27. The form in which DNA is packaged most of the time

   A. chromosome
   B. chromatin
   C. gene
   D. nuclear envelope
   E. anucleate
   F. nucleolus

Comprehensive Review (Chapters 1–6)

Answer the following questions using what you have learned so far in this book.

28. *True or False.* A person can only stay focused on a task for about 50–60 minutes. _____

29. The simplest type of sugar is a(n) _____.

30. Untested factors in an experiment are called _____.

31. Which of the following is the largest unit of measurement?

   A. millimeter   C. centimeter

   B. kilometer   D. meter

32. What is the function of cholesterol in the plasma membrane? _____

_____

33. The word part that means "loving" is _____.

Section 6.4 Endoplasmic Reticulum and Golgi

Outside the nucleus, in the cytoplasm of a cell, several organelles are attached to or associated with the nuclear envelope. These organelles—the endoplasmic reticulum and Golgi—perform important functions in the cell.

The terms below are some of those that will be introduced in Section 6.4. To become familiar with these terms, reproduce each word on the line beside it. Pronounce each term as you write it. You will learn the definitions of these words as you complete this section.

1. endoplasmic reticulum (ER)_____

2. smooth endoplasmic reticulum (SER) _____

3. rough endoplasmic reticulum (RER) _____

4. transport vesicle_____

5. ribosome_____

6. Golgi _____

7. secretory vesicle_____

Concept 1: Endoplasmic Reticulum

endoplasmic reticulum (ER) a network of membranes attached to the nuclear envelope

Attached at one end to the nuclear envelope is a network of membranes known as the *endoplasmic reticulum (ER)*. **Figure 6.10** shows the placement of the endoplasmic reticulum. The membranes of the endoplasmic reticulum are responsible for moving materials within a cell. These materials may be needed inside the cell or outside of the cell. The endoplasmic reticulum can also process, store, or digest some materials.

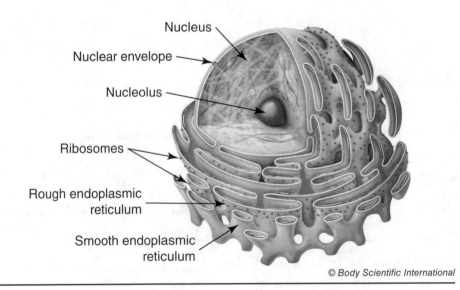

Nucleus

Nuclear envelope

Nucleolus

Ribosomes

Rough endoplasmic reticulum

Smooth endoplasmic reticulum

© Body Scientific International

Figure 6.10   The endoplasmic reticulum surrounds the nucleus.

Recall Activity

1. The membranes of the _____ move materials within a cell.

2. The endoplasmic reticulum can also _____, _____, or _____ some materials.

Concept 2: Types of Endoplasmic Reticulum

There are two types of endoplasmic reticulum: smooth and rough. The rough endoplasmic reticulum (RER) has ribosomes on the membrane surface. The smooth endoplasmic reticulum (SER) has a smooth surface that contains no ribosomes. The rough and smooth endoplasmic reticulum are connected.

Recall Activity

1. List the two types of endoplasmic reticulum. _____

_____

2. The rough and smooth endoplasmic reticulum are _____.

Concept 3: Smooth Endoplasmic Reticulum

The *smooth endoplasmic reticulum (SER)* has smooth membranes that are not studded with ribosomes. The SER resembles a set of semicircular tubes. In liver cells, the SER breaks down drugs, alcohol, and lipids. In small intestine cells, the SER transports fats, and in muscle cells, the SER stores calcium. Not all cells contain SER.

smooth endoplasmic reticulum (SER) a network of smooth membranes that are not studded with ribosomes

Recall Activity

1. The _____ resembles a set of semicircular tubes.

2. The SER in liver cells breaks down _____, _____, and _____.

3. The SER in muscle cells stores _____.

4. The SER in small intestine cells transports _____.

5. Not all cells contain _____.

Concept 4: Rough Endoplasmic Reticulum

rough endoplasmic reticulum (RER) a network of membranes studded with ribosomes

transport vesicle a sack that moves a product to another location inside the cell

The *rough endoplasmic reticulum (RER)* is a network of flat canals covered with small bumps. The bumps on the RER are ribosomes, which make proteins. Proteins made in the RER leave the RER via transport vesicles. A *transport vesicle* is a sack that moves a product to another location inside the cell. Cells that make products for export out of the cell, such as white blood cells that make antibodies and stomach cells that make digestive enzymes, have more RER.

Recall Activity

1. The _____ is a network of flat canals covered with small bumps.

2. The bumps on the RER are _____.

3. Proteins made in the RER leave the RER via _____.

Concept 5: Ribosomes

ribosome a structure that assembles amino acids into specific proteins

Ribosomes stud the RER and play an active role in protein synthesis. A *ribosome* is a structure that assembles amino acids into specific proteins. Ribosomes may be free or bound. *Free ribosomes* are found in a cell's cytoplasm, and *bound ribosomes* are attached to the nuclear envelope or RER.

Recall Activity

1. A(n) _____ assembles amino acids into specific proteins.

2. Free ribosomes are found in a cell's _____.

3. Bound ribosomes are attached to the _____ or _____.

Concept 6: Ribosome Structure

Ribosomes are made of ribosomal RNA and proteins produced by the nucleoli in the nucleus. A ribosome has no membrane (**Figure 6.11**). Cells that produce enzymes, such as pancreatic and liver cells, may have millions of ribosomes. The proteins produced by ribosomes may be used inside the cell or shipped out of the cell. Ribosomes in beta cells of the pancreas make insulin.

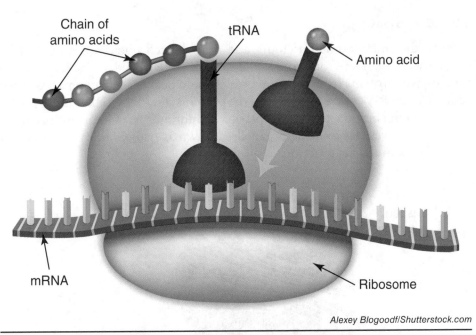

Chain of amino acids

tRNA

Amino acid

mRNA

Ribosome

Figure 6.11 A ribosome, composed of ribosomal RNA and proteins, assembles amino acids into a protein based on instructions sent from the nucleus.

Recall Activity

1. Ribosomes are made of ribosomal RNA and proteins produced by the _____ in the nucleus.

2. Cells that produce _____ may have millions of ribosomes.

Concept 7: Ribosome Proteins

In protein synthesis, a ribosome assembles a chain of amino acids based on instructions sent from the nucleus. Free ribosomes make proteins that stay within a cell. Bound ribosomes make proteins that leave a cell or become part of the plasma membrane. Ribosomes can switch between being free or bound. For example, a ribosome may be bound to ER to assemble a certain protein, then detach and become free to assemble a different protein.

Recall Activity

1. _____ ribosomes make proteins that stay within a cell.

2. _____ ribosomes make proteins that leave a cell or become part of a plasma membrane.

Concept 8: Golgi

Golgi an organelle that receives proteins from transport vesicles and packages them into secretory vesicles

secretory vesicle a sack that moves proteins out of the cell

Next to the endoplasmic reticulum and near the cell nucleus is an organelle called the *Golgi*. The Golgi looks like a stack of flattened sacks. This structure receives proteins from transport vesicles and packages them into secretory vesicles. *Secretory vesicles* then move the proteins out of the cell. Other vesicles from the Golgi become part of the plasma membrane. The Golgi also packages enzymes into vesicles to make organelles known as *lysosomes*. Lysosomes will be discussed in the next section.

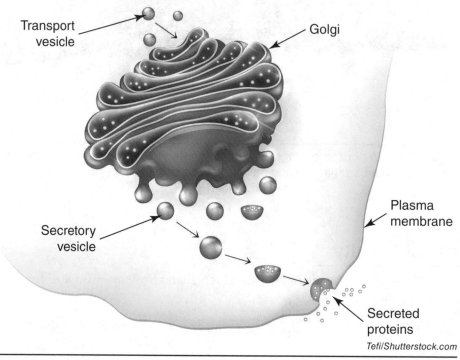

Transport vesicle

Golgi

Secretory vesicle

Plasma membrane

Secreted proteins

Tefi/Shutterstock.com

Figure 6.12 The Golgi packages proteins for transport out of the cell.

Recall Activity

1. The _____ looks like a stack of flattened sacks.

2. The Golgi receives proteins from _____ vesicles and packages them into _____ vesicles.

3. Some vesicles from the Golgi become part of the _____.

4. The Golgi packages enzymes into vesicles to make _____.

Section 6.4 Reinforcement

Answer the following questions using what you learned in this section.

1. _____ vesicles leave the Golgi.

2. SER resembles a set of semicircular _____.

3. *True or False.* Rough and smooth ER are connected. _____

4. Unscramble the letters: turmulice. Define the word that is formed. _____

   _____

5. SER has smooth membranes that are not studded with _____.

6. Does a ribosome have a membrane? _____

7. Write the letters backward: emosobir. Define the word that is formed. _____

   _____

8. SER in liver cells breaks down _____, _____, and

   _____.

9. In protein synthesis, a(n) _____ assembles a chain of amino acids.

10. *True or False.* Ribosomes can be free or bound. _____

11. Which type of ER has ribosomes on the membrane surface? _____

12. Unscramble the letters: lgiog. Define the word that is formed. _____

    _____

13. Proteins are transported via _____ vesicles from the ER to the Golgi.

14. The ER membranes move materials _____ a cell.

15. Ribosomes are made of ribosomal _____ and proteins produced by the nucleoli in the nucleus.

16. _____ in some cells of the pancreas make insulin.

17. *True or False.* The ER can process, store, or digest some materials. _____

18. _____ ribosomes make proteins that leave a cell.

19. The _____ packages enzymes into vesicles to make lysosomes.

20. *True or False.* All vesicles from the Golgi become part of the plasma membrane. _____

21. Which of the following words are misspelled?
    - A. vessicle
    - B. Golge
    - C. endoplasmic
    - D. ribosome

Match the following terms with their definitions.

_____ 22. A network of membranes containing ribosomes

_____ 23. A structure that assembles proteins

_____ 24. A sack that transports proteins out of the cell

_____ 25. A network of membranes containing no ribosomes

_____ 26. A structure that packages proteins for transport out of the cell

A. smooth endoplasmic reticulum

B. rough endoplasmic reticulum

C. ribosome

D. Golgi

E. secretory vesicle

Comprehensive Review (Chapters 1–6)

Answer the following questions using what you have learned so far in this book.

27. The helium atom contains _____ proton(s) and _____ electron(s).

28. What do cubic units measure?_____

29. A scientific law is a general statement of _____.

30. The prefix *peri-* means "_____."

31. How many nuclei does an anucleate cell have? _____

32. Which of the following will help you remember words?

    A. writing   C. speaking

    B. reading   D. All of the above.

Section 6.5 Cytoplasm

All the material inside a cell except for the nucleus is known as *cytoplasm*. As you have learned, cytoplasm is composed of cytosol and organelles. In this section, you will learn about additional components of cytoplasm.

The terms below are some of those that will be introduced in Section 6.5. To become familiar with these terms, reproduce each word on the line beside it. Pronounce each term as you write it. You will learn the definitions of these words as you complete this section.

1. mitochondrion_____

2. lysosome_____

3. peroxisome _____

4. cytoskeleton _____

5. microfilament_____

6. intermediate filament _____

7. microtubule_____

Concept 1: Mitochondria

The cytoplasm of a cell is full of organelles. One such organelle is the mito-chondrion (plural *mitochondria*). The *mitochondrion* is the site of cell respira-tion and the powerhouse of the cell. During cell respiration, just outside and inside a mitochondrion, the energy from glucose and other molecules is used to make adenosine triphosphate (ATP), which is the energy storage molecule in the cell. The number of mitochondria in a cell varies by cell type. Cells that use a lot of energy, such as muscle cells, have many mitochondria. Cells that do not use much energy, such as some blood cells, have few mitochondria.

mitochondrion the powerhouse of the cell and the site of cell respiration

Recall Activity

1. The _____ are sites of cell respiration.

2. Which type of cell would have more mitochondria: a muscle cell or a blood cell?_____

3. _____ is the energy storage molecule in the cell.

Concept 2: Mitochondria Structure

The mitochondria in a cell are shaped like kidney beans. Each mitochondrion has two membranes: an outer membrane and a highly convoluted inner mem-brane. The surface of the inner membrane is called the *cristae* (**Figure 6.13**). Mitochondria are found in a cell's cytoplasm.

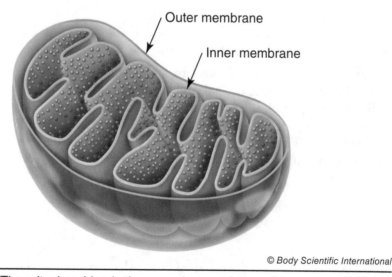

Outer membrane

Inner membrane

© Body Scientific International

Figure 6.13 The mitochondrion is the powerhouse of the cell.

Recall Activity

1. The mitochondria are shaped like _____.

2. The surface of the mitochondrion's inner membrane is called the _____.

Concept 3: Lysosomes

lysosome a large bag of enzymes; prevents enzymes from harming the cell and releases them to destroy bacteria

Another organelle found in the cytoplasm is the lysosome. A *lysosome* is a large bag of enzymes. Because these enzymes would dissolve the cell if they were released from the bag, the membrane of the lysosome prevents enzymes from harming the cell.

Lysosomes play a role in your body's immune response. In your body, white blood cells surround and engulf bacteria. A bacterium is brought into a cell inside a vesicle. Once the vesicle enters the cell, the membrane of a lysosome fuses with the vesicle containing the bacterium and releases enzymes into the vesicle to destroy the bacterium. Lysosomes also break down worn-out cell parts (for example, worn-out mitochondria). Lysosomes are produced by the Golgi.

Recall Activity

1. A(n) _____ is a large bag of enzymes.

2. The membrane of the lysosome prevents _____ from harming the cell.

Concept 4: Peroxisomes

peroxisome a small bag containing enzymes that break down chemicals and free radicals

Organelles known as *peroxisomes* are small bags containing enzymes that break down chemicals, such as alcohol, and harmful molecules called *free radicals*. Free radicals damage molecules by stealing electrons. To break down free radicals, peroxisomes release the enzymes oxidase and catalase, which change free radicals into water. The cells of the liver and kidneys, which destroy harmful chemicals, contain many peroxisomes. Peroxisomes are found in a cell's cytoplasm.

Recall Activity

1. _____ are small bags containing enzymes that break down chemicals.

2. To break down free radicals, peroxisomes release the enzymes _____ and _____, which change free radicals into water.

Concept 5: Cytoskeleton

The skeleton of a cell is not made of bones. However, like bones support the body, the *cytoskeleton* does support the cell. The building blocks of the cytoskeleton are

- microfilaments
- intermediate filaments
- microtubules

These components are listed from the smallest in diameter to the largest in diameter and are illustrated in **Figure 6.14**.

cytoskeleton the structure that supports the cell; includes microfilaments, intermediate filaments, and microtubules

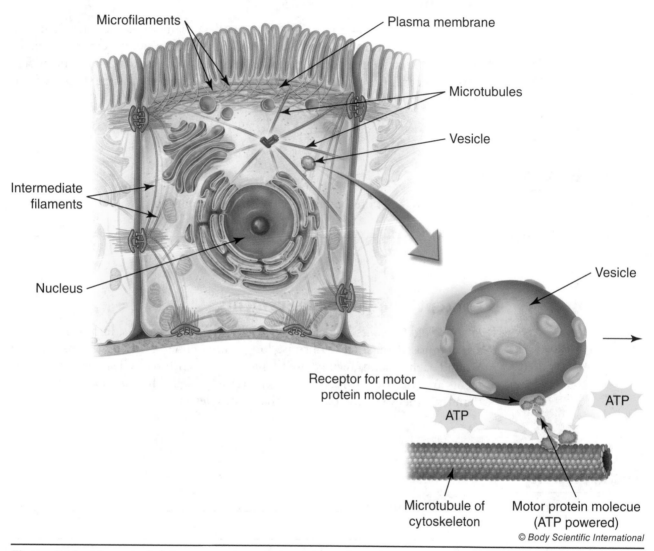

Figure 6.14 The cytoskeleton supports and strengthens the cell.

Recall Activity

1. Is the cytoskeleton made of bones? _____

2. Arrange these components from smallest to largest: intermediate filaments, microfilaments, and microtubules. _____

3. Which component of the cytoskeleton has the largest diameter? _____

Concept 6: Microfilaments

microfilament a structure that forms a net on the inside of the plasma membrane

The cytoskeleton component with the smallest diameter is the microfilament. *Microfilaments* form a net on the inside of the plasma membrane; they are made of two globular (round) protein chains wrapped around each other. The microfilament net reinforces the plasma membrane and helps it change shape. Microfilaments are assembled and disassembled as needed.

Recall Activity

1. _____ form a net on the inside of the plasma membrane.

2. What are microfilaments made of? _____

Concept 7: Intermediate Filaments

intermediate filament a structure that holds organelles in position

Intermediate filaments hold some organelles, like the nucleus, in position. They are composed of several fibrous, long, and slender protein strands twisted around each other. Intermediate filaments also reinforce cell shape. These filaments are not readily disassembled and reassembled. They are more permanent than the other building blocks of the cytoskeleton.

Recall Activity

1. List two functions of intermediate filaments. _____

_____

2. Intermediate filaments are not readily _____.

Concept 8: Microtubules

microtubule a structure that organelles attach to and that forms the roadway on which organelles are moved throughout the cell

The cytoskeleton component with the largest diameter is the microtubule. *Microtubules* are made of globular proteins called *tubulins*. Tubulins are assembled in a coil to form a hollow tube. The microtubules grow out of the central area in the cytoplasm of the cell.

Microtubules form an internal structure for organelle attachment. The outside surfaces of the microtubules serve as roadways. Motor proteins move organelles like mitochondria around the cell along the roadway. The roadway is quickly assembled and disassembled as needed. Microtubules also form the structures of cilia and flagella and guide the movement of chromatids during cell division. You will learn more about cilia and flagella in the next section.

Recall Activity

1. The _____ grow out of the central area in the cytoplasm of the cell.

2. Microtubules are made of globular proteins called _____.

3. The outside surfaces of the microtubules serve as _____.

Section 6.5 Reinforcement

Answer the following questions using what you learned in this section.

1. Which of the following cytoskeleton components is the most permanent?
   A. intermediate filaments
   B. microfilaments
   C. microtubules

2. Oxidase and catalase enzymes, released from _____, change free radicals into water.

3. Lysosomes are produced by the _____.

4. Unscramble the letters: thoonimacrid. Define the word that is formed. _____
   _____

5. _____ are composed of several fibrous, long, and slender protein strands twisted around each other.

6. _____ hold some organelles, like the nucleus, in position.

7. *True or False.* Organelles move inside the microtubules. _____

8. What are the three components of the cytoskeleton? _____
   _____

9. Write the letters backward: emmososyl. Define the word that is formed. _____
   _____

10. *True or False.* The word *mitochondria* is singular. _____

11. Microfilaments form a net on the inside of the _____.

12. Unscramble the letters: stocktyleeno. Define the word that is formed. _____
    _____

13. _____ are involved in breaking down alcohol.

14. Which components of the cytoskeleton are assembled and disassembled as needed? _____

_____

15. A(n) _____ is shaped like a kidney bean.

16. _____ form the structures of cilia and flagella.

17. *True or False.* The cytoskeleton is not made of bones and does not support the cell. _____

18. The powerhouse of the cell is the _____.

19. Which component of the cytoskeleton is made of globular protein? _____

20. *True or False.* Microtubules are hollow. _____

21. Which of the following words are misspelled?

    A. motochondria   C. filament

    B. lysososme   D. perixoisome

Match the following terms with their definitions.

_____ 22. A structure that supports the cell

_____ 23. An organelle that breaks down cell parts

_____ 24. An organelle that breaks down chemicals

_____ 25. The powerhouse of the cell

    A. mitochondrion
    B. lysosome
    C. peroxisome
    D. cytoskeleton

Comprehensive Review (Chapters 1–6)

Answer the following questions using what you have learned so far in this book.

26. If a circle is divided into 16 red and blue parts, and 7 parts are red, what fraction of the circle is blue?

_____

27. A lipid with one double bond is a(n) _____ fat.

28. A fact is a(n) _____ observation.

29. *Dors/o* is to "back" as _____ is to "belly."

30. The membranes of the endoplasmic reticulum are responsible for moving materials _____ a cell.

31. A(n) _____ is based on a phenomenon that you have witnessed, detected, or read about.

Section 6.6 Outside the Cell

Outside of a cell, membrane extensions aid in cell movement and absorption. Membrane junctions bind cells together. In this section, you will learn about the types of membrane extensions and junctions.

The terms below are some of those that will be introduced in Section 6.6. To become familiar with these terms, reproduce each word on the line beside it. Pronounce each term as you write it. You will learn the definitions of these words as you complete this section.

1. cilia _____

2. flagella _____

3. microvilli _____

4. membrane junction _____

5. tight junction _____

6. desmosome _____

7. gap junction _____

Concept 1: Membrane Extensions

Several structures outside the cell aid in cell function. These structures extend from the plasma membrane into the surrounding interstitial fluid. Extensions of the plasma membrane include cilia, flagella, and microvilli. Cilia and flagella are involved with movement, and microvilli aid the cell in absorption.

Recall Activity

1. _____ and _____ are involved with movement.

2. _____ aid the cell in absorption.

Concept 2: Cilia

Cilia (singular *cilium*) look like hairs on the outside of the cell (**Figure 6.15**). Cilia do not *move* a cell; a cell is stationary. Rather, cilia move objects or liquids around a cell. Cilia contain groups of paired microtubules. Bending of the microtubules causes the cilia to wave.

cilia hairs on the outside of a cell that move objects or liquid around the cell

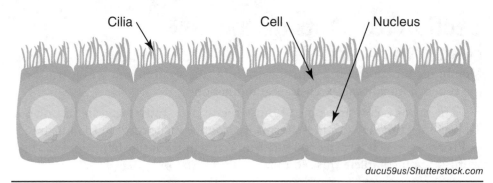

Cilia   Cell   Nucleus

ducu59us/Shutterstock.com

Figure 6.15   Cilia look like small hairs.

Only a few types of cells in your body have cilia. Cells lining your windpipe have cilia. These cilia use a coordinated waving motion to move layers of mucus over the surfaces of windpipe cells. The layers of mucus trap dust particles, preventing particle entry into the lungs. Cilia in the fallopian tubes move an egg cell from the ovary into the uterus.

Recall Activity

1. Cilia look like _____ on the outside of the cell.

2. Cilia contain groups of paired _____.

3. Which cells in the human body have cilia?_____

Concept 3: Flagella

flagella whip-like structures that propel a cell forward

Flagella (singular *flagellum*) are whip-like and are longer than cilia. The only human cells with a flagellum are sperm cells (**Figure 6.16**). The whirring motion of the flagellum propels a sperm cell through the body of a female in search of an egg cell. Malformed sperm may have two or more flagella. Flagella are also composed of groups of paired microtubules.

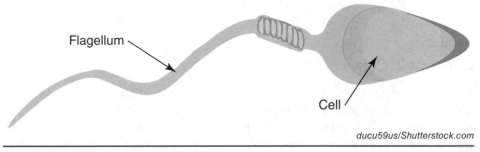

Flagellum

Cell

ducu59us/Shutterstock.com

Figure 6.16   A flagellum is whip-like.

Recall Activity

1. _____ are whip-like.

2. Which is longer: a cilium or a flagellum?_____

Concept 4: Microvilli

Microvilli (singular *microvillum*) are not involved in movement. Microvilli are finger-like projections of the plasma membrane that increase the surface area of the cell to allow for more absorption (**Figure 6.17**). For example, since the small intestine absorbs digested macromolecules, cells lining the small intestine have microvilli that allow more macromolecules to enter. The lining of the small intestine is called the *brush border* due to the presence of microvilli.

microvilli finger-like projections of the plasma membrane that increase the surface area of the cell to allow for more absorption

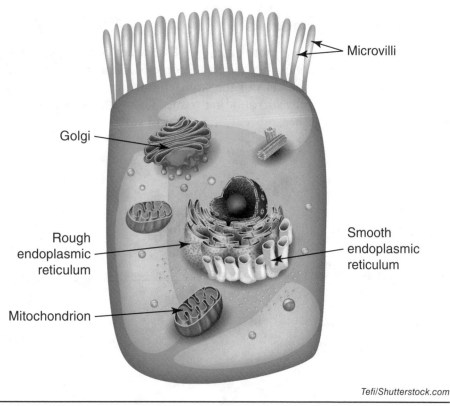

Tefi/Shutterstock.com

Figure 6.17 Microvilli increase the surface area of a cell.

Recall Activity

1. _____ increase the surface area of the cell to allow for more

_____.

2. The lining of the small intestine is called the _____ due to the presence of microvilli.

Concept 5: Membrane Junctions

membrane junction the attachment between nearby cells

In the body, most cells are attached to other nearby cells. This attachment is formed through *membrane junctions*. There are three types of membrane junctions: tight junctions, desmosomes, and gap junctions.

Recall Activity

1. *True or False*. Most cells in the body are unattached._____

2. What are the three membrane junctions? _____

_____

Concept 6: Tight Junctions

tight junction a membrane junction that binds adjacent cells together to form an impermeable barrier

Tight junctions are made by proteins and bind adjacent cells together to form an impermeable barrier. This barrier prevents the movement of liquid between the cells. For example, the cells of the stomach must prevent acids inside the stomach from leaking into surrounding tissue. Tight junctions hold the cells lining the stomach together, preventing leakage of stomach acid.

Recall Activity

1. _____ bind adjacent cells together to form a(n) _____
   barrier.

2. The barrier formed by tight junctions prevents the movement of _____
   between cells.

3. Cells lining the _____ have tight junctions.

Concept 7: Desmosomes

Like spot welds that join panels on a car, *desmosomes* are locking joints between adjacent cells. Desmosomes consist of interlinked, anchoring proteins and hold cells together to prevent them from being torn away from each other by force. For example, cells in the skin are subject to abrasion when the skin is scraped. Desmosomes hold skin cells together, preventing damage. As another example, as the heart beats, muscle cells of the heart stretch, but do not separate from one another due to the anchoring strength of desmosomes.

desmosome a locking joint between adjacent cells that prevents cells from being separated by force

Recall Activity

1. _____ are locking joints between adjacent cells.

2. *True or False.* Desmosomes consist of interlinked, anchoring proteins. _____

3. _____ prevent cells from separating by force.

Concept 8: Gap Junctions

A *gap junction* contains communication tunnels between adjacent cells. These tunnels, called *connexons*, are made of protein. Ions can flow from one cell to another through gap junctions. For example, the movement of ions through muscle cells, such as in the heart muscle, coordinates contraction.

gap junction a membrane junction that contains communication tunnels between adjacent cells

Recall Activity

1. _____ are communication tunnels between cells.

2. A(n) _____ contains communication tunnels between cells.

3. _____ can flow from one cell to another through gap junctions.

Section 6.6 Reinforcement

Answer the following questions using what you learned in this section.

1. *True or False.* Connexons are made of protein._____

2. Unscramble the letters: glumlafle. Define the word that is formed. _____

_____

3. Which of the following words is plural?
   A. cilium   C. microvilli
   B. flagellum

4. List the extensions of the plasma membrane. _____

_____

5. Which of the following membrane junctions forms an impermeable barrier?
   A. tight junctions   C. desmosomes
   B. gap junctions

6. Which of the following words are misspelled?
   A. cilia   C. desomosome
   B. flagellem   D. tight junction

7. *True or False.* Desmosomes prevent heart muscle cells from separating. _____

8. Unscramble the letters: emossdome. Define the word that is formed._____

_____

9. Which of the following structures is involved in absorption?
   A. desmosome   C. tight junction   E. flagella
   B. microvilli   D. cilia   F. gap junction

10. *True or False.* A flagellum is hair-like and is longer than a cilium._____

11. Cilia look like _____ on the outside of the cell.

12. The lining of the small intestine is called the *brush border* due to the presence of

_____.

13. Which of the following does *not* belong in this group?
    A. cilia   C. desmosome
    B. flagella   D. microvilli

14. Which membrane junction allows for ion flow between cells?_____

15. Write the letters backward: illivorcim. Define the word that is formed. _____

_____

16. Which is larger: a gap junction or a connexon?_____

17. Which of the following cells have cilia?

    A. small intestine cells   C. fallopian tube cells

    B. windpipe cells   D. stomach cells

18. List the membrane junctions._____

_____

19. Which of the following structures are involved in moving a cell?

    A. microvilli   C. cilia

    B. flagellum

20. Which of the following structures are made of proteins?

    A. tight junctions   C. gap junctions

    B. desmosomes

21. *True or False.* Desmosomes prevent leakage into a cell._____

Match the following terms with their definitions.

_____ 22. Membrane extensions that aid in absorption

_____ 23. Membrane extensions that are whip-like

_____ 24. Membrane extensions that are hair-like

_____ 25. Membrane junctions that prevent leakage between cells

_____ 26. Membrane junctions that contain communication tunnels

_____ 27. Membrane junctions that prevent cells from separating

A. cilia
B. flagella
C. microvilli
D. tight junctions
E. desmosomes
F. gap junctions

Comprehensive Review (Chapters 1–6)

Answer the following questions using what you have learned so far in this book.

28. _____ seeks natural explanations to phenomena.

29. The prefix of the term *submucosa* means "_____."

30. A disaccharide has _____ sugar(s).

31. How many milliliters are in 1 liter?_____

32. List the building blocks of the cytoskeleton._____

_____

33. The _____ portion of a hypothesis is the independent variable.

Answer the following questions using what you learned in this chapter.

1. The structure of muscle cells allows them to _____ or
   _____.

2. The _____ are specialized structures that perform specific functions inside
   the cell.

3. The _____ is the barrier that keeps molecules inside or outside of the cell.

4. *True or False.* The plasma membrane is like a hard shell. _____

5. Morphology is the study of _____ or _____.

6. The cell is the basic unit of _____.

7. *True or False.* A phospholipid has two lipid heads. _____

8. A glycolipid is a(n) _____ chain attached to a(n)
   _____.

9. *True or False.* The number of activities that can occur inside a cell is limited by the surface area of
   the cell. _____

10. Is the phosphate head of a phospholipid hydrophilic or hydrophobic? Explain. _____
    _____

11. Where are ribosomes made? _____

12. Cells reproduce by a process known as _____.

13. *True or False.* DNA is wrapped around proteins called *nucleoli*. _____

14. List the three basic parts of the cell. _____
    _____

15. *True or False.* Ribosomes assemble amino acids to make proteins. _____

16. Microtubules are made of globular proteins called _____.

17. *True or False.* Cells with no nucleus are called *multinucleate*. _____

18. Globular proteins form _____ that allow select molecules to pass through
    the plasma membrane.

19. *True or False.* A ribosome has no membrane. _____

20. Which of the following structures packages materials?
    A. nucleus   C. Golgi
    B. ribosome   D. nucleolus

21. *True or False.* The membrane of the RER is studded with ribosomes. _____

22. Which of the following structures packages enzymes into vesicles to make lysosomes?

A. Golgi

C. cytoskeleton

B. nucleolus

D. smooth endoplasmic reticulum

23. *True or False.* All cells contain smooth endoplasmic reticulum. _____

24. _____ are made of two globular (round) protein chains wrapped around each other.

25. ATP is the _____ storage molecule in the cell.

26. Which cell structure breaks down worn-out cell parts? _____

27. Bending of the _____ causes the cilia to wave.

28. *True or False.* A gap junction contains communication tunnels between cells. _____

29. The outside surfaces of the microtubules serve as _____.

30. *True or False.* Microvilli help a cell move. _____

31. Which of the following cells has a flagellum?

A. small intestine cell

C. stomach cell

B. sperm cell

D. egg cell

32. _____ are locking joints between adjacent cells.

Comprehensive Review (Chapters 1–6)

Using what you have learned so far in this book, match the following terms with their definitions.

_____ 33. A chain of nucleotides

_____ 34. A small bag in a cell containing enzymes that break down chemicals and free radicals

_____ 35. A combining form that means "back (of the body)"

_____ 36. A test of a hypothesis

_____ 37. The "then" part of a hypothesis

_____ 38. A large bag of enzymes in a cell that prevents enzymes from harming the cell and releases them to destroy bacteria

_____ 39. The study of body parts

_____ 40. Testable and observable

_____ 41. A combining form that means "cell"

_____ 42. The longest measurement across a circle

_____ 43. A combining form that means "belly side (of the body)"

A. nucleic acid

B. dors/o

C. dependent variable

D. peroxisome

E. experiment

F. lysosome

G. anatomy

H. cyt/o

I. natural

J. diameter

K. ventr/o

Chapter 7
Cell Physiology

Introduction

Many processes that sustain the body take place inside the cell. Understanding the processes that happen inside the cell is essential to understanding body function. In this chapter, you will look at how the plasma membrane acts as a gatekeeper to regulate the movement of materials into and out of the cell. Other functions of the cell explained in this chapter include cell respiration, the maintenance of homeostasis, protein synthesis, and cell division.

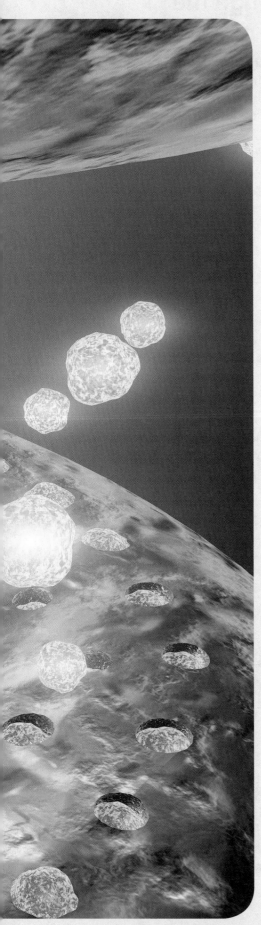

Objectives

After completing this chapter, you will be able to

- explain how materials enter and exit the cell
- understand a concentration gradient
- explain diffusion, facilitated diffusion, and osmosis
- list the steps of cell respiration
- explain active transport, endocytosis, and exocytosis
- describe how homeostasis is maintained in the cell
- explain protein synthesis
- understand cell division

Key Terms

The following terms and phrases will be introduced and explained in Chapter 7. Read through the list to become familiar with the words.

active transport	lactic acid
anabolic reaction	lipid barrier
aquaporin	lyse
carrier	meiosis
catabolic reaction	mitosis
cell respiration	nonpolar
concentration gradient	osmosis
crenation	phagocytosis
diffusion	pinocytosis
diploid	polar
downhill reaction	polypeptide
endocytosis	protein buffer
equilibrium	protein synthesis
exocytosis	receptor-mediated endocytosis
facilitated diffusion	replication
gamete	sense strand
haploid	sodium-potassium pump
high-energy bond	soluble
homeostasis	solute pump
hypertonic	transcription
hypotonic	translation
interphase	uphill reaction
isotonic	zygote

Section 7.1 Movement Through the Plasma Membrane

The plasma membrane is responsible for keeping molecules inside or outside of the cell. In this section, you will learn more about the plasma membrane's selective permeability. You will learn about molecules the plasma membrane allows through and about the structures that move molecules through the plasma membrane.

The terms below are some of those that will be introduced in Section 7.1. To become familiar with these terms, reproduce each word on the line beside it. Pronounce each term as you write it. You will learn the definitions of these words as you complete this section.

1. polar _____

2. nonpolar _____

3. lipid barrier _____

4. soluble _____

5. aquaporin _____

6. carrier _____

7. solute pump _____

Concept 1: Selective Permeability

You learned in Section 6.2 that the plasma membrane of a cell is composed of the phospholipid bilayer. The phospholipid bilayer is *selectively permeable*, meaning that only certain materials can pass through it. This is important for cell function. If the wrong materials enter or leave a cell, this could harm the cell. The plasma membrane must allow the correct molecules to move through and prevent the wrong molecules from gaining passage.

Recall Activity

1. The phospholipid bilayer is selectively _____.

2. If the wrong materials enter or leave a cell, this could _____ the cell.

Concept 2: Molecules Entering the Cell

Materials that must enter a cell include oxygen, glucose, amino acids, and ions. The oxygen you breathe is transported by your blood cells from the lungs to your body cells. Blood also transports glucose and amino acids from the digestive system to the body cells. Glucose, oxygen, and some amino acids are used in cell respiration, which you will learn about later in this chapter. Most amino acids are assembled to make proteins in a process known as *protein synthesis*. Ions also need to enter a cell and are essential in maintaining homeostasis.

Recall Activity

1. What molecules need to enter the cell? _____

_____

2. Oxygen, glucose, and amino acids are transported to body cells via the _____.

Concept 3: Molecules Exiting the Cell

Waste and products must exit a cell. For example, carbon dioxide is a waste product that moves out of the cell into the blood and then to the lungs. Nitrogen waste also moves out of the cell through the plasma membrane. Some cells are like factories and produce products like enzymes and hormones. These products must pass through the plasma membrane for delivery to the rest of the body. Ions also need to leave a cell to maintain homeostasis.

Recall Activity

1. _____ and _____ are waste products that must exit the cell.

2. Some cells are like _____ and produce products like

_____ and _____.

Concept 4: Polarity of Molecules

Molecules can be polar or nonpolar. A *polar* substance has a charge. This could be a positive or negative charge (such as an ion) or opposite charges at either end of a molecule (such as water). Polar substances are attracted to other polar substances. For example, the Na^+ and Cl^- ions in salt dissolve in water because they are attracted to the charges of the water molecules. A *nonpolar* substance has no charge. An example of a nonpolar substance is oil. A nonpolar substance can dissolve in another nonpolar substance (for example, oil dissolves in benzene). However, a nonpolar substance is not attracted to and cannot dissolve in a polar substance. This is why oil (nonpolar) and water (polar) do not mix. The polarity of a molecule affects whether it can pass through a cell's phospholipid bilayer.

polar having a charge

nonpolar having no charge

Recall Activity

1. A(n) _____ substance has a charge and is attracted to other

_____ substances.

2. A(n) _____ substance has no charge.

3. The _____ of a molecule affects whether it can pass through a cell's phospho-lipid bilayer.

Concept 5: Lipid Solubility

When entering or exiting a cell, some molecules can pass directly through the phospholipid bilayer due to their lipid solubility. The phospholipid bilayer of the plasma membrane only allows certain molecules to pass through, and the lipid portion of the phospholipid bilayer acts as a *lipid barrier* to molecules that are not lipid soluble.

If a molecule is *soluble*, this means it is capable of dissolving. A *lipid-soluble* molecule is capable of dissolving in a nonpolar substance. Hydrophobic molecules and nonpolar molecules are lipid soluble. Hydrophilic molecules and polar molecules, like ions, are *not* lipid soluble.

lipid barrier the lipid portion of the phospholipid bilayer that prevents molecules that are not lipid soluble from passing through

soluble capable of dissolving

Recall Activity

1. The lipid portion of the phospholipid bilayer acts as a(n) _____ to molecules that are not lipid soluble.

2. Hydrophobic molecules and _____ molecules are lipid soluble.

3. Hydrophilic molecules and polar molecules, like ions, are *not* lipid _____.

Concept 6: Passing Through the Lipid Barrier

Lipid-soluble, nonpolar, and hydrophobic molecules—such as oxygen, carbon dioxide, and lipid-soluble vitamins—can pass through the lipid barrier and move directly through the phospholipid bilayer (**Figure 7.1**). Hydrophilic and polar molecules, however, are *not* lipid soluble, and thus are prevented from moving through the phospholipid bilayer. An exception to this rule is water molecules, which can pass through the lipid barrier despite their polarity.

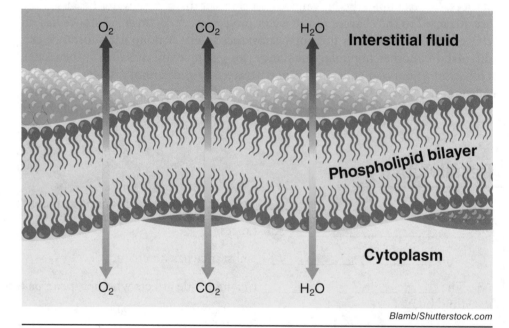

Figure 7.1 Oxygen, carbon dioxide, and water can move through the lipid barrier.

Recall Activity

1. What molecules can move through the lipid barrier? _____

   _____

2. What molecules are prevented from moving through the lipid barrier? _____

   _____

3. _____ molecules can pass through the lipid barrier despite their polarity.

Concept 7: Protein Channels

While they cannot pass directly through the phospholipid bilayer, molecules that are not lipid soluble can enter or exit a cell through protein channels (**Figure 7.2**). As you have learned, some globular proteins in the plasma membrane form channels that allow select molecules to move through the plasma membrane. These proteins form tubes that span the two layers of the phospholipid bilayer, pushing aside the phospholipids and creating a tunnel. Small, polar molecules, such as sodium ions, calcium ions, chloride ions, and potassium ions, move through the plasma membrane in this fashion.

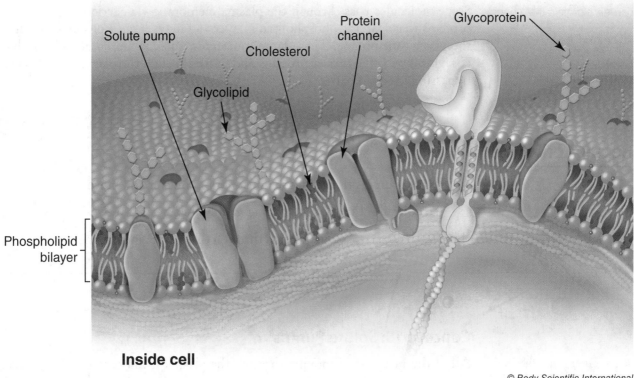

© Body Scientific International

Figure 7.2 Protein channels allow polar molecules to pass through the plasma membrane. Solute pumps use energy to push ions or molecules into or out of a cell.

Recall Activity

1. Globular proteins form _____ that allow select molecules to move through the plasma membrane.

2. What molecules move through the plasma membrane via protein channels? _____

_____

Concept 8: Aquaporin Channels

aquaporin a protein tunnel embedded in the phospholipid bilayer that helps water move into or out of the cell

Water molecules move through the lipid barrier as well as through aquaporins when entering or exiting a cell. *Aquaporins* are proteins embedded in the phospholipid bilayer. Aquaporins form tunnels that help water move into or out of the cell. The aquaporin tunnel helps protect water molecules—which are polar, charged, and hydrophilic—from the lipid barrier.

Recall Activity

1. _____ form tunnels that help water move into or out of the cell.

2. Aquaporin tunnels help protect water molecules from the _____.

Concept 9: Carrier Proteins

carrier a protein that spans the phospholipid bilayer and moves large molecules, such as amino acids and glucose, through the plasma membrane

Some molecules pass through the plasma membrane via carriers. *Carriers* are proteins that span the phospholipid bilayer and move large molecules through the plasma membrane. These large molecules, such as amino acids and glucose, bind with the carrier proteins and move through the plasma membrane, bypassing the lipid barrier.

Recall Activity

1. _____ are proteins that span the phospholipid bilayer and move

_____ molecules through the plasma membrane.

2. Which large molecules bind with carrier proteins to pass through the plasma membrane?

_____

Concept 10: Solute Pumps

solute pump a protein in the phospholipid bilayer that uses energy to move specific ions into or out of a cell

All of the methods of moving through the plasma membrane that have been discussed so far do not require energy. Sometimes, however, molecules require energy to enter or exit a cell. These molecules enter or exit through *solute pumps*. Solute pumps are proteins and are similar to carrier proteins in size. They are

located in the phospholipid bilayer and use energy to move specific ions into
or out of a cell (Figure 7.2).

Recall Activity

1. Sometimes molecules require _____ to enter or exit a cell.

2. _____ are located in the phospholipid bilayer and use energy to move specific ions into or out of a cell.

Section 7.1 Reinforcement

Answer the following questions using what you learned in this section.

1. Unscramble the letters: runparaqoi. Define the word that is formed. _____

   _____

2. Aquaporins are tunnels that help _____ move into or out of a cell.

3. Which of the following molecules are lipid soluble?

   A. oxygen   C. carbon dioxide   E. glucose

   B. sodium ion   D. amino acid

4. List two molecules that bind with carrier proteins to bypass the lipid barrier. _____

   _____

5. *True or False.* Hydrophobic and nonpolar molecules are lipid soluble. _____

6. The _____ bilayer is selectively permeable.

7. *True or False.* Some globular proteins form channels that allow movement into or out of the cell. _____

8. The _____ portion of the phospholipid bilayer acts as a barrier to molecules that are not lipid soluble.

9. Which of the following molecules are hydrophilic?

   A. calcium ion   C. lipid-soluble   D. carbon dioxide

   B. chloride ion   vitamin

10. *True or False.* Nonpolar and hydrophobic molecules can move through the lipid barrier. _____

11. Which of the following is a waste product that exits a cell?

    A. ion   C. carbon dioxide

    B. oxygen   D. glucose

12. Can hydrophobic molecules move through the lipid barrier? Explain. _____

    _____

13. Which of the following channels allows ions to enter and exit the cell?

    A. aquaporin   C. carrier

    B. protein channel

14. The glucose that enters a cell is used in _____.

15. Which of the following is *not* a waste product that moves out of the cell?
    A. carbon dioxide   C. glucose
    B. nitrogen

16. Which of the following words are misspelled?
    A. hydorphillic   C. soluble
    B. aquaporin   D. permiable

17. *True or False.* Large, polar molecules pass through the plasma membrane via protein channels. _____

18. Nitrogen waste must move _____ the cell through the plasma membrane.

19. Unscramble the letters: dryhcholipi. Define the word that is formed. _____
    _____

20. Because the plasma membrane is selectively _____, only certain materials can enter or leave the cell.

21. Molecules that are _____ soluble can pass through the lipid barrier.

22. _____ use energy to move specific ions into or out of a cell.

Match the following terms with their definitions.

_____ 23. Proteins that help water enter or exit a cell

_____ 24. Capable of being dissolved

_____ 25. Proteins that allow large molecules to move through the plasma membrane

_____ 26. Proteins that use energy to pump ions into or out of a cell

A. soluble
B. carriers
C. aquaporins
D. solute pumps

Comprehensive Review (Chapters 1–7)

Answer the following questions using what you have learned so far in this book.

27. The liquid inside a cell's nucleus is called _____.

28. Identify and define the prefix in the term *homogeneous*. _____

29. *True or False.* In a nucleotide, purine bases always pair with other purine bases. _____

30. What is the mass of 250 mL of water in kilograms? _____

31. In what four ways can molecules that are not lipid soluble pass through the plasma membrane?
    _____

32. A fact is a(n) _____ observation.

33. Science utilizes different types of _____, or facts that relate to a possible cause.

Section 7.2 Areas of High and Low Concentration

Movement through the plasma membrane operates on the principle that atoms move from areas of high concentration to areas of low concentration. In this section, you will review concentration and learn about downhill and uphill reactions.

The terms below are some of those that will be introduced in Section 7.2. To become familiar with these terms, reproduce each word on the line beside it. Pronounce each term as you write it. You will learn the definitions of these words as you complete this section.

1. concentration gradient _____

2. downhill reaction _____

3. equilibrium _____

4. uphill reaction _____

Concept 1: Reviewing Concentration

In Section 4.8, you learned about the concept of concentration. *Concentration* refers to the number of atoms per one unit of volume. The drawings in **Figure 7.3** represent beakers filled with water (one unit of volume). The purple dots represent atoms dissolved in the water, illustrating concentration.

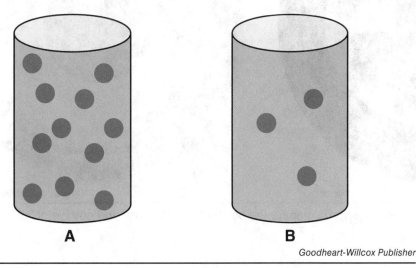

A   B

Goodheart-Willcox Publisher

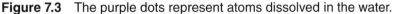

Figure 7.3 The purple dots represent atoms dissolved in the water.

Recall Activity

Concept 2: Comparing Concentrations

Cell functions depend on the concentration of atoms *inside* the cell compared to the concentration of atoms *outside* the cell. To help visualize this, imagine concentration as air pressure. *Air pressure* is the concentration of atoms (primarily nitrogen) that make up air. The pressure of air at sea level is 14.7 lbs/in². However, in a tire, an air compressor concentrates atoms so that the inside of the tire has an air pressure of 32 lbs/in². The air pressure inside the tire is greater than the air pressure outside the tire. In this analogy, the tire is the cell's plasma membrane (**Figure 7.4**).

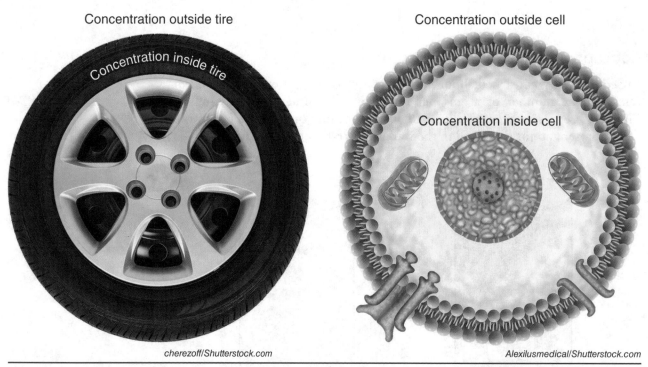

Concentration outside tire

Concentration inside tire

Concentration outside cell

Concentration inside cell

cherezoff/Shutterstock.com

Alexilusmedical/Shutterstock.com

Figure 7.4 In discussing cell functions, you compare the concentrations inside and outside of a cell. The cell can be visualized as a tire.

Recall Activity

1. The air pressure outside a tire is _____, and the air pressure inside the tire is

   _____.

2. In this analogy, the tire is the cell's _____.

Concept 3: Concentration Gradient

The difference between concentrations inside the plasma membrane and outside the plasma membrane is called the *concentration gradient*. You can picture the concentration gradient as a hill, with high concentration at the top of the hill and low concentration at the bottom of the hill (**Figure 7.5**). The greater the difference in concentration, the steeper the gradient will be.

concentration gradient the difference between concentrations inside the plasma membrane and outside the plasma membrane

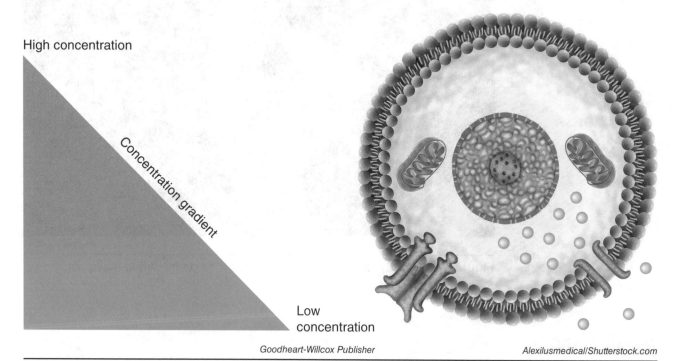

High concentration

Concentration gradient

Low concentration

Goodheart-Willcox Publisher

Alexilusmedical/Shutterstock.com

Figure 7.5   The air pressure inside a tire is greater than the air pressure outside the tire. The larger this difference, the steeper the concentration gradient is. Similarly, the greater the difference between concentrations inside the plasma membrane and outside the plasma membrane, the steeper the concentration gradient will be. In the case of this cell, concentration is higher inside the plasma membrane than outside.

Recall Activity

1. What is the concentration gradient? _____

   _____

2. At the top of the hill, the concentration is _____ than at the bottom of the hill.

Concept 4: Moving Between Concentrations

In the analogy of the tire, air is in high concentration inside the tire and in low concentration outside the tire. Because of this, opening a tire's valve causes air to move *out* of the tire, from high concentration inside the tire to low concentration outside the tire (**Figure 7.6**). This same concept is true of the cell's plasma membrane. Atoms tend to move through the plasma membrane from areas of *high* concentration to areas of *low* concentration.

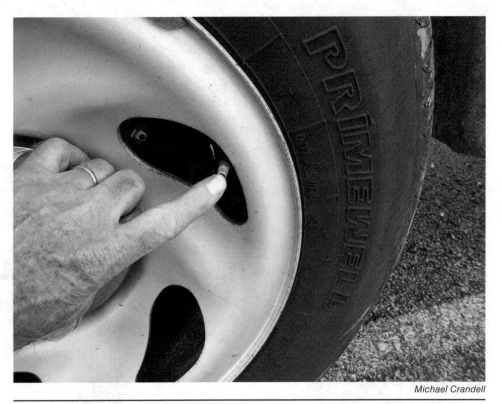

Michael Crandell

Figure 7.6 Opening a tire's valve allows the air inside the tire to move out.

Recall Activity

1. Opening a tire's valve causes air to move _____ the tire.

2. Atoms tend to move through the plasma membrane from areas of _____ concentration to areas of _____ concentration.

Concept 5: High to Low Concentration

As you learned in Section 4.8, atoms are constantly moving and colliding. If there is nothing preventing the movement of atoms, atoms will always move from areas where there are more of them (areas of high concentration) to areas where there are fewer of them (areas of low concentration). This movement down the concentration gradient, from high concentration to low concentration, is a *downhill reaction* (**Figure 7.7**). Because atoms naturally tend to move from areas of high concentration to areas of low concentration, no energy input is required for this type of reaction.

downhill reaction the movement of atoms down the concentration gradient, from high concentration to low concentration; does not require energy

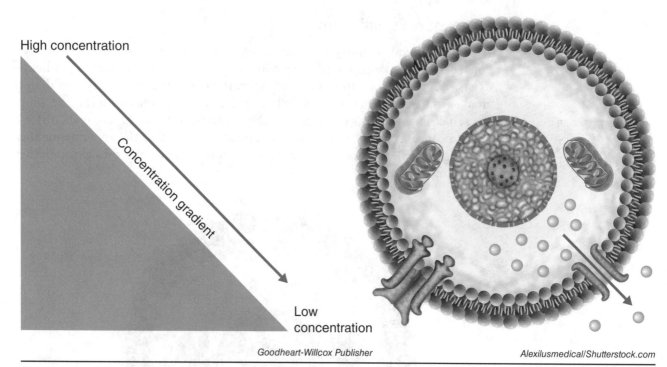

Figure 7.7 In a downhill reaction, atoms move *down* the concentration gradient—from areas of high concentration to areas of low concentration.

Recall Activity

1. In the space below, draw a concentration gradient and label the high and low concentrations. Draw an arrow to illustrate a downhill reaction.

2. Movement from an area of high concentration to an area of low concentration is called a(n) _____ reaction.

3. Because atoms naturally tend to move from areas of high concentration to areas of low concentration, no _____ is required for this type of reaction.

Concept 6: Equilibrium

Atoms will tend to move from areas of high concentration to areas of low concentration as long as a difference in concentration (concentration gradient) exists. As time passes and as atoms move, the concentration gradient will get smaller until the concentrations on both sides of the plasma membrane become the same. This state is known as *equilibrium*. In equilibrium, there is *no* difference in concentration between the area inside the cell and the area outside the cell (**Figure 7.8**). As such, there will be no net movement of atoms through the plasma membrane.

equilibrium a state in which concentrations on both sides of the plasma membrane are equal

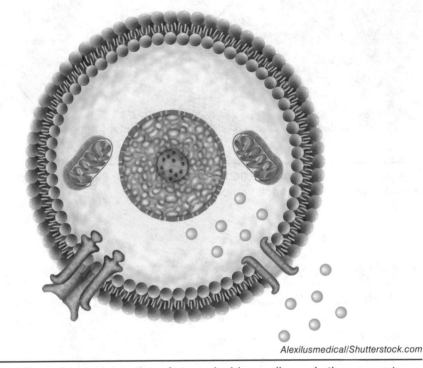

Alexilusmedical/Shutterstock.com

Figure 7.8 Once the concentration of atoms inside a cell equals the concentration of atoms outside the cell, equilibrium has been achieved.

Recall Activity

1. Atoms will move from areas of high concentration to areas of low concentration as long as a(n) _____ in concentration exists.

2. In _____, the concentrations on both sides of the plasma membrane are equal.

Concept 7: Low to High Concentration

If you are standing at the top of a hill and want to get to the bottom, it takes no energy input to roll to the bottom. However, if you are at the bottom of a hill and want to get to the top, you must exert energy. You cannot lie down at the bottom of the hill and expect to roll up.

The same is true for atoms. Because atoms tend to move from areas of high concentration to areas of low concentration, a downhill reaction requires no energy input. Energy input is, however, required for atoms to move from areas of *low* concentration to areas of *high* concentration. When atoms move from areas of low concentration to areas of high concentration, this is an *uphill reaction*. You will learn more about uphill reactions in Section 7.6.

uphill reaction the movement of atoms up the concentration gradient, from low concentration to high concentration; requires energy

Recall Activity

1. In the space below, draw a concentration gradient and label the high and low concentrations. Draw an arrow to illustrate an uphill reaction.

2. If you are at the bottom of a hill and want to get to the top, you must exert _____.

3. It takes energy input for atoms to move from areas of _____ concentration to areas of _____ concentration.

Section 7.2 Reinforcement

Answer the following questions using what you learned in this section.

1. *True or False.* If there is no difference between concentrations inside the cell and outside the cell, atoms will not tend to move through the plasma membrane. _____

2. Moving from an area of _____ concentration to an area of _____ concentration is an *uphill reaction.*

3. Compared to air pressure outside a tire, is air pressure inside the tire higher or lower? _____
_____

4. _____ refers to the number of atoms or molecules per one unit of volume.

5. In a concentration gradient, high concentration is represented at the _____ of the hill.

6. Which of the following words are misspelled?

   A. gradeint   C. concentration

   B. equalibrium

7. Atoms are constantly _____ and _____.

8. _____ is achieved when concentrations on both sides of the plasma membrane are the same.

9. Moving from an area of high concentration to an area of low concentration is called a(n) _____ reaction.

10. *True or False.* Atoms will stop moving once a difference in concentration exists. _____

11. Unscramble the letters: liquibrimue. Define the word that is formed. _____

    _____

12. *True or False.* No energy input is required to move from an area of low concentration to an area of high concentration. _____

13. It takes energy input to move _____ a hill.

14. In equilibrium, concentrations on both sides of the plasma membrane are _____.

15. Concentration refers to the number of atoms or molecules per one unit of _____.

16. Unscramble the letters: nedritag. Define the word that is formed. _____

    _____

17. *True or False.* Energy input is required for a downhill reaction. _____

18. The difference between concentrations inside a cell and outside a cell is known as a(n)

    _____.

19. Atoms naturally tend to move from areas of _____ concentration to areas of _____ concentration.

20. Energy input is required for a(n) _____ reaction.

Match the following terms with their definitions.

_____ 21. Moving from high to low concentration

_____ 22. A state in which concentrations are equal on either side of the plasma membrane

_____ 23. A difference in concentration

_____ 24. The number of atoms or molecules per one unit of volume

_____ 25. Moving from low to high concentration

A. concentration

B. concentration gradient

C. downhill reaction

D. uphill reaction

E. equilibrium

Comprehensive Review (Chapters 1–7)

Answer the following questions using what you have learned so far in this book.

26. How many protons are in a sulfur atom? _____

27. Which of the following word parts means "belly side (of the body)"?
    A. ventr/o   C. meso-
    B. dors/o   D. medi/o

28. *True or False.* The metric unit of volume is the meter. _____

29. Ions can enter or leave a cell through _____ channels.

30. List the three extensions of the plasma membrane. _____

_____

31. The _____ portion of a hypothesis is the independent variable.

32. Scientific explanations require the support of _____.

Section 7.3 Diffusion

Atoms tend to move from areas of high concentration to areas of low concentration. When atoms make this movement and spread out into areas of low concentration, this is known as *diffusion*. In this section, you will learn about diffusion and facilitated diffusion.

The terms below are some of those that will be introduced in Section 7.3. To become familiar with these terms, reproduce each word on the line beside it. Pronounce each term as you write it. You will learn the definitions of these words as you complete this section.

1. diffusion _____

2. facilitated diffusion _____

Concept 1: What Is Diffusion?

No energy input is required for atoms to move from areas of high concentration to areas of low concentration. In *diffusion*, atoms spread out from areas of high concentration into areas of low concentration. Diffusion does not require any energy—only a difference in concentration. Diffusion can happen in semisolid substances, liquids, or gases. For example, smoke atoms rise from a candle in high concentration, but as they spread out into the surrounding air, they become less concentrated and eventually are no longer visible (**Figure 7.9**). In a cell, diffusion happens when oxygen, carbon dioxide, and water move through the plasma membrane from an area of high concentration to an area of low concentration.

diffusion the spreading out of atoms from areas of high concentration into areas of low concentration

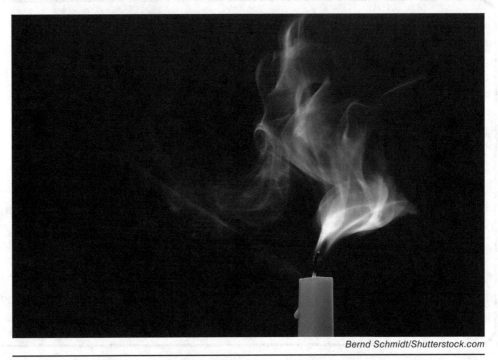

Figure 7.9 As smoke atoms disperse into the air, they become less visible.

Recall Activity

1. No energy input is required for atoms to move from areas of _____ concentration to areas of _____ concentration.

2. _____ can happen in semisolid substances, liquids, or gases.

3. As smoke atoms spread out into the air, they become _____ concentrated.

4. In a cell, diffusion happens when _____, _____, and _____ move through the plasma membrane from an area of high concentration to an area of low concentration.

Concept 2: Uniform Distribution

In diffusion, atoms spread out until they achieve *uniform distribution*, which is another way of describing equilibrium. For example, when a drop of dye is added to water, dye atoms are highly concentrated in the drop, and the surrounding water has a low concentration. Due to the constant motion of atoms, dye atoms will begin to spread out into the water (**Figure 7.10**). The dye atoms will continue to spread out until they are uniformly distributed in the water. After uniform distribution has been achieved, the dye atoms will continue to move (because atoms are constantly moving), but there will be no net movement or difference in the color of the solution because the atoms will be in equilibrium.

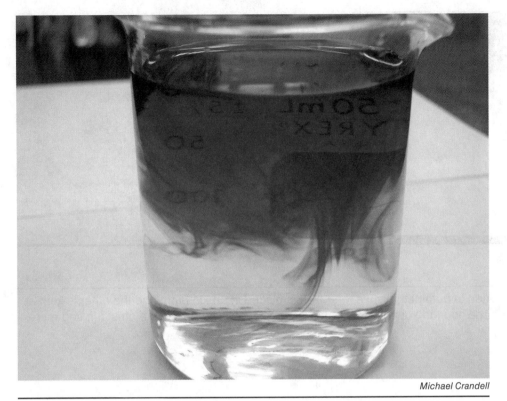

Michael Crandell

Figure 7.10 The dye atoms are spreading out into the water.

Recall Activity

1. In a drop of dye, dye atoms are _____ concentrated in the drop, and the surrounding water has a(n) _____ concentration.

2. Dye atoms will continue to spread out until they are _____ distributed in the water.

Concept 3: Effect of Temperature on Diffusion

The speed at which atoms diffuse depends on temperature. In high temperatures, atoms diffuse more quickly. In low temperatures, atoms diffuse more slowly.

The experiment in **Figure 7.11** demonstrates this phenomenon. In the experiment, dye is added to the middles of two petri dishes filled with agar (a semisolid substance through which dye can move). Once added, the dye atoms begin to spread out. One petri dish is placed in an ice bath, and the other dish is kept at room temperature. After one hour, the amount of dye movement is measured. As you can see, in the dish kept at room temperature, the dye spreads out more quickly than in the dish placed in the ice bath. This is because low temperatures cause atoms to move, and thus diffuse, more slowly.

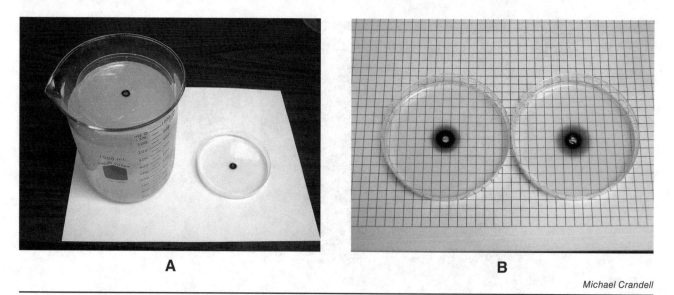

A   B

Figure 7.11 After dye is added to both petri dishes, one dish is placed in an ice bath, and the other is kept at room temperature (A). After one hour, the dishes are compared (B), revealing which dye atoms diffused more quickly.

Recall Activity

1. The speed at which atoms diffuse depends on _____.

2. In _____ temperatures, atoms diffuse more quickly.

3. In _____ temperatures, atoms diffuse more slowly.

4. In the petri dish kept at a higher temperature, the dye atoms spread out more
   _____.

5. In the petri dish kept at a lower temperature, the dye atoms spread out more
   _____.

Concept 4: Effect of Size on Diffusion

The speed at which atoms spread out also depends on size. Small atoms (atoms with small atomic masses) will diffuse more quickly than larger atoms (atoms with larger atomic masses). Similarly, small molecules containing fewer atoms will diffuse more quickly than larger molecules containing more atoms.

The experiment in **Figure 7.12** demonstrates this difference. In this experiment, three different dyes (containing molecules of different sizes) were added to one petri dish. After one hour, the dyes containing larger molecules diffused more slowly than the dyes containing smaller molecules.

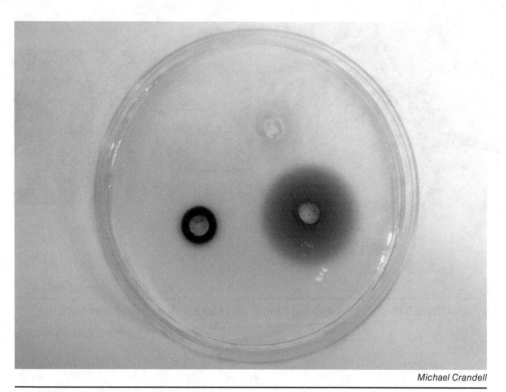

Figure 7.12 These three dyes have different molecular weights. In one hour, the dye with the smallest molecular weight spread the most quickly.

Recall Activity

1. Molecules with fewer atoms diffuse _____ than molecules with more atoms.

2. The speed at which atoms spread out depends on _____.

3. Which atom would diffuse more quickly: lithium or magnesium?_____

4. In the experiment in Figure 7.12, which dye diffused most quickly?_____

5. In the experiment in Figure 7.12, which dye diffused most slowly?_____

Concept 5: Diffusion in the Lungs

To better understand diffusion, you can envision the type of diffusion that takes place in the lungs. When you inhale, two layers of thin cells separate the air you breathe in from the blood in your lungs. Oxygen and carbon dioxide molecules easily move through these layers of cells.

Compared to your blood, the air in your lungs has a *high* concentration of oxygen. Therefore, oxygen moves from the air in your lungs into your blood. Compared to your blood, the air in your lungs has a *low* concentration of carbon dioxide. Therefore, carbon dioxide moves from your blood into the air in your lungs (**Figure 7.13**). Once this exchange has taken place, you exhale the air in your lungs, breathing out carbon dioxide.

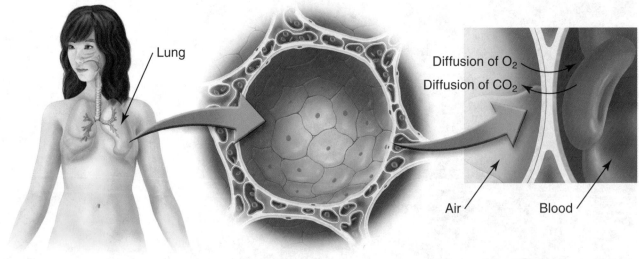

Diffusion of O₂

Diffusion of CO₂

Lung

Air

Blood

© Body Scientific International

Figure 7.13 In the lungs, oxygen diffuses from the air into the blood, and carbon dioxide diffuses from the blood into the air.

Recall Activity

1. Carbon dioxide moves from an area where it is _____ concentrated to an area where it is _____ concentrated.

2. Oxygen moves from an area where it is _____ concentrated to an area where it is _____ concentrated.

3. In the lungs, carbon dioxide diffuses from the _____ into the _____, and oxygen diffuses from the _____ into the _____.

Concept 6: Facilitated Diffusion

facilitated diffusion the spreading out of atoms from areas of high concentration into areas of low concentration through protein channels and carrier proteins in the plasma membrane

Molecules that cannot pass through the lipid barrier of the plasma membrane also diffuse in a process known as facilitated diffusion. In *facilitated diffusion*, protein channels and carrier proteins in the plasma membrane allow certain molecules to enter or leave the cell. No energy is required in facilitated diffusion because molecules are moving from areas of high concentration to areas of low concentration. Molecules that enter or leave a cell using facilitated diffusion include charged ions, such as sodium, calcium, chloride, and potassium ions, and some large molecules.

Recall Activity

1. In _____, protein channels and carrier proteins in the plasma membrane allow certain molecules to enter or leave the cell.

2. What molecules enter or leave a cell using facilitated diffusion? _____

_____

Section 7.3 Reinforcement

Answer the following questions using what you learned in this section.

1. Diffusion can happen in _____ substances, liquids, or gases.

2. *True or False.* Atoms stop moving altogether once they are uniformly distributed. _____

3. Which will diffuse more slowly: a small molecule or a large molecule? _____

4. Unscramble the letters: delittafica. Define the word that is formed. _____
_____

5. Is energy input required for atoms to move from areas of high concentration to areas of low concentration? Explain. _____

6. List two factors that affect the speed of diffusion. _____

7. *True or False.* In the lungs, carbon dioxide moves from the blood into the air. _____

8. In facilitated diffusion, _____ channels and _____ proteins in the plasma membrane allow certain molecules to enter or leave the cell.

9. As smoke atoms spread out from a candle into the surrounding air, they become less concentrated and thus less _____.

10. *True or False.* When dye atoms are uniformly distributed in water, there is no net movement of atoms in the solution. _____

11. What is the difference between diffusion and facilitated diffusion?_____
_____

12. Which atom would diffuse more quickly: hydrogen or sodium? _____

13. In the lungs, carbon dioxide moves _____ the blood _____ the air.

14. *True or False.* Ions require facilitated diffusion to move through the plasma membrane. _____

15. When a drop of dye is added to water, dye atoms are more highly concentrated in the _____ than in the water.

16. Oxygen and carbon dioxide move between the blood and the air in the lungs in a process known as _____.

17. *True or False.* Molecules containing fewer atoms diffuse more quickly than molecules containing more atoms. _____

18. No energy input is required when atoms move from areas of _____ concentration to areas of _____ concentration.

19. Which of the following words is misspelled?
    A. facilitated   C. aquaporin
    B. diffussion   D. energy

20. In the lungs, _____ moves from the air into the blood.

21. Unscramble the letters: suffinoid. Define the word that is formed. _____

_____

22. In which process do protein channels and carrier proteins in the plasma membrane allow certain molecules to enter or leave the cell? _____

23. Why does facilitated diffusion not require energy? _____

_____

Comprehensive Review (Chapters 1–7)

Answer the following questions using what you have learned so far in this book.

24. Can scientific laws be proven false? Explain. _____

_____

25. What type of bond exists between the oxygen and hydrogen atoms in a water molecule?_____

26. If 42% of people in a 200-person survey said "yes," how many people said "yes"?_____

27. Using context, you can determine that the term *hydrocephalus* refers to
_____ on the brain.

28. Which of the following is *not* a liquid?

   A. nucleoplasm   C. cytosol

   B. mitochondria   D. interstitial fluid

29. Atoms naturally tend to move from areas of _____ concentration to areas of
_____ concentration.

30. Physics, chemistry, geology, and biology are _____ of science.

Section 7.4 Osmosis

In osmosis, water passes through the plasma membrane. In this section, you will learn about osmosis and about comparing solute and solvent concentrations on either side of the plasma membrane.

The terms below are some of those that will be introduced in Section 7.4. To become familiar with these terms, reproduce each word on the line beside it. Pronounce each term as you write it. You will learn the definitions of these words as you complete this section.

1. osmosis _____   4. hypotonic_____

2. hypertonic_____   5. crenation _____

3. isotonic _____   6. lyse _____

Concept 1: What Is Osmosis?

Osmosis refers to the diffusion of water molecules through the plasma membrane. As you have learned, to enter or exit a cell, water molecules move through the phospholipid bilayer and aquaporins of a cell's plasma membrane. Atoms move from areas of high concentration to areas of low concentration. Thus, in osmosis, water molecules move through the phospholipid bilayer and aquaporins from areas with a *high* concentration of water to areas with a *low* concentration of water. As a type of diffusion, osmosis requires no energy.

osmosis a type of diffusion in which water molecules move through the phospholipid bilayer and aquaporins

Recall Activity

1. To enter or exit a cell, water molecules move through the _____ and _____ of a cell's plasma membrane.

2. In osmosis, water molecules move from areas with a(n) _____ concentration of water to areas with a(n) _____ concentration of water.

3. Why does osmosis require no energy? _____

_____

Concept 2: Solute and Solvent Concentrations

As you learned in Section 4.8, a *solution* is comprised of a solute and a solvent. The *solute* is the atoms dissolved in the solution, and the *solvent* is the liquid in which the atoms are dissolved. One example of a solution is salt water. In salt water, the solute is salt, and the solvent is water.

The concentration of a solution can be broken into the proportional concentrations of the solute and solvent. When added together, the proportional concentrations of the solute and solvent equal 100%. In the example of salt water, if the solution is 2% salt, then it will be 98% water. Salt water is present inside a cell and around a cell (**Figure 7.14**). To understand osmosis, you will compare the salt water concentrations inside and outside a cell.

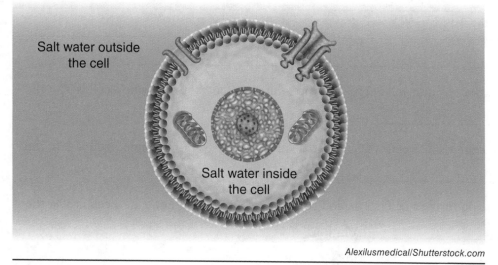

Salt water outside the cell

Salt water inside the cell

Alexilusmedical/Shutterstock.com

Figure 7.14 There is salt water inside the cell and outside the cell.

Recall Activity

1. If the solute accounts for 3% of a solution's concentration, the solvent accounts for

   _____.

2. If the solute accounts for _____ of a solution's concentration, the solvent accounts for 93%.

3. To understand osmosis, you compare the salt water concentrations _____

   and _____ a cell.

Concept 3: Hypertonic, Isotonic, and Hypotonic Solutions

The solution of salt water outside the cell can be classified as hypertonic, isotonic, or hypotonic. As you have learned, the prefix *hyper-* means "above." The combining form *is/o* means "same," and the prefix *hypo-* means "below." Knowing these word parts will help you remember the three types of solutions.

hypertonic a type of solution outside a cell that has a higher solute concentration than the solution inside a cell

isotonic a type of solution outside a cell that has the same solute concentration as the solution inside a cell

hypotonic a type of solution outside a cell that has a lower solute concentration than the solution inside a cell

The solution outside a cell is *hypertonic* if it has a solute concentration *higher* than the solute concentration inside the cell. For example, if the solute concentration inside a cell is 2%, and the solute concentration outside a cell is 4%, the cell is in a hypertonic solution. The solution outside a cell is *isotonic* if it has a solute concentration *equal to* the solute concentration inside the cell. If the solute concentration inside a cell is 2%, and the solute concentration outside a cell is 2%, the cell is in an isotonic solution. Finally, the solution outside a cell is *hypotonic* if it has a solute concentration *lower* than the solute concentration inside the cell. If the solute concentration inside a cell is 2%, and the solute concentration outside a cell is 1%, the cell is in a hypotonic solution.

Recall Activity

1. Write the meanings of the following word parts.

   hypo- _____

   is/o _____

   hyper- _____

2. If the solute concentration inside a cell is 3%, and the solute concentration outside a cell is 5%, the

   cell is in a(n) _____ solution.

3. If the solute concentration inside a cell is 3%, and the solute concentration outside a cell is 2%, the

   cell is in a(n) _____ solution.

4. If the solute concentration inside a cell is 3%, and the solute concentration outside a cell is 3%, the

   cell is in a(n) _____ solution.

Concept 4: Comparing Solute and Solvent Concentrations

If you know the solute concentration of a solution, you can calculate the solvent concentration. As you have learned, the proportional concentrations of the solute and solvent, when added together, equal 100%. If a solution has a solute concentration of 2%, the solvent concentration will be 98%. You can also write this concentration as 2/98 (solute concentration/solvent concentration). The higher the concentration of solute, the lower the solvent concentration will be.

Recall Activity

1. A solution that is 5% salt has a concentration of 5/_____.

2. A solution that is 92% water has a concentration of _____/92.

3. In the concentration 3/97, the 3 represents _____ concentration, and the 97 represents _____ concentration.

Concept 5: Movement of Water During Osmosis

During osmosis, water moves *down* the concentration gradient—that is, from areas of high water concentration to areas of low water concentration (**Figure 7.15**). For example, imagine that the salt water concentration inside a cell is 2/98, and the salt water concentration outside the cell is 4/96. The cell is in a *hypertonic* solution because the solute concentration is higher outside the cell. The water concentration inside the cell is 98%, and the water concentration outside the cell is 96%. Because of this, water will move *out of* the cell, into the area of lower water concentration. If the salt water concentration were 2/98 inside the cell and 1/99 outside the cell, water would move *into* the cell. If the salt water concentration were 2/98 inside the cell and 2/98 outside the cell, there would be no net water movement through the plasma membrane.

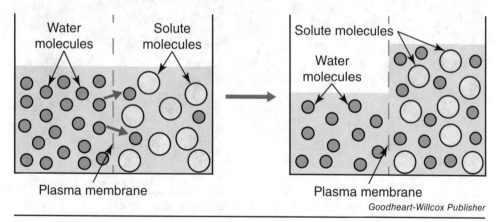

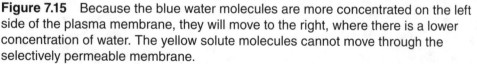

Goodheart-Willcox Publisher

Figure 7.15 Because the blue water molecules are more concentrated on the left side of the plasma membrane, they will move to the right, where there is a lower concentration of water. The yellow solute molecules cannot move through the selectively permeable membrane.

Recall Activity

1. If the salt water concentration is ²⁄₉₈ inside a cell and ³⁄₉₇ outside the cell, the cell is in a(n)

   _____ solution, and water will move _____ the cell.

2. If the salt water concentration is ²⁄₉₈ inside a cell and ¹⁄₉₉ outside the cell, the cell is in a(n)

   _____ solution, and water will move _____ the cell.

3. If the salt water concentration is ²⁄₉₈ inside a cell and ²⁄₉₈ outside the cell, the cell is in a(n)

   _____ solution, and there will be no _____ water

   movement.

4. Which of the following represents the highest water concentration?

   A. ³⁄₉₇   C. ⁶⁄₉₄

   B. ⁴⁄₉₆   D. ¹⁄₉₉

Concept 6: Effect of Osmosis on Cell Size

crenation the shrinking of a cell due to water leaving it

lyse to burst after swelling past maximum size; can occur in cells as water enters them

In osmosis, water leaves or enters a cell. If a cell is in a hypertonic solution, water will leave the cell. When water leaves a cell, the cell shrinks. This is called *crenation*. If a cell is in a hypotonic solution, water will enter the cell. When water enters a cell, the cell swells (**Figure 7.16**). However, the cell can only swell to a maximum size. If more water enters the cell after this point, the cell *lyses* (bursts).

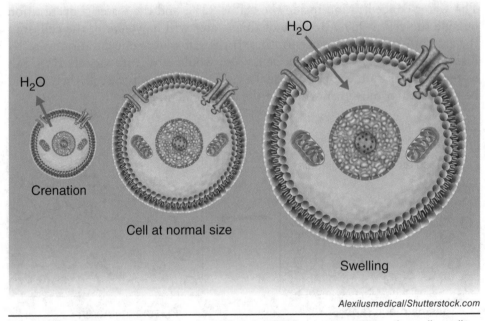

H₂O

H₂O

Crenation

Cell at normal size

Swelling

Alexilusmedical/Shutterstock.com

Figure 7.16 When water leaves, the cell shrinks. When water enters, the cell swells.

Recall Activity

1. If a cell is in a hypotonic solution, water _____ the cell.

2. Water entering a cell causes _____.

3. If a cell is in a hypertonic solution, water _____ the cell.

4. Water leaving a cell causes _____.

Section 7.4 Reinforcement

Answer the following questions using what you learned in this section.

1. Which of the following concentrations does *not* represent a solution?

   A. $\frac{2}{98}$ C. $\frac{1}{98}$

   B. $\frac{0}{100}$

2. Crenation occurs when water _____ a cell.

3. Which of the following is *not* a possible concentration for a solution?

   A. $\frac{3}{97}$ C. $\frac{2}{97}$ E. $\frac{6}{94}$

   B. $\frac{4}{96}$ D. $\frac{9}{91}$

4. Unscramble the letters: ronphicyte. Define the word that is formed. _____

   _____

5. Which of the following concentrations represents a solution hypertonic to $\frac{4}{96}$?

   A. $\frac{3}{97}$ C. $\frac{4}{96}$

   B. $\frac{6}{94}$

6. Osmosis refers to the movement of water molecules through the _____ and

   _____.

7. *True or False.* When water leaves a cell, the cell shrinks. _____

8. The combining form _____ means "same."

9. Which of the following concentrations represent solutions hypotonic to $\frac{5}{95}$?

   A. $\frac{3}{97}$ C. $\frac{4}{96}$

   B. $\frac{6}{94}$

10. *True or False.* If a cell is in a hypertonic solution, water will leave the cell. _____

11. The prefix *hyper-* means "_____."

12. Water is to solvent as salt is to _____.

13. Which of the following concentrations represents a solution isotonic to $\frac{4}{96}$?

    A. $\frac{3}{97}$ C. $\frac{4}{96}$

    B. $\frac{6}{94}$

14. In the concentration $\frac{3}{97}$, the 3 represents the concentration of the _____.

15. A cell in a hypotonic solution will gain water, causing it to _____.

16. The prefix _____ means "below."

17. *True or False.* A cell in a hypotonic solution may lyse. _____

18. To enter or exit a cell, water molecules move through the _____ and _____ of a cell's plasma membrane.

19. In the concentration 7⁄93, the 93 represents the concentration of the_____.

20. *True or False.* If a cell is in an isotonic solution, there is no concentration gradient._____

21. A solution that is 96% water has a concentration of _____/96.

22. *True or False.* Osmosis does not require energy.

Match the following terms with their definitions.

_____ 23. A solution that has a lower solute concentration as compared to another solution

_____ 24. The shrinking of a cell

_____ 25. A solution that has the same solute concentration as another solution

_____ 26. To burst

_____ 27. The water in a salt water solution

_____ 28. The salt in a salt water solution

_____ 29. A channel that helps water molecules pass through the plasma membrane

_____ 30. A solution that has a higher solute concentration as compared to another solution

A. aquaporin
B. solute
C. solvent
D. hypertonic
E. isotonic
F. hypotonic
G. lyse
H. crenation

Comprehensive Review (Chapters 1–7)

Answer the following questions using what you have learned so far in this book.

31. Calculate the surface area of a circle with a diameter 4 cm long. _____

32. Untested factors that could affect the dependent variable in an experiment are known as _____.

33. How is diffusion different from osmosis?_____

_____

34. Which of the following atoms has the largest number of electron shells?
    A. hydrogen   C. phosphorus
    B. carbon   D. nitrogen

35. *True or False.* Intermediate filaments are the most permanent part of the cytoskeleton. _____

36. The prefix *micro-* is to "small" as the prefix *hemi-* is to "_____."

37. Biology is the science that studies _____.

Section 7.5 Cell Respiration

Cell respiration is the process by which a cell produces ATP. ATP is the energy storage molecule inside a cell. In this section, you will learn about the process of cell respiration and how energy is transformed for use in a cell.

The terms below are some of those that will be introduced in Section 7.5. To become familiar with these terms, reproduce each word on the line beside it. Pronounce each term as you write it. You will learn the definitions of these words as you complete this section.

1. anabolic reaction _____

2. catabolic reaction _____

3. cell respiration _____

4. high-energy bond _____

5. lactic acid _____

Concept 1: Anabolic and Catabolic Reactions

Molecules, which are combinations of atoms, can be joined together or broken apart. Joining molecules together requires energy, whereas breaking molecules apart releases energy. In an *anabolic reaction*, molecules are joined together in a process that *requires* energy. In a *catabolic reaction*, molecules are broken apart in a process that *releases* energy (**Figure 7.17**).

anabolic reaction a reaction in which molecules are joined together, requiring energy

catabolic reaction a reaction in which molecules are broken apart, releasing energy

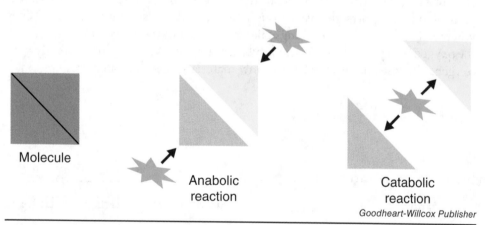

Molecule

Anabolic
reaction

Catabolic
reaction

Goodheart-Willcox Publisher

Figure 7.17 Molecules are joined together in an anabolic reaction. Molecules are broken apart in a catabolic reaction.

Recall Activity

1. Joining molecules together _____ energy, whereas breaking molecules apart

   _____ energy.

2. Molecules are joined together in a(n) _____ reaction, and molecules are

   broken apart in a(n) _____ reaction.

Concept 2: Energy Transformation

The carbohydrates you eat contain energy. Your cells and your life depend on this energy. However, this form of energy (stored in the bonds of carbohydrate molecules) cannot be used directly by a cell. In many ways, this type of energy is like a different currency. If you tried to use U.S. dollars in Japan, stores would not take your money. If you transformed your U.S. dollars into Japanese currency, however, you could make a purchase at a store. Similarly, energy from the carbohydrates you eat must be transformed for use in cells. This transformation, known as *cell respiration*, takes place around and inside the mitochondria in cells.

Recall Activity

1. If you _____ your U.S. dollars into another currency, you could make a purchase at a store in a different country.

2. Cell respiration transforms energy from the _____ you eat into a form usable by a cell.

3. Cell respiration takes place around and inside the _____ in cells.

Concept 3: Glucose and Oxygen

Cell respiration requires glucose and oxygen. When you eat carbohydrates, the cells of your digestive system break down the carbohydrates into glucose, and your blood transports glucose throughout the body to supply every cell. When you breathe, the cells of your lungs take oxygen out of the air you breathe and put the oxygen into your blood. Your blood then supplies every cell in your body with oxygen. Glucose and oxygen are two raw materials essential for cell respiration.

Recall Activity

1. Your digestive system breaks down the carbohydrates you eat into _____.

2. _____ and _____ are two raw materials essential for cell respiration.

cell respiration the process of adding one phosphate molecule (P) to one adenosine diphosphate (ADP) molecule to create adenosine triphosphate (ATP); occurs around or inside the mitochondria

high-energy bond the bond with the third phosphate molecule in ATP; is broken when the cell requires energy

Concept 4: ADP to ATP

Cell respiration is the process of creating ATP, the energy storage molecule in cells. In cell respiration, the energy from glucose is used to add one phosphate molecule (P) to one adenosine diphosphate (ADP) molecule. Adding one P to ADP forms adenosine triphosphate (ATP), and the newly formed bond with the added phosphate molecule is a *high-energy bond* (**Figure 7.18**). Transforming ADP into ATP is an anabolic reaction because, using energy, two molecules (P and ADP) are joined to form one larger molecule (ATP).

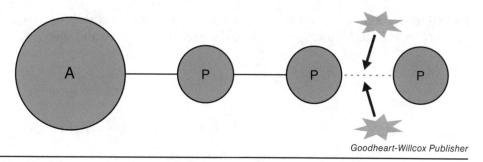

Figure 7.18 In cell respiration, ADP is transformed into ATP in an anabolic reaction. The newly formed bond (shown in red) is a high-energy bond.

Recall Activity

1. In cell respiration, one P is added to ADP, forming _____.

2. Joining P and ADP together to form ATP is a(n) _____ reaction.

Concept 5: Steps in Cell Respiration

The basic reaction of cell respiration creates ATP by adding one P to ADP. This reaction occurs in several stages. The steps of cell respiration are

- glycolysis
- prep reaction
- citric acid cycle
- electron transport chain

During *glycolysis*, glucose is broken down. At this point, cell respiration will only continue if oxygen is present. The next two steps—*prep reaction* and *citric acid cycle*—produce carbon dioxide. Carbon dioxide then leaves the cell, enters the blood, and is exhaled from the lungs. At the end of cell respiration, during the *electron transport chain* step, oxygen is used to produce water.

Recall Activity

1. The basic reaction of cell respiration creates _____ by adding one P to

_____.

2. What are the steps of cell respiration? _____

_____

3. Cell respiration will only continue past the first step if _____ is present.

Concept 6: No Oxygen

As you have learned, cell respiration cannot continue past the first step if oxygen is not present. During heavy exercise with a high demand for ATP, for example, the cardiovascular system may not be able to supply muscle cells with enough oxygen

lactic acid a product of cell respiration that begins without oxygen; can cause tiredness and soreness in muscles

for cell respiration. In this situation, muscle cells will undergo glycolysis only and produce *lactic acid*. A buildup of lactic acid makes muscles tired and sore.

Recall Activity

1. Cell respiration _____ continue past the first step if oxygen is not present.

2. A buildup of _____ makes muscles tired and sore.

Concept 7: Other Energy Sources

The primary source of energy that you consume is carbohydrates. However, cells can also use the energy in fats and protein during some steps of cell respiration. Cells use fats as a primary source of energy only when a person has not consumed enough carbohydrates, and cells use protein as a primary source of energy only if carbohydrate and fat sources are lacking.

Recall Activity

1. In addition to carbohydrates, cells can use the energy in _____ and _____ during some steps of cell respiration.

2. When will cells use protein as a primary source of energy? _____

_____

Concept 8: ATP to ADP

As you have learned, the process of cell respiration (adding one P to ADP to create ATP) forms a new phosphate bond. This newly formed phosphate bond in ATP is called a *high-energy bond*. When a cell needs energy to push atoms from areas of *low* concentration to areas of *high* concentration (uphill reaction), the high-energy bond in ATP is broken. This catabolic reaction releases energy, which pushes atoms up the concentration gradient (**Figure 7.19**). The uphill reactions fueled by this energy are important for muscle contraction and nerve impulse transmission, among other functions.

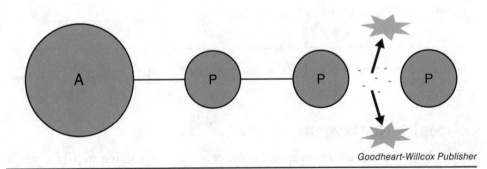

Goodheart-Willcox Publisher

Figure 7.19 When cells need energy for uphill reactions, the high-energy bond formed during cell respiration is broken, releasing energy.

Recall Activity

1. When energy is required, the _____ bond in ATP is broken.

2. Breaking one of ATP's bonds is a(n) _____ reaction.

Section 7.5 Reinforcement

Answer the following questions using what you learned in this section.

1. The raw materials needed for cell respiration include one adenosine diphosphate molecule, one phosphate molecule, _____, and _____.

2. What happens to molecules in an anabolic reaction? _____

   _____

3. Which of the following is *not* a step in cell respiration?
   - A. glycolysis
   - B. prep reaction
   - C. breaking the high-energy bond
   - D. citric acid cycle

4. The _____ required for cell respiration comes from the air you breathe.

5. *True or False.* Joining molecules together requires energy, and breaking molecules apart releases energy. _____

6. A catabolic reaction _____ energy.

7. *True or False.* Cell respiration takes place inside the mitochondria of some, but not all, cells. _____

8. Your digestive system breaks down the _____ you consume into glucose.

9. In a(n) _____ reaction, molecules are broken apart.

10. *True or False.* Adding one P to ADP to create ATP is a catabolic reaction. _____

11. Breaking molecules apart _____ energy.

12. If muscle cells begin to undergo cell respiration without enough oxygen, they will produce _____.

13. An anabolic reaction is to requiring energy as a(n) _____ is to releasing energy.

14. When energy is required for uphill reactions, ATP is broken apart into _____ and _____.

15. List the steps in cell respiration. _____

   _____

16. *True or False.* Oxygen is required to transform ADP into ATP. _____

17. List two effects of lactic acid on muscles. _____

18. Joining ADP and P forms ATP, and the newly formed bond with the added P is a(n) _____ bond.

19. *True or False.* After being produced by cell respiration, carbon dioxide leaves the cell, enters the blood, and is exhaled from the lungs. _____

20. *True or False.* Cells use fats as a primary source of energy only if protein sources are lacking. _____

21. The energy from the carbohydrates you eat is used to make ATP by joining _____ and _____.

22. Breaking the high-energy bond in ATP releases energy, which pushes atoms _____ the concentration gradient.

Match the following terms with their definitions.

_____ 23. Breaking a molecule apart

_____ 24. A product of muscle cells undergoing glycolysis only

_____ 25. Joining molecules together

A. anabolic reaction
B. catabolic reaction
C. lactic acid

Comprehensive Review (Chapters 1–7)

Answer the following questions using what you have learned so far in this book.

26. *True or False.* There is one universal scientific method. _____

27. The chemical formula $2C_6H_{14}$ represents _____ carbon atom(s) and _____ hydrogen atom(s).

28. What is the function of solute pumps in the plasma membrane? _____
_____

29. What are the three basic parts of a cell? _____

30. Which of the following prefixes represents the smallest number?
    A. tetra-   C. hexa-
    B. tri-   D. di-

31. When using a graduated cylinder, you should read the measurement at the _____ of the meniscus.

32. If you are having trouble concentrating, try _____ your study location, time, duration, or method.

Section 7.6 Energy-Required Reactions

Thus far in this chapter, you have learned about movement through the plasma membrane that requires no energy. In this section, you will learn about movement through the plasma membrane that *does* require energy.

The following terms are some of those that will be introduced in Section 7.6. To become familiar with these terms, reproduce each word on the line beside it. Pronounce each term as you write it. You will learn the definitions of these words as you complete this section.

1. active transport _____

2. exocytosis _____

3. endocytosis _____

4. phagocytosis _____

5. pinocytosis _____

6. receptor-mediated endocytosis _____

Concept 1: Uphill Reactions

As you learned in Section 7.2, an *uphill reaction* occurs when atoms move from areas of *low* concentration to areas of *high* concentration. Because atoms naturally tend to do the opposite of this, energy is required to move up the concentration gradient (**Figure 7.20**).

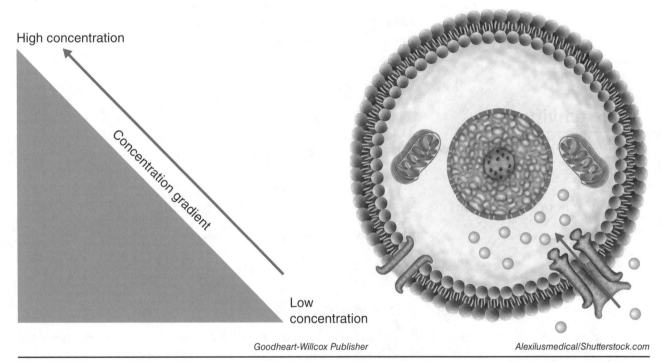

High concentration

Concentration gradient

Low concentration

Goodheart-Willcox Publisher   Alexilusmedical/Shutterstock.com

Figure 7.20 An uphill reaction occurs when atoms move from areas of low concentration to areas of high concentration.

The energy required for an uphill reaction is produced by breaking a phosphate bond on adenosine triphosphate (ATP). ATP consists of one adenosine molecule plus three phosphates (A-P-P-P). Breaking one of ATP's phosphate bonds results in the molecule ADP (A-P-P) plus one phosphate. This catabolic reaction releases energy to push atoms from areas of low concentration to areas of high concentration.

Recall Activity

1. _____ is required for atoms to move from areas of low concentration to areas of high concentration.

2. The energy required for an uphill reaction is produced by _____ a(n) _____ bond on ATP.

3. ATP consists of one _____ molecule plus three _____.

4. What molecule is formed when one of ATP's phosphate bonds is broken? _____

Concept 2: Active Transport

active transport the movement of atoms from areas of low concentration to areas of high concentration using solute pumps; requires energy

As you have learned, energy is not required for diffusion, facilitated diffusion, or osmosis. Energy is, however, required for atoms to move from areas of low concentration to areas of high concentration. In *active transport*, a cell moves atoms uphill (from areas of low concentration to areas of high concentration) using solute pumps, which require energy to operate.

One example of active transport is the pumping of Ca^{++} ions, which are involved in muscle cell contraction. Solute pumps in muscle cells use energy from breaking ATP to push Ca^{++} ions uphill, into a storage area where they are in high concentration. Another example of active transport is the sodium-potassium pump, which you will learn about in the next section.

Recall Activity

1. In active transport, a cell moves atoms _____ using _____.

2. Solute pumps in muscle cells use _____ from breaking _____ to push Ca^{++} ions uphill.

Concept 3: Exocytosis

exocytosis a type of energy-required reaction in which atoms are moved out of a cell

Another reaction that requires energy is exocytosis. In *exocytosis*, atoms are moved out of a cell. One example of exocytosis is the movement of proteins out of a cell. Inside the cell, proteins are produced and transported to the *Golgi*. The Golgi packages proteins into *secretory vesicles*, which then travel toward the plasma membrane. The membrane of the secretory vesicle fuses with the plasma membrane, and then the phospholipids of the plasma membrane and the vesicle membrane separate, releasing the contents of the vesicle (proteins) outside the cell (**Figure 7.21**).

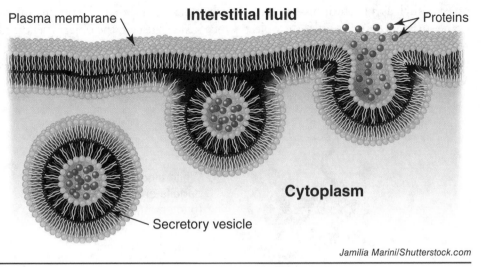

Plasma membrane

Interstitial fluid

Proteins

Cytoplasm

Secretory vesicle

Jamilia Marini/Shutterstock.com

Figure 7.21 In exocytosis, materials are moved out of a cell.

Recall Activity

1. Atoms are moved out of a cell in _____.

2. *True or False.* Exocytosis requires energy. _____

3. To release proteins, the phospholipids of the plasma membrane and the vesicle membrane fuse and then _____.

Concept 4: Endocytosis

Energy is also required for endocytosis. In *endocytosis*, atoms are brought into a cell. There are three types of endocytosis:

- phagocytosis
- pinocytosis
- receptor-mediated endocytosis

In the next few concepts, you will learn about the types of endocytosis.

endocytosis a type of energy-required reaction in which atoms are brought into a cell

Recall Activity

1. In _____, atoms are brought into a cell.

2. Endocytosis requires _____.

3. What are the three types of endocytosis? _____

_____

Concept 5: Phagocytosis

The first type of endocytosis is phagocytosis. *Phagocytosis* is also known as *cell eating*. In phagocytosis, a cell forms a pocket in its plasma membrane. An

phagocytosis a type of endocytosis in which the plasma membrane of a cell surrounds and engulfs an object; also known as *cell eating*

object—such as a bacterium—is fitted into the pocket, and then the plasma membrane surrounds and engulfs the object. Once inside the cell, the object is encased within a membrane, where it is broken down by enzymes and then expelled out of the cell (**Figure 7.22**). One example of a cell that uses phagocytosis is a *phagocyte*. Your blood contains phagocytes, which protect your body by eating bacteria.

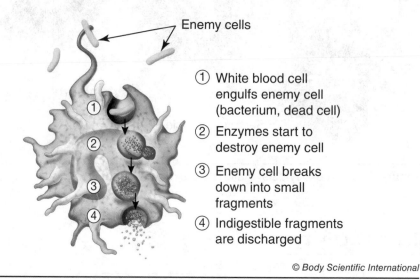

1. White blood cell engulfs enemy cell (bacterium, dead cell)
2. Enzymes start to destroy enemy cell
3. Enemy cell breaks down into small fragments
4. Indigestible fragments are discharged

© Body Scientific International

Figure 7.22 In phagocytosis, materials move into a cell, where they are broken down and then expelled.

Recall Activity

1. Phagocytosis is also known as _____.

2. In phagocytosis, the cell forms a(n) _____ to surround and engulf an object.

3. Your blood contains _____, which protect your body by eating bacteria.

pinocytosis a type of endocytosis in which the plasma membrane of a cell surrounds and engulfs a liquid containing atoms; also known as *cell drinking*

Concept 6: Pinocytosis

Another type of endocytosis is pinocytosis. In *pinocytosis*, a liquid containing atoms is brought inside a cell. Pinocytosis is similar to phagocytosis in that the plasma membrane forms a pocket and surrounds the liquid, encasing the liquid in a membrane within the cell. Pinocytosis is also called *cell drinking*.

Recall Activity

1. In pinocytosis, a(n) _____ containing atoms is brought inside a cell.

2. How is pinocytosis similar to phagocytosis? _____

_____

_____

3. Pinocytosis is also called _____.

Concept 7: Receptor-Mediated Endocytosis

The third type of endocytosis is receptor-mediated endocytosis. In *receptor-mediated endocytosis*, only certain substances can enter a cell. To enter, a substance must bind with a specific protein within a pit in the phospholipid bilayer. Once the substance binds, the neck of the pit closes and creates a vesicle inside the cell. Substances that can bind to these proteins and enter a cell include iron, enzymes, and insulin. Some disease-causing agents, such as viruses and bacterial toxins, may also enter this way.

receptor-mediated endocytosis a type of endocytosis in which a substance binds to a specific protein in a pit of the phospholipid bilayer and is brought into the cell inside a vesicle

Recall Activity

1. In _____, only certain substances can enter a cell.

2. To enter, a substance must bind with a specific protein within a(n) _____ in the phospholipid bilayer.

3. List the three types of endocytosis. _____

_____

Section 7.6 Reinforcement

Answer the following questions using what you learned in this section.

1. ATP consists of one _____ molecule plus three _____.

2. *True or False.* In endocytosis, atoms are moved out of a cell. _____

3. Which of the following is *not* a type of endocytosis?

   A. pinocytosis   C. exocytosis

   B. phagocytosis

4. _____ pumps in muscle cells use _____ from breaking ATP to push Ca^{++} ions uphill.

5. Phagocytosis is a type of _____.

6. _____ is also called *cell eating*.

7. *True or False.* Active transport requires energy. _____

8. Unscramble the letters: stoondycise. Define the word that is formed. _____

_____

9. List the three types of endocytosis. _____

_____

10. *True or False.* Atoms are moved out of a cell in exocytosis. _____

11. Which of the following words are misspelled?

    A. endocytosis   C. pintocyotis

    B. entocytosis   D. exocytoses

12. Pinocytosis is also called *cell* _____.

13. How is receptor-mediated endocytosis different from phagocytosis and pinocytosis? _____
    _____
    _____

14. How is active transport different from facilitated diffusion? _____
    _____

15. Substances bind to proteins in a pit of the phospholipid bilayer during _____
    endocytosis.

16. Pinocytosis is type of _____.

17. In exocytosis, the Golgi packages proteins into _____ to leave a cell.

18. The energy released by breaking one of ATP's _____ bonds pushes atoms
    from areas of low concentration to areas of high concentration.

Match the following terms with their definitions.

_____ 19. An energy-required reaction of moving atoms into a cell

_____ 20. A type of endocytosis in which certain atoms bind to
             proteins in the pit of the phospholipid bilayer

_____ 21. Cell eating

_____ 22. Cell drinking

_____ 23. An energy-required reaction of moving atoms out of a cell

_____ 24. The movement of atoms from areas of low concentration
             to areas of high concentration using solute pumps

A. active transport
B. exocytosis
C. endocytosis
D. phagocytosis
E. pinocytosis
F. receptor-mediated
   endocytosis

Comprehensive Review (Chapters 1–7)

Answer the following questions using what you have learned so far in this book.

25. The "then" portion of a hypothesis is the _____ variable.

26. If a platform scale reads 200 g, 70 g, and 2.3 g, the mass of the object being weighed is
    _____.

27. *True or False.* The mitochondrion is the powerhouse of a cell. _____

28. Atoms that have donated or accepted electrons so that the numbers of protons and electrons are
    unequal are called _____.

29. *True or False.* The prefixes *tetra-* and *quadri-* both mean "four." _____

30. What happens during osmosis? _____
    _____

31. A(n) _____ is a word or phrase that can help you recall information.

Section 7.7 Maintaining Homeostasis

For a cell to survive, it must maintain a state of relative stability, known as *homeostasis*. Many of the physiological processes you have learned about so far in this chapter help the cell maintain homeostasis. In this section, you will learn about homeostasis and how it is achieved.

The terms below are some of those that will be introduced in Section 7.7. To become familiar with these terms, reproduce each word on the line beside it. Pronounce each term as you write it. You will learn the definitions of these words as you complete this section.

1. homeostasis _____

2. sodium-potassium pump _____

3. protein buffer _____

Concept 1: Homeostasis

A major function of a cell's physiology is maintaining homeostasis. The cell is the basic unit of life, but life can only exist within a narrow range of circumstances. For life to continue, cells must maintain *homeostasis*, which is a state of relative stability. The environment around a cell can constantly change, but the internal state of a cell must remain *constant* for the cell to live. Cells maintain homeostasis by adjusting the concentrations of certain ions inside the cell.

homeostasis a state of relative stability

Recall Activity

1. _____ is a state of relative stability.

2. The internal state of a cell must remain _____ for the cell to live.

3. Cells maintain homeostasis by _____ the concentrations of certain ions inside the cell.

Concept 2: Sodium and Potassium in Homeostasis

For a cell to function, it must maintain homeostasis in the concentrations of sodium ions (Na^+) and potassium ions (K^+) inside the cell. In homeostasis, sodium ions are in high concentration outside a cell and in low concentration inside a cell. Potassium ions are in high concentration inside a cell and in low concentration outside a cell (**Figure 7.23**). However, facilitated diffusion causes sodium ions to enter a cell (moving from high to low concentration) and potassium ions to leave a cell (moving from high to low concentration). The gain of sodium ions and the loss of potassium ions disrupt the homeostasis of sodium and potassium concentrations inside the cell.

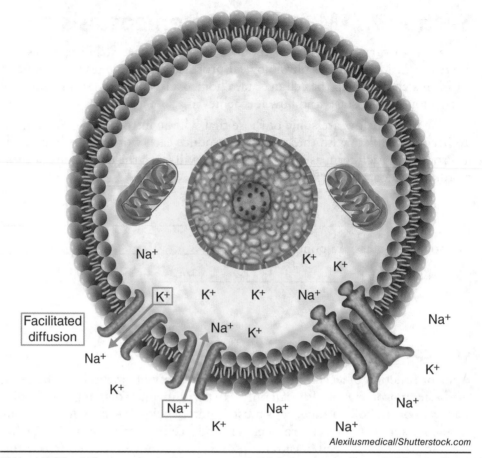

Figure 7.23 In homeostasis, Na⁺ ions are in high concentration outside a cell, but low concentration inside a cell. K⁺ ions are in high concentration inside a cell, but low concentration outside a cell. Facilitated diffusion, however, causes sodium ions to enter a cell and potassium ions to leave a cell.

Recall Activity

1. Because of facilitated diffusion, sodium ions _____ a cell, and potassium ions _____ a cell.

2. In facilitated diffusion, both sodium and potassium ions move from areas of _____ concentration to areas of _____ concentration.

3. In homeostasis, sodium ions are in high concentration _____ the cell, and potassium ions are in high concentration _____ the cell.

4. The gain of sodium ions and the loss of potassium ions disrupt the _____ of sodium and potassium concentrations inside the cell.

Concept 3: Sodium-Potassium Pump

With sodium ions constantly entering and potassium ions constantly leaving a cell, you can see that the cell must do something to maintain homeostasis.

A cell maintains proper concentrations of sodium and potassium with the *sodium-potassium pump*, which uses energy to push sodium ions *out* of the cell and potassium ions *into* the cell (**Figure 7.24**). Because sodium and potassium ions are constantly diffusing through protein channels in the plasma membrane, the sodium-potassium pump must constantly pump ions uphill to maintain homeostasis inside the cell.

sodium-potassium pump a solute pump in the plasma membrane that uses energy to pump sodium ions out of a cell and potassium ions into a cell

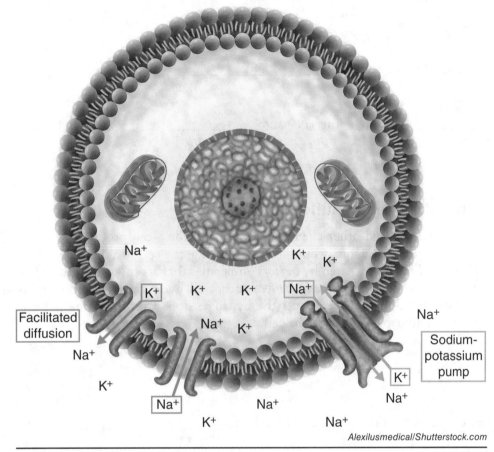

Alexilusmedical/Shutterstock.com

Figure 7.24 The sodium-potassium pump maintains homeostasis inside the cell.

Recall Activity

1. If the sodium-potassium pump does not pump, as time passes, will the number of sodium ions inside the cell increase or decrease? _____

2. If the sodium-potassium pump does not pump, as time passes, will the number of potassium ions inside the cell increase or decrease? _____

3. *True or False.* The sodium-potassium pump must constantly pump to maintain homeostasis. _____

4. Does pushing sodium ions out of the cell and potassium ions into the cell require energy? _____

Concept 4: pH in Homeostasis

Another concentration that must remain constant inside a cell is pH. As you have learned, *pH* is the measurement of acid or base in a liquid. In homeostasis, the pH inside a cell is between 7.0 and 7.4. The numbers of hydrogen ions (H^+) and hydroxide ions (OH^-) inside a cell affect pH.

Recall Activity

1. In homeostasis, the pH inside a cell is between _____ and _____.

2. The numbers of _____ ions (H^+) and _____ ions (OH^-) inside a cell affect pH.

Concept 5: Protein Buffers

protein buffer a protein molecule that accepts all hydrogen ions produced by chemical reactions inside a cell

Cell respiration and other chemical reactions inside a cell produce hydrogen ions. In excess, these ions would lower pH inside the cell to a dangerous level below 7.0. This is prevented by *buffers* (molecules that accept or donate hydrogen ions). Inside a cell, *protein buffers* accept all hydrogen ions produced in chemical reactions. This prevents the hydrogen ions from lowering pH and maintains homeostasis inside the cell.

Recall Activity

1. Cell respiration and other chemical reactions inside a cell produce _____ ions.

2. In excess, hydrogen ions would _____ pH inside the cell to a dangerous level _____ 7.0.

3. Inside a cell, protein buffers accept all _____ ions produced in _____.

Section 7.7 Reinforcement

Answer the following questions using what you learned in this section.

1. What is homeostasis? _____

2. Life can only exist within a(n) _____ range of circumstances.

3. In homeostasis, the pH inside a cell is between _____ and _____.

4. Unscramble the letters: frubef. Define the word that is formed. _____

_____

5. Which of the following words are misspelled?
   A. homeostasis
   B. protien
   C. potasium
   D. concentration

6. Because of facilitated diffusion, sodium ions are constantly _____ a cell.

7. *True or False.* Energy is required to pump potassium ions out of a cell. _____

8. In homeostasis, sodium ions are in _____ concentration outside a cell and in _____ concentration inside a cell. Potassium ions are in _____ concentration inside a cell and in _____ concentration outside a cell.

9. Inside a cell, _____ buffers accept all hydrogen ions produced in chemical reactions.

10. *True or False.* In homeostasis, the pH inside a cell is between 6.0 and 6.4. _____

11. Does adding hydrogen ions to a liquid lower or raise the pH value? _____

12. Write the letters backward: sisatsoemoh. Define the word that is formed. _____

_____

13. How does facilitated diffusion disrupt the homeostasis of sodium and potassium concentrations inside a cell? _____

_____

14. Cells maintain _____ by adjusting the concentrations of certain ions inside the cell.

15. The environment around a cell can constantly change, but the internal state of a cell must remain _____ for the cell to live.

16. The sodium-potassium pump uses energy to push sodium ions _____ the cell and potassium ions _____ the cell.

17. *True or False.* Energy is not required for a cell to maintain homeostasis in the concentrations of sodium and potassium ions. _____

18. Would too few or too many hydrogen ions lower the pH inside a cell to a dangerous level below 7.0?

_____

19. *True or False.* The sodium-potassium pump pumps only when homeostasis has been severely disrupted. _____

20. Sodium and potassium ions diffuse through _____ in the plasma membrane.

21. Protein _____ maintain the homeostasis of pH inside a cell.

Match the following terms with their definitions.

_____ 22. A molecule that can accept or donate hydrogen ions

_____ 23. The process by which sodium ions enter a cell and potassium ions leave a cell

_____ 24. A state of relative stability

_____ 25. The solute pump that pushes potassium ions into a cell and sodium ions out of a cell

_____ 26. An ion that, in homeostasis, is in low concentration inside a cell

_____ 27. An ion that, in homeostasis, is in high concentration inside a cell

A. homeostasis
B. buffer
C. sodium ion
D. potassium ion
E. facilitated diffusion
F. sodium-potassium pump

Comprehensive Review (Chapters 1–7)

Answer the following questions using what you have learned so far in this book.

28. Which subatomic particle is involved in bonding? _____

29. *True or False.* Chromosomes and chromatin are different forms of the same DNA. _____

30. Which of the following prefixes mean "toward"?
    A. ad-   C. ex-   E. ef-
    B. epi-   D. af-

31. Which of the following does *not* require energy?
    A. facilitated diffusion   C. receptor-mediated endocytosis
    B. exocytosis   D. pinocytosis

32. A(n) _____ is a brief summary of a scientific article.

33. If a circle has a surface area of 3.14 cm², what is the diameter of the circle? _____

34. *True or False.* Students tend to like subjects at which they excel. _____

Section 7.8 Protein Synthesis

An important function of the cell is protein synthesis. Proteins are important to the maintenance of the human body, and cells play a vital role in assembling proteins for the body's use. In this section, you will learn about proteins and the steps in protein synthesis.

The terms below are some of those that will be introduced in Section 7.8. To become familiar with these terms, reproduce each word on the line beside it. Pronounce each term as you write it. You will learn the definitions of these words as you complete this section.

1. polypeptide _____

2. protein synthesis _____

3. transcription _____

4. sense strand _____

5. translation _____

Concept 1: Types of Proteins

Protein synthesis is an important cell function. Some cells are like factories that produce proteins. For example, some pancreatic cells make *enzymes* (a class of proteins). Once enzymes are produced, they are transported through the plasma membrane and to the digestive system, where they help break down food.

To understand protein synthesis, recall the types of proteins. Your body contains two types of proteins: structural proteins and functional proteins. *Structural proteins* provide support for body tissues. For example, the structural protein collagen supports bones, tendons, and ligaments. The structural protein keratin makes up your hair and fingernails. *Functional proteins* orchestrate activities in cells. Examples of functional proteins are enzymes, hemoglobin, antibodies, and some hormones.

Recall Activity

1. Your body contains two types of proteins: _____ proteins and _____ proteins.

2. Functional proteins orchestrate _____ in cells.

Concept 2: Chains of Amino Acids

As you have learned, a protein is a chain of amino acids. There are 20 different types of amino acids, and different proteins are unique combinations of these 20 building blocks. Proteins contain at least 50 and up to thousands of amino acids. Though not proteins, combinations of 10–49 amino acids are called *polypeptides*. For a protein or polypeptide to function properly, the unique order of amino acids must be correct (**Figure 7.25**).

polypeptide a combination of 10–49 amino acids

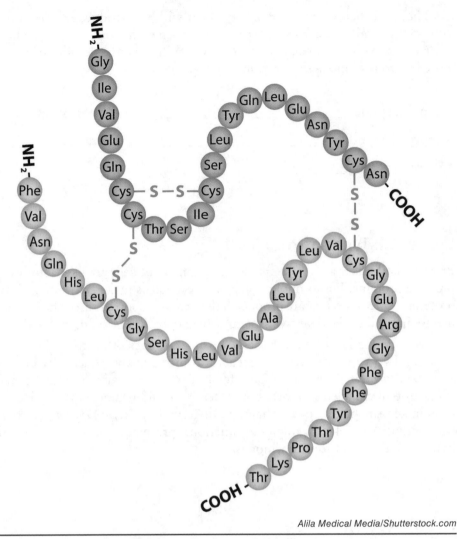

Figure 7.25 These two chains of amino acids make up the hormone insulin. Notice the unique sequence of amino acids in each chain.

Recall Activity

1. A(n) _____ is a chain of amino acids.

2. There are _____ different types of amino acids.

3. Proteins contain at least _____ and up to thousands of amino acids. Combinations of 10–49 amino acids are called _____.

Concept 3: Synthesis

protein synthesis the process of placing amino acids in the proper sequence to form a specific protein

Synthesis refers to the assembly of a substance or structure. In *protein synthesis*, amino acids are placed in the proper sequence to form a specific protein. The organelles involved are the nucleus and ribosomes. A cell's nucleus sends a set of assembly instructions to a ribosome. The ribosome then assembles amino acids in the order specified by the assembly instructions. In the next few concepts, you will learn about the process of protein synthesis and the roles played by amino acids, DNA, and RNA.

Recall Activity

1. What happens in protein synthesis? _____

   _____

2. The two cell structures most involved in protein synthesis are the _____ and

   _____.

3. A cell's _____ sends a set of assembly instructions to a(n)

   _____.

4. The _____ assembles amino acids in the _____ specified by the assembly instructions.

Concept 4: Receiving Amino Acids

The amino acids used in protein synthesis come from the foods you eat. When you eat foods containing protein (meat and many types of plants), your digestive system breaks down the protein into amino acids. Your blood then carries the amino acids to your body cells. Once amino acids enter your cells, they are assembled into proteins or broken down for energy.

Recall Activity

1. List two types of food that contain protein. _____

2. Once amino acids enter your cells, they are _____ into proteins or broken

   down for _____.

Concept 5: The Role of DNA

As you have learned, chromosomes are made of DNA. Chromosomes never leave the nucleus of a cell, and each chromosome houses hundreds to thousands of genes. Each gene, or segment of DNA, contains the instructions to assemble amino acids into a particular protein. The role of DNA in protein synthesis is to provide the instructions for assembling proteins.

Recall Activity

1. Do chromosomes leave the nucleus of a cell?_____

2. Each _____ contains the instructions to assemble amino acids into a particular protein.

Concept 6: The Role of RNA

Three types of RNA are involved in protein synthesis. These include

- messenger RNA (mRNA)
- transfer RNA (tRNA)
- ribosomal RNA (rRNA)

mRNA is a copy of DNA made in the nucleus. tRNA carries amino acids to their correct locations. rRNA makes up ribosomes.

Recall Activity

1. What are the three types of RNA involved in protein synthesis?_____

_____

2. _____ carries amino acids to their correct locations.

Concept 7: Steps in Protein Synthesis

There are two steps in protein synthesis: transcription and translation. Transcription takes place in the cell's nucleus, and translation takes place at the ribosome. During *transcription*, a gene is copied. The copy is in the form of *mRNA*. In *translation*, mRNA specifies the order in which amino acids are assembled (**Figure 7.26**).

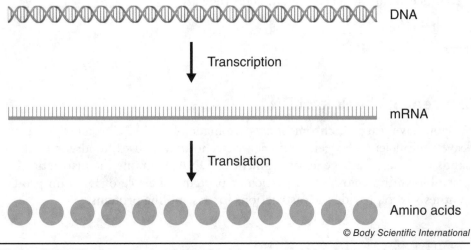

© *Body Scientific International*

Figure 7.26 The steps in protein synthesis are transcription followed by translation.

Recall Activity

1. The two steps in protein synthesis are _____ and

   _____.

2. _____ takes place in the nucleus, and _____ takes place at the ribosome.

Concept 8: Transcription

The process of *transcription* happens in a cell's nucleus. During transcription, one strand of a gene's DNA is copied. This strand is called the *sense strand*. To make the copy, RNA bases line up next to the complementary DNA bases of the sense strand. Once the chain of RNA bases is complete, the RNA copy of the DNA sense strand is known as *mRNA*. After mRNA has been formed, it leaves the nucleus and travels to a ribosome.

transcription the first stage of protein synthesis in which the sense strand of DNA is copied to make mRNA in a cell's nucleus

sense strand the strand of DNA containing assembly instructions for a specific protein; is copied to make mRNA during transcription

Recall Activity

1. During transcription, the _____ strand of a gene's DNA is copied.

2. After _____ has been formed, it leaves the nucleus and travels to a(n)

   _____.

Concept 9: Translation

The process of *translation* happens at the ribosome. Once mRNA reaches the ribosome, it is used as a template to assemble amino acids in the correct order. tRNA positions amino acids at the correct locations, as dictated by the mRNA. Once the amino acids are assembled, peptide bonds form between them, creating the protein.

translation the second stage of protein synthesis in which a ribosome assembles amino acids in the order dictated by mRNA

Recall Activity

1. mRNA is used as a(n) _____ to assemble amino acids in the correct order.

2. _____ bonds form between amino acids, creating the protein.

Concept 10: Movement Out of the Cell

Once proteins have been assembled, some stay in the cell, and others are moved out of the cell. Energy is required to move proteins out of the cell. Proteins that move out of a cell are assembled by ribosomes in the *rough endoplasmic reticulum* (*RER*). Proteins leave the RER in *transport vesicles*, which are received by the *Golgi*. The Golgi then packages the proteins into *secretory vesicles*, which travel toward the plasma membrane and release the proteins outside the cell by exocytosis.

Recall Activity

1. Proteins that move out of a cell are assembled by ribosomes in the _____ endoplasmic reticulum.

2. Proteins leave the RER in _____ vesicles, which are received by the _____.

3. The Golgi packages proteins into _____ vesicles.

Section 7.8 Reinforcement

Answer the following questions using what you learned in this section.

1. Once mRNA has been formed, it leaves the _____ and travels to a ribosome.

2. *True or False.* Hemoglobin is a functional protein. _____

3. For a protein or polypeptide to function properly, the unique _____ of amino acids must be correct.

4. Which type of RNA positions amino acids at the correct locations, as dictated by mRNA?

   _____

5. Your body contains two types of proteins: _____ proteins and _____ proteins.

6. Which of the following is *not* a type of RNA involved in protein synthesis?
   A. mRNA   C. wRNA
   B. rRNA   D. tRNA

7. *True or False.* The process of transcription takes place at a ribosome. _____

8. List the three types of RNA involved in protein synthesis. _____

   _____

9. A protein is a chain of _____.

10. *True or False.* In protein synthesis, the DNA sense strand leaves the nucleus. _____

11. Once amino acids enter your cells, they are _____ into proteins or _____ for energy.

12. Unscramble the letters: sarrpittcinno. Define the word that is formed. _____

    _____

13. The end product of transcription is a copy of the DNA sense strand, known as _____.

14. Is collagen a structural or functional protein? _____

15. Which types of proteins orchestrate activities in all cells? _____

16. Unscramble the letters: netshissy. Define the word that is formed. _____
_____

17. Which of the following words are misspelled?
   A. animo acid   C. structual   E. chromosome
   B. transcription   D. translation

18. During _____, a gene containing assembly instructions is copied.

19. In protein synthesis, amino acids are placed in the proper _____ to form a(n)
_____ protein.

20. *True or False.* Peptide bonds join amino acids. _____

21. There are _____ different types of amino acids, and different
_____ are unique combinations of these building blocks.

22. Explain how proteins are transported out of the cell. _____
_____
_____
_____

Match the following terms with their definitions.

_____ 23. The copying of the sense strand of DNA

_____ 24. A bond that joins amino acids

_____ 25. The process of assembling a structure or substance

_____ 26. The assembly of amino acids as dictated by mRNA

_____ 27. A combination of 10–49 amino acids

A. polypeptide
B. synthesis
C. transcription
D. translation
E. peptide bond

Comprehensive Review (Chapters 1–7)

Answer the following questions using what you have learned so far in this book.

28. The combining form *chlor/o* means "_____."

29. How many meters are in 12 kilometers? _____

30. *True or False.* Scientific methods are used to obtain opinions. _____

31. If a liquid contains many more OH⁻ ions than H⁺ ions, the liquid is a strong
_____.

32. *True or False.* Cell respiration is the process of breaking the high-energy bond in ATP. _____

33. In the phospholipid bilayer, the _____ face *toward* the interstitial fluid or
cytosol, and the _____ face *away* from the interstitial fluid or cytosol.

34. Your _____ is your way of feeling, thinking about, and viewing a situation.

Section 7.9 Cell Division

In your body, old cells die and are replaced by new cells. New cells form through the process of cell division. There are two types of cell division: mitosis and meiosis. In this section, you will learn about diploid and haploid cells and the process of cell division.

The terms below are some of those that will be introduced in Section 7.9. To become familiar with these terms, reproduce each word on the line beside it. Pronounce each term as you write it. You will learn the definitions of these words as you complete this section.

1. diploid _____

2. haploid _____

3. gamete _____

4. zygote _____

5. replication _____

6. interphase _____

7. mitosis _____

8. meiosis _____

Concept 1: Diploid and Haploid Cells

Most of the cells in your body have one or more nuclei, and as you learned in Section 6.3, the nucleus of a cell contains *chromosomes* (**Figure 7.27**). Almost all cells in the human body have a nucleus containing 23 pairs of chromosomes (46 total chromosomes). These cells are considered *diploid* (2N) because their chromosomes are paired. A few cells in your body, however, are *haploid* (N), meaning they contain just one chromosome from each pair for a total of 23 individual chromosomes (**Figure 7.28**). Only reproductive cells (eggs in females and sperm in males), called *gametes*, are haploid.

diploid a human cell containing 23 pairs of chromosomes (46 total chromosomes)

haploid a human cell containing 23 total chromosomes

gamete a human reproductive cell containing 23 total chromosomes; egg in females and sperm in males

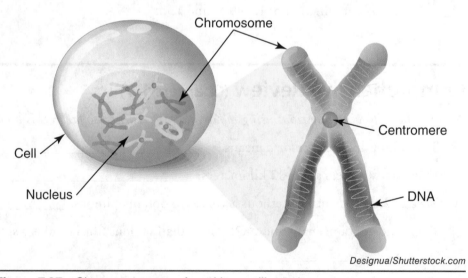

Designua/Shutterstock.com

Figure 7.27 Chromosomes are found in a cell's nucleus.

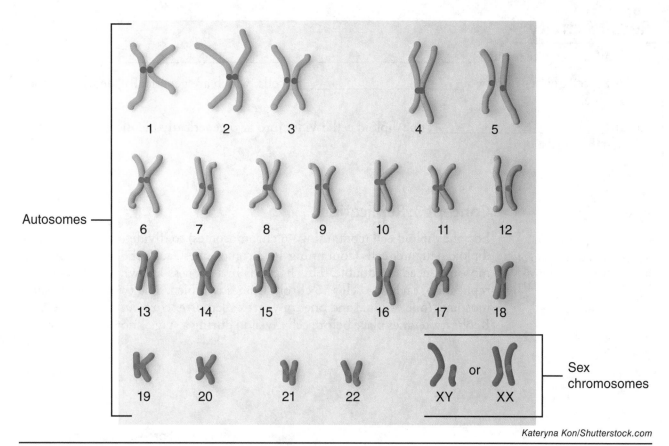

Figure 7.28 A diploid cell has 46 total chromosomes. A haploid cell has 23 total chromosomes.

Recall Activity

1. Almost all cells in the human body have a nucleus containing 23 _____ of chromosomes.

2. _____ cells contain 23 pairs of chromosomes for a total of _____ chromosome(s).

3. _____ cells contain a total of 23 individual chromosomes.

4. Which cells in the human body are haploid? _____

Concept 2: The Beginning of the Human Life Cycle

The human life cycle begins with one cell: a *zygote*, which is formed by the fusion of an egg and a sperm. The zygote divides into two *daughter cells*, which are genetically identical to the zygote. This type of cell division, in which one diploid cell divides into two genetically identical diploid daughter cells, is called *mitosis*. You will learn more about mitosis later in this section. This type of cell division explains how a human grows from one cell to the trillions of cells that make up an adult. Your body grows by increasing its number of cells.

zygote the first cell of the human life cycle formed by the fusion of an egg and a sperm

Recall Activity

1. How is a zygote formed? _____

2. A zygote divides into two _____ cells, which are genetically identical to the zygote.

3. In _____, one diploid cell divides into two genetically identical diploid daughter cells.

Concept 3: Replication

replication the copying of a cell's 46 chromosomes to create 92 total chromatids; takes place during interphase before cell division

For one diploid cell (containing 46 chromosomes) to divide into two identical diploid daughter cells (containing 46 chromosomes each), the number of chromosomes needs to double. This happens in a process known as *replication*. In replication, each of a cell's 46 chromosomes is copied. The two identical chromosomes (one original and one copy) are called *sister chromatids* (**Figure 7.29**). Replication takes place before cell division during a stage known as *interphase*.

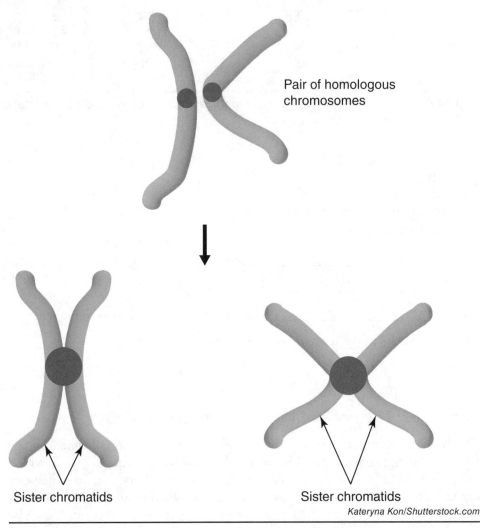

Pair of homologous chromosomes

Sister chromatids

Sister chromatids

Kateryna Kon/Shutterstock.com

Figure 7.29 In replication, each chromosome in a pair is copied.

Recall Activity

1. In _____, each of a cell's 46 chromosomes is copied.

2. Replication takes place _____ cell division.

3. After replication, the two identical chromosomes are called _____.

4. After replication, how many individual chromatids will a cell have? _____

Concept 4: Interphase

The life cycle of a cell has two major phases: interphase and mitosis. During *interphase*, the cell continues to perform its specific functions and does not divide, though it is preparing for cell division. The length of interphase depends on the type of cell. Interphase may be as short as a few minutes or as long as many years. Replication takes place during interphase.

interphase a phase in which a cell continues to perform its specific functions and does not divide, though it is preparing for cell division

Recall Activity

1. The life cycle of a cell has two major phases: _____ and mitosis.

2. What happens during interphase? _____

   _____

3. Replication takes place during _____.

Concept 5: Mitosis

Mitosis is the process by which one diploid cell divides into two genetically identical diploid daughter cells. Almost all cells in the human body undergo mitosis at some point in their life cycles. Mitosis can be divided into four stages (**Figure 7.30**).

mitosis the process by which one diploid cell divides into two genetically identical diploid daughter cells; has four stages and happens in most cells

1. *Prophase.* During *prophase*, the first stage of mitosis, the nuclear envelope around the nucleus dissolves, and spindle fibers (which will pull sister chromatids apart) begin to grow.

2. *Metaphase.* In *metaphase*, the 46 pairs of sister chromatids line up in the center of the cell.

3. *Anaphase.* During *anaphase*, the sister chromatids are separated and pulled to opposite ends of the cell by spindle fibers.

4. *Telophase.* In *telophase*, the sister chromatids have migrated to opposite ends of the cell. The cell divides down the middle in a process called *cytokinesis* (the division of cytoplasm). This creates two daughter cells containing 46 chromatids each. The chromatids are called *chromosomes* once mitosis is complete.

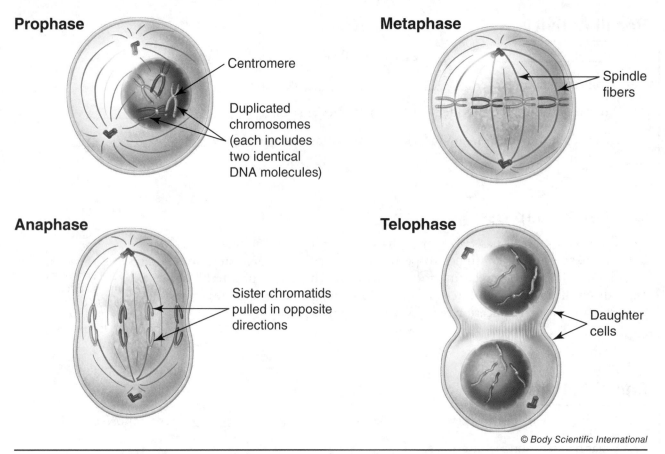

Prophase

Centromere

Duplicated chromosomes (each includes two identical DNA molecules)

Metaphase

Spindle fibers

Anaphase

Sister chromatids pulled in opposite directions

Telophase

Daughter cells

© Body Scientific International

Figure 7.30 Mitosis results in two identical diploid daughter cells.

Recall Activity

1. List the stages of mitosis._____

_____

2. Mitosis is the process by which one _____ cell divides into

_____ genetically identical diploid daughter cell(s).

3. The nuclear envelope dissolves during the _____ stage of mitosis.

4. During which stage of mitosis are sister chromatids pulled to opposite ends of the cell by spindle

fibers? _____

Concept 6: Meiosis

meiosis the process by which one diploid cell undergoes two sets of cell division to produce haploid cells; happens only in the testes and ovaries

Most cells in the human body divide by mitosis. However, in some specialized organs, cells divide by a process known as *meiosis*. Meiosis takes place in the cells of the testes (in males) and ovaries (in females). In meiosis, a diploid cell undergoes two sets of cell division to produce haploid cells (one egg or four sperm).

Meiosis has two stages. In the first stage, one diploid cell divides into two haploid daughter cells. In the second stage, each of the two daughter cells divides into two more haploid daughter cells (**Figure 7.31**). In males, meiosis begins at puberty and continues until death. In females, meiosis begins before birth and ends at menopause.

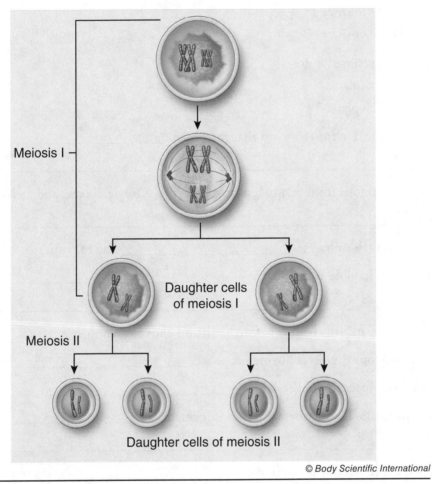

© Body Scientific International

Figure 7.31 In meiosis, a diploid cell undergoes two sets of cell division to produce haploid cells.

Recall Activity

1. Meiosis takes place in the cells of the _____ (in males) and _____ (in females).

2. Meiosis has _____ stage(s).

3. When does meiosis begin and end in males and females? _____

_____

Section 7.9 Reinforcement

Answer the following questions using what you learned in this section.

1. What are the two types of cell division? _____

2. Which of the following terms refers to the division of cytoplasm?
   A. metaphase   C. cytokinesis
   B. zygote   D. meiosis

3. Which of the following is *not* a stage of mitosis?
   A. prophase   C. anaphase
   B. zygote   D. telophase

4. Unscramble the letters: helpsatoe. Define the word that is formed. _____
   _____

5. Arrange the following stages of mitosis from first to last: anaphase, prophase, telophase, and metaphase.
   _____

6. The life cycle of a cell has two major phases: _____ and mitosis.

7. *True or False.* Meiosis produces haploid cells. _____

8. When does replication take place? _____

9. In _____, meiosis begins before birth and ends at menopause.

10. *True or False.* The nuclear envelope dissolves during prophase. _____

11. Which type of cell division produces diploid cells? _____

12. Unscramble the letters: dormthaci. Define the word that is formed. _____
    _____

13. Sister chromatids line up at the center of the cell in the _____ stage of mitosis.

14. What is a cell doing during interphase? _____
    _____

15. Diploid cells contain 23 pairs of chromosomes, or _____ total chromosome(s).

16. _____ cells contain a total of 23 chromosomes.

17. Which type of cell division occurs only in the testes and ovaries? _____

18. *True or False.* Your body grows by increasing the sizes of its cells. _____

19. List the steps of mitosis in alphabetical order. _____

_____

20. Mitosis produces two genetically _____ diploid daughter cells.

21. The human life cycle begins with one cell, called a(n) _____.

22. Which of the following words are misspelled?
   A. mytosis   C. zygote   E. chromatid
   B. meiois   D. haploid   F. dipoid

Match the following terms with their definitions.

_____ 23. A cell formed by the fusion of an egg and a sperm

_____ 24. The duplication of chromosomes

_____ 25. A cell containing 23 pairs of chromosomes

_____ 26. A type of cell division that produces haploid cells

_____ 27. A cell containing 23 individual chromosomes

_____ 28. A type of cell division that produces diploid cells

A. haploid
B. diploid
C. zygote
D. replication
E. mitosis
F. meiosis

Comprehensive Review (Chapters 1–7)

Answer the following questions using what you have learned so far in this book.

29. *True or False.* An enzyme is a protein catalyst._____

30. Explain the difference between free and bound ribosomes. _____

_____

_____

31. The prefix of the term *subnasal* means "_____."

32. In a graph, which axis is vertical?_____

33. A scientific _____ is a general statement of fact.

34. What are the steps in protein synthesis? _____

35. Scientific explanations require the support of _____.

Chapter 7 Review

Answer the following questions using what you learned in this chapter.

1. In _____, each of a cell's 46 chromosomes is copied.

2. Does facilitated diffusion require energy? Why or why not? _____
   _____

3. Which of the following does *not* require energy?
   A. exocytosis   C. osmosis
   B. pinocytosis   D. phagocytosis

4. In translation, a(n) _____ assembles amino acids in the order specified by
   _____ RNA.

5. Where in the cell does cell respiration take place? _____

6. In _____, atoms spread out from areas of high concentration into areas of
   low concentration.

7. Where is mRNA assembled during protein synthesis? _____

8. *True or False.* In the lungs, oxygen moves from the blood into the air. _____

9. What happens during translation, and where does translation occur? _____
   _____

10. In cell respiration, the energy from _____ is used to add one
    _____ molecule to one adenosine _____ molecule.

11. Proteins that move out of a cell are assembled by ribosomes in the rough _____.

12. Describe the difference between downhill reactions and uphill reactions. Give an example of each.
    _____
    _____

13. In a downhill reaction, atoms move *down* the concentration gradient, from areas of
    _____ concentration to areas of _____ concentration.

14. Cells maintain _____ by adjusting the concentrations of ions inside the cell.

15. *True or False.* Atoms tend to move from areas of low to high concentration. _____

16. What is the function of the Golgi in transporting proteins out of a cell? _____
    _____

17. *True or False.* Haploid cells contain 23 pairs of chromosomes. _____

18. List the four steps in cell respiration. _____
    _____

19. Breaking the high-energy bond in ATP is a(n) _____ reaction, meaning it
    _____ energy.

20. _____ refers to the movement of water molecules through the phospholipid
    bilayer and aquaporins.

21. Because of facilitated _____, sodium ions are constantly moving into a cell.

22. In a(n) _____ reaction, molecules are joined together.

23. Describe the difference between mitosis and meiosis. _____

_____

_____

24. *True or False.* Water molecules move through the plasma membrane via aquaporins because they cannot pass through the phospholipid bilayer. _____

25. Combinations of 10–49 amino acids are called _____.

26. How does a cell maintain homeostasis in sodium and potassium concentrations? _____

_____

27. Which of the following atoms will diffuse most quickly?
    A. lithium   C. carbon
    B. aluminum   D. helium

Comprehensive Review (Chapters 1–7)

Using what you have learned so far in this book, match the following terms with their definitions.

_____ 28. An atomic bond in which electrons are shared

_____ 29. A combining form that means "triangular"

_____ 30. A combining form that means "middle"

_____ 31. A prediction about the outcome of an experiment

_____ 32. An atomic bond in which the partial charges of water molecules attract

_____ 33. A molecule that can accept or donate hydrogen ions to resist changes in pH

_____ 34. The spreading out of atoms from areas of high concentration into areas of low concentration

_____ 35. The amount of matter in an object

_____ 36. A membrane junction that binds adjacent cells together to form an impermeable barrier

_____ 37. A membrane junction that contains communication tunnels between adjacent cells

_____ 38. A type of endocytosis in which the plasma membrane surrounds and engulfs an object

_____ 39. The best explanation today of why a phenomenon occurs

A. hydrogen bond
B. gap junction
C. covalent bond
D. buffer
E. delt/o
F. tight junction
G. diffusion
H. hypothesis
I. medi/o
J. mass
K. scientific theory
L. phagocytosis

Chapter 8

Human Body Tissues

Introduction

The human body is composed of many cells working together. When cells work together, they make up a tissue. There are several types of tissue in the human body. In this chapter, you will learn about the different types of cells that make up tissues and about the four types of tissue found in the human body. Your knowledge of cell parts and physiology will help you understand the tissues and their functions.

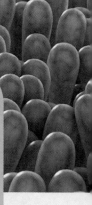

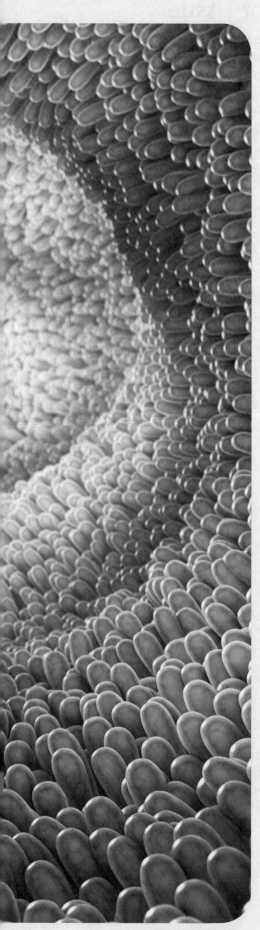

Objectives

After completing this chapter, you will be able to

- explain the characteristics of tissue
- list the four types of tissue found in the human body
- describe the composition and types of epithelial tissue
- know the types of connective tissue proper
- understand the properties of bone, cartilage, and blood
- list the types of muscle tissue
- understand the components of nerve tissue

Key Terms

The following terms and phrases will be introduced and explained in Chapter 8. Read through the list to become familiar with the words.

action potential	ligament
apical surface	loose connective tissue
avascular tissue	mucus
basal surface	muscle tissue
basement membrane	myocyte
bone	nerve tissue
cartilage	neuroglia
chondrocyte	neuron
collagen fiber	neurotransmitter
columnar cell	organ
compact bone	osteoblast
connective tissue	osteoclast
connective tissue proper	osteocyte
cuboidal cell	plasma
dense connective tissue	pseudostratified arrangement
elastic fiber	reticular fiber
endocrine gland	simple arrangement
epithelial tissue	spongy bone
excitable tissue	squamous cell
exocrine gland	stratified arrangement
extracellular matrix	tendon
fibroblast	tissue
gland	transitional cell
involuntary muscle	vascular tissue
lacuna	voluntary muscle

Section 8.1 Characteristics of Tissue

Tissues are groups of cells that work together to perform a specific task. There are four types of tissue in the human body, and tissues may be vascular or avascular. Understanding the characteristics and types of tissue is important for comprehending organ structures and functions. In this section, you will learn about tissue characteristics, tissue types, and organs.

The terms below are some of those that will be introduced in Section 8.1. To become familiar with these terms, reproduce each word on the line beside it. Pronounce each term as you write it. You will learn the definitions of these words as you complete this section.

1. tissue _____

2. organ _____

3. vascular tissue _____

4. avascular tissue _____

Concept 1: What Are Tissues?

Cells fulfill many functions in the body and are specialized to perform specific tasks. For example, a muscle cell contracts. A group of muscle cells contracts together. When cells work together to do a job, they are considered a *tissue*. Muscle tissue is a group of muscle cells contracting together.

tissue a group of cells that work together to do a job

Recall Activity

1. Cells are _____ to perform specific tasks.

2. When cells work together to do a job, they are considered a(n) _____.

Concept 2: Types of Tissue

There are four types of tissue in the human body:

- epithelial tissue
- connective tissue
- muscle tissue
- nerve tissue

The four types of tissue have different compositions and functions. Epithelial tissue makes up the surfaces and internal linings of the body. Connective tissue provides structure and protection for the body. Muscle and nerve tissue are excitable tissues that produce electrical charges when stimulated.

Recall Activity

1. What are the four types of tissue in the human body?_____

_____

2. _____ tissue makes up the surfaces and internal linings of the body.

3. Connective tissue provides _____ and _____ for the body.

4. _____ and _____ tissue are excitable tissues that pro-duce _____ charges when stimulated.

Concept 3: Tissues Make Up Organs

When cells work together to do a job, they are considered a *tissue*. When tissues work together to perform a specific function, they are considered an *organ*. Organs are made of different types of tissue working together to do a job. An organ is composed of different tissue types.

organ a group of different types of tissue that work together to do a job

Recall Activity

1. When tissues work together to perform a specific function, they are considered a(n) _____.

2. *True or False.* An organ is composed of one type of tissue._____

Concept 4: Blood Supply for Tissues

All cells in the human body require oxygen to survive. Oxygen enters the body through the lungs and diffuses into the blood. The blood then circulates oxygen to the rest of the body. To receive adequate oxygen, all tissues in the human body need access to a blood supply (blood vessels). This blood supply also removes the waste produced by cells. How tissues achieve access to a blood supply depends on whether they are vascular or avascular.

Recall Activity

1. All cells in the human body require _____ to survive.

2. To receive adequate oxygen, all tissues in the human body need access to a(n) _____.

Concept 5: Vascular Tissue

vascular tissue a type of tissue that has direct access to a blood supply; is permeated by blood vessels

Vascular tissue has direct access to a blood supply. Blood vessels permeate vascular tissue, delivering nutrients and oxygen and removing waste from the group of cells (**Figure 8.1**). Examples of vascular tissue include muscle tissue and tissue in the lungs.

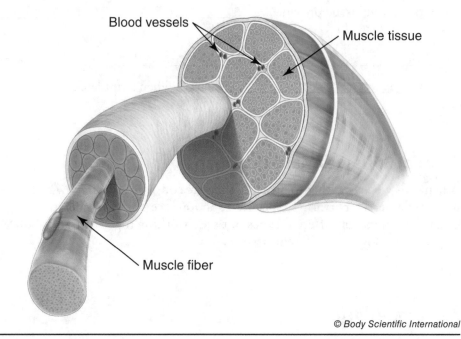

© Body Scientific International

Figure 8.1 Vascular tissue, such as this muscle tissue, is permeated by blood vessels.

Recall Activity

1. Vascular tissue has _____ access to a blood supply.

2. What are two examples of vascular tissue? _____

Concept 6: Avascular Tissue

avascular tissue a type of tissue that does not have direct access to a blood supply

Avascular tissue does *not* have direct access to a blood supply. Blood vessels do not permeate avascular tissue. Instead, avascular tissue receives oxygen and nutrients and removes waste via diffusion through adjacent tissue. Epithelial tissue is an example of avascular tissue. In epithelial tissue, a basement membrane lies beneath the tissue and is in contact with vascular tissue. Nutrients and waste diffuse through the basement membrane between epithelial tissue and the vascular tissue.

Recall Activity

1. Avascular tissue receives oxygen and nutrients and removes waste via _____ through adjacent tissue.

2. Epithelial tissue is an example of _____ tissue.

3. A(n) _____ membrane lies beneath epithelial tissue and is in contact with vascular tissue.

4. Nutrients and waste diffuse through the basement membrane between _____ tissue and _____ tissue.

Section 8.1 Reinforcement

Answer the following questions using what you learned in this section.

1. *True or False.* Epithelial tissue is avascular. _____

2. Which of the following words is misspelled?
   A. vascular   C. organ
   B. anvascular   D. tissue

3. Explain the difference between a tissue and an organ. _____

   _____

4. *True or False.* A tissue is a group of cells that work together to do a job. _____

5. What are the four types of tissue in the human body? _____

   _____

6. Write the letters backward: ralucsav. Define the word that is formed. _____

   _____

7. _____ tissue makes up the surfaces and internal linings of the body.

8. *True or False.* Avascular tissue does not have direct access to a blood supply. _____

9. A(n) _____ is made of different types of tissue working together to do a job.

10. To receive adequate oxygen, all tissues in the human body need access to a(n)

    _____.

11. *True or False.* Connective tissue produces an electrical charge when stimulated. _____

12. Blood vessels permeate _____ tissue, delivering nutrients and oxygen and removing waste from the group of cells.

13. Which of the following types of tissue provides structure and protection for the body?
    A. connective tissue   C. epithelial tissue
    B. nerve tissue   D. muscle tissue

14. Nutrients and waste _____ through the basement membrane between epithelial tissue and vascular tissue.

15. Unscramble the letters: seiuts. Define the word that is formed. _____

_____

16. Oxygen enters the body through the _____ and diffuses into the

_____.

17. *True or False.* Cells are specialized to perform specific tasks. _____

18. List the four types of tissue in the human body in alphabetical order. _____

_____

19. Give one example of avascular tissue. _____

Comprehensive Review (Chapters 1–8)

Answer the following questions using what you have learned so far in this book.

20. A hypothesis is a prediction about the _____ of an experiment.

21. What does the prefix *hyper-* mean? _____

22. How many millimeters are in 1 centimeter? _____

23. Which part of the cytoskeleton forms roadways on which organelles are moved around a cell?

_____

24. Which of the following subatomic particles is *not* located in the core of an atom?
    A. proton   C. electron
    B. neutron

25. *True or False.* No energy input is required to move from an area of low concentration to an area of high concentration. _____

26. A(n) _____ is a physically observable fact or event.

27. What are two examples of vascular tissue? _____

Section 8.2 Epithelial Tissue

Epithelial tissue covers and lines the outer and inner surfaces of the body. The outermost layer of your skin is an example of epithelial tissue. In this section, you will learn about epithelial tissue composition and types.

The following terms are some of those that will be introduced in Section 8.2. To become familiar with these terms, reproduce each word on the line beside it. Pronounce each term as you write it. You will learn the definitions of these words as you complete this section.

1. epithelial tissue _____

2. apical surface _____

3. basal surface _____

4. basement membrane _____

5. squamous cell _____

6. cuboidal cell _____

7. columnar cell _____

8. transitional cell _____

9. simple arrangement _____

10. stratified arrangement_____

11. pseudostratified arrangement

    _____

12. mucus _____

13. gland _____

14. exocrine gland _____

15. endocrine gland _____

Concept 1: Epithelium

The first type of tissue in the human body is *epithelial tissue*, which is also called *epithelium*. Epithelial tissue covers the surfaces of the body and lines the body's internal hollow tubes and cavities. As a covering and as a lining, epithelial tissue acts as a border, either within the body or between the body and the outside environment. You can think of most epithelial tissue as sheets of tightly packed cells. These sheets can be thin (one layer of cells) or thick (multiple layers of cells), and cells in some of these sheets can secrete products or absorb nutrients. Glands, which are not sheets of cells, are another type of epithelium.

epithelial tissue a type of tissue that covers the surfaces of the body and lines the body's internal hollow tubes and cavities; also called *epithelium*

Recall Activity

1. _____ covers the surfaces of the body and lines the body's internal hollow tubes and cavities.

2. You can think of most epithelial tissue as _____ of tightly packed cells.

3. Which type of epithelium is not a sheet of cells? _____

Concept 2: Layers of Epithelial Tissue

Epithelial tissue covers both hollow and nonhollow surfaces. For a hollow organ (like the small intestine), both the outermost and innermost layers of cells are epithelial tissue (**Figure 8.2**). For an organ that is not hollow (like the liver) and for the skin, only the outermost layer of cells is epithelial tissue. Underneath the epithelial tissue is connective tissue.

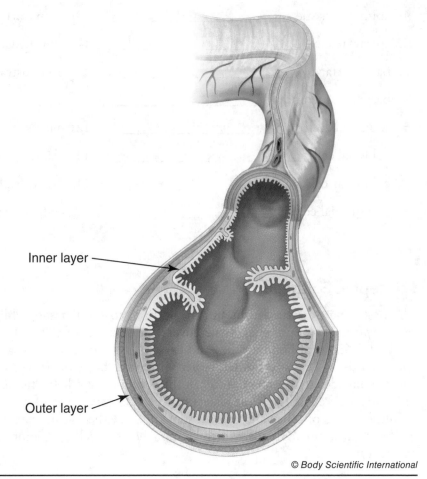

Inner layer

Outer layer

© Body Scientific International

Figure 8.2 The inner and outer layers of this hollow organ are epithelial tissue.

Recall Activity

1. For hollow organs, both the _____ and _____ layers of cells are epithelial tissue.

2. Underneath the epithelial tissue of the skin is _____ tissue.

3. For an organ that is not hollow, only the outermost layer of cells is _____.

apical surface the top layer of epithelial tissue that has contact with open space

basal surface the bottom layer of epithelial tissue that has contact with the basement membrane

basement membrane the acellular membrane beneath epithelial tissue through which nutrients and waste diffuse

Concept 3: Apical and Basal Surfaces

Epithelial tissue always has an *apical surface* and a *basal surface*, or a top and a bottom. Because epithelial tissue forms a border, one of its surfaces is always in contact with open space. This surface is the *apical surface*. The other surface of epithelial tissue is the base, or *basal surface*. The basal surface is attached to a *basement membrane* (**Figure 8.3**).

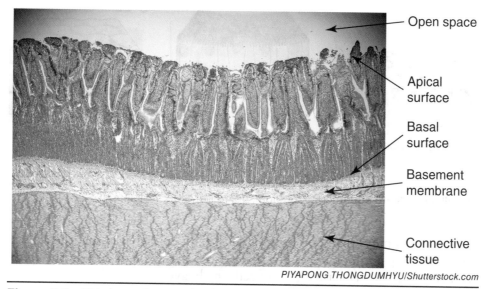

Open space

Apical surface

Basal surface

Basement membrane

Connective tissue

Figure 8.3 This is a micrograph of epithelial tissue. The apical surface of epithelial tissue is exposed to open space. The basal surface is attached to a basement membrane. The basement membrane lies on top of connective tissue.

You can think of epithelial tissue as a house. The apical surface is the roof, which has contact with open space. The basal surface is the foundation, and the foundation is attached to a basement membrane, which is in contact with the ground.

Recall Activity

1. The _____ surface of epithelial tissue is in contact with open space.

2. The _____ surface of epithelial tissue is attached to a basement membrane.

Concept 4: Epithelial Cell Shapes

Cells that make up epithelial tissue come in four different shapes: squamous, cuboidal, columnar, and transitional (**Figure 8.4**). *Squamous cells* are flat and are so thin that macromolecules can move through them. *Cuboidal cells* are square, and *columnar cells* are tall. Cuboidal and columnar cells are not as thin as squamous cells. *Transitional cells* can stretch or relax, changing shape and thickness as needed.

squamous cell a flat epithelial cell; is so thin that macromolecules can move through it

cuboidal cell a square epithelial cell

columnar cell a tall epithelial cell

transitional cell an epithelial cell that can stretch or relax, changing shape and thickness as needed

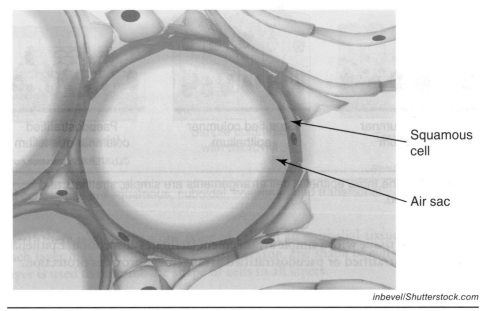

Squamous cell

Air sac

Figure 8.6   Squamous cells make up the air sacs in your lungs.

Recall Activity

1. The thinnest sheet of tissue in the human body is _____.

2. Molecules can easily _____ through simple squamous epithelium.

3. When you take a breath, the oxygen molecules you inhale move into the

   _____ in your lungs and then diffuse through the simple squamous epithe-

   lium into your _____.

Concept 7: Simple Cuboidal Epithelium

Simple cuboidal epithelium is an epithelial tissue consisting of one layer of square cells. The kidney's tubules are composed of simple cuboidal epithelium (**Figure 8.7**). These epithelial cells are involved in *secretion* (moving products out of the blood) and *absorption* (bringing products into the blood). The kidney's tubules sort what materials will be returned to the blood (glucose, some ions, and water) and what materials will be put into urine (nitrogen waste, other ions, and water), depending on the body's requirements.

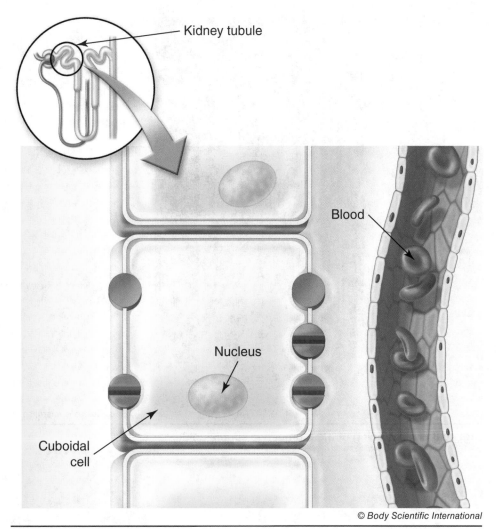

Kidney tubule

Blood

Nucleus

Cuboidal
cell

© Body Scientific International

Figure 8.7 Notice the square shapes of cuboidal cells in the kidney's tubule.

Recall Activity

1. Simple cuboidal epithelium is an epithelial tissue consisting of _____ layer(s)
   of _____ cells.

2. The kidney's tubules are composed of simple _____ epithelium.

Concept 8: Simple Columnar Epithelium

Epithelial tissue with one layer of tall cells is *simple columnar epithelium*.
The lining of the digestive tract, from the stomach to the intestines, is simple
columnar epithelium (**Figure 8.8**). The columnar epithelial cells of the small
intestine have microvilli that facilitate the absorption of digested molecules.
Simple columnar epithelium is also found in the fallopian tubes of the female
reproductive system. In the fallopian tubes, epithelial cells are ciliated, and
cilia move egg cells from the ovary to the uterus.

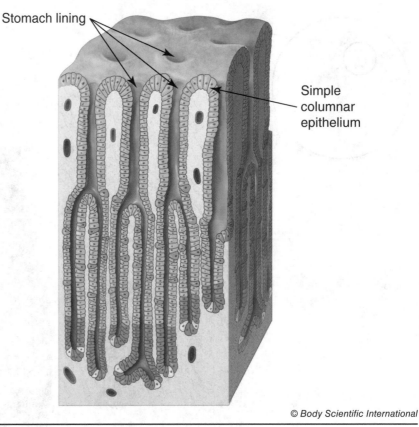

Stomach lining

Simple columnar epithelium

© Body Scientific International

Figure 8.8   The lining of the stomach is simple columnar epithelium.

Recall Activity

1. Where in the body is simple columnar epithelium found?_____

_____

2. Epithelial tissue with one layer of tall cells is _____ epithelium.

Concept 9: Pseudostratified Columnar Epithelium

Epithelial tissue consisting of one layer of cells of varying sizes is *pseudostratified columnar epithelium*. Your trachea, or windpipe, is lined with ciliated pseudostratified columnar epithelium. Among the columnar cells are *goblet cells*, which secrete *mucus* (a substance that coats and moistens linings in the body). Mucus traps dust particles that move through the windpipe with each breath. Cilia move mucus out of the windpipe and toward the esophagus, protecting the lungs from dust.

mucus a substance that coats and moistens linings in the body

Recall Activity

1. The windpipe is also called the _____.

2. The windpipe is lined with _____ epithelium.

Concept 10: Stratified Squamous Epithelium

Stratified squamous epithelium is epithelial tissue made of multiple layers of flat cells. This type of epithelium protects underlying tissues. The surface of the skin and the lining of the mouth and throat are stratified squamous epithelium. Stratified squamous epithelium is adapted to wear. The epithelial cells of the basal layer continually reproduce, and the epithelial cells of the apical layer are shed by abrasion (rubbing or scraping). Cells of the basal layer gradually replace apical cells as the apical cells are shed (**Figure 8.9**).

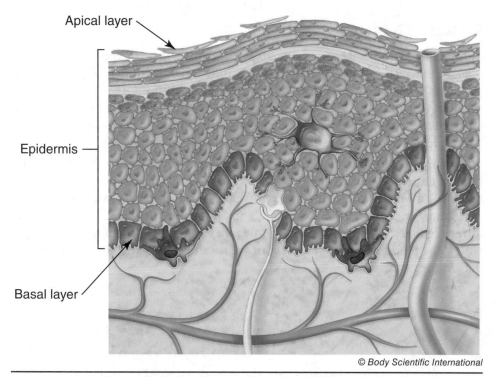

Figure 8.9 The epidermis is made of stratified squamous epithelium.

Recall Activity

1. _____ epithelium is made of multiple layers of flat cells.

2. The epithelial cells of the basal layer continually _____.

Concept 11: Transitional Epithelium

Transitional epithelial cells can change in shape and size. *Transitional epithelium*, which is made of transitional epithelial cells, is a type of epithelial tissue that expands and shrinks as needed. The urinary bladder contains transitional epithelium, which allows it to expand and recoil as it is filled and emptied.

Recall Activity

1. _____ epithelium, which is made of _____ epithelial cells, is a type of epithelial tissue that expands and shrinks as needed.

2. The urinary bladder contains transitional epithelium, which allows it to _____ and _____ as it is filled and emptied.

Concept 12: Glands

gland an epithelial tissue that produces and secretes products

exocrine gland a gland that releases a product through a duct

endocrine gland a gland that releases a product into the interstitial fluid surrounding a cell; also called *ductless gland*

While they are not sheets of cells, glands are also a type of epithelial tissue. A *gland* is an epithelial tissue that produces and secretes products. Glands release products either through a duct or into interstitial fluid. Glands that release a product (for example, oil) through a duct are called *exocrine glands*. Glands that release a product (for example, a hormone) into the interstitial fluid surrounding a cell are called *endocrine glands* or *ductless glands*.

Examples of exocrine glands include goblet cells, salivary glands, and oil glands. Exocrine glands may be *unicellular* (having one cell; for example, goblet cells) or *multicellular* (having many cells; for example, salivary glands and oil glands). Examples of endocrine glands include the thyroid, pituitary, and adrenal glands. These glands make hormones and release them into interstitial fluid. The blood then picks up the hormones and transports them to their targets in the body.

Recall Activity

1. _____ glands release a product into the interstitial fluid surrounding a cell.

2. _____ glands release a product through a duct.

3. What type of gland is the adrenal gland? _____

4. Exocrine glands may be _____ (having one cell) or _____ (having many cells).

Section 8.2 Reinforcement

Answer the following questions using what you learned in this section.

1. A gland is an epithelial tissue that _____ and _____ products.

2. Where in the body is ciliated pseudostratified columnar epithelium found? _____

3. Give an example of a unicellular exocrine gland. _____

4. Which of the following contain stratified squamous epithelium?
   A. surface of the skin
   B. lungs
   C. trachea
   D. lining of the mouth

5. Which type of epithelial tissue expands and shrinks as needed? _____

6. *True or False.* The apical surface of epithelial tissue is in contact with open space. _____

7. Write the three arrangements of epithelial cells in alphabetical order. _____

_____

8. What is the difference between exocrine and endocrine glands? _____

_____

9. *True or False.* The kidney's tubules are composed of simple squamous epithelium. _____

10. The base, or _____ surface of epithelial tissue, is attached to a(n)

_____ membrane.

11. The surface of the skin contains _____ squamous epithelium.

12. *True or False.* Stratified squamous epithelium is composed of multiple layers of flat cells._____

13. Which of the following cell arrangements have one layer?
    A. stratified
    B. simple
    C. pseudostratified

14. *True or False.* Molecules can easily diffuse through simple squamous epithelium. _____

15. Describe the shape of columnar epithelial cells._____

16. The thyroid, pituitary, and adrenal glands produce and secrete _____.

17. Unscramble the letters: umaqusso. Define the word that is formed. _____

_____

18. A simple cell arrangement facilitates _____.

19. If there are multiple layers of cells in an epithelial tissue, the shape of cells in the

_____ layer is used to describe the shape of cells in all layers.

20. Which of the following words are misspelled?
    A. transtional
    B. epithelium
    C. squamous
    D. stratufied

21. Goblet cells in the windpipe secrete _____.

22. Name and briefly describe the four epithelial cell shapes. _____

_____

23. In stratified squamous epithelium, cells of the _____ layer gradually replace

apical cells as the apical cells are _____.

Comprehensive Review (Chapters 1–8)

Answer the following questions using what you have learned so far in this book.

24. A logical process used to evaluate the natural world is known as a(n) _____.

25. *True or False.* The most basic skill in learning science is understanding the words. _____

26. If 24 people say "yes," and 26 people say "no," what percentage of people said "yes"? _____

27. The prefix *endo-* means "_____."

28. *True or False.* Avascular tissue has direct access to a blood supply. _____

29. Which of the following membrane junctions forms an impermeable barrier?
    A. desmosome   C. gap junction
    B. tight junction

30. In the concentration ³⁄₉₇, does the 97 represent solute or solvent concentration?_____

31. The chemical formula $2C_5H_{12}$ represents _____ carbon atom(s) and
    _____ hydrogen atom(s).

Section 8.3 Connective Tissue Proper

Connective tissue is responsible for connecting body structures and supporting and protecting the body. In this section, you will learn about one category of connective tissue: connective tissue proper.

The terms below are some of those that will be introduced in Section 8.3. To become familiar with these terms, reproduce each word on the line beside it. Pronounce each term as you write it. You will learn the definitions of these words as you complete this section.

1. connective tissue _____

2. connective tissue proper_____

_____

3. extracellular matrix _____

_____

4. collagen fiber _____

5. elastic fiber_____

6. reticular fiber _____

7. fibroblast _____

8. loose connective tissue _____

_____

9. dense connective tissue_____

_____

10. tendon_____

11. ligament _____

Concept 1: Connective Tissue

Connective tissue, the second type of tissue in the human body, fulfills the important functions of connection, support, and protection. Several types of tissue are gathered together under the category of connective tissue. Some types of connective tissue connect body structures. Others support body parts, and still others protect the body. Connective tissue underlies and supports epithelial tissue. The two main categories of connective tissue are *connective tissue proper* (loose and dense connective tissue) and bone, cartilage, and blood. You will learn about bone, cartilage, and blood in Section 8.4.

connective tissue a type of tissue that fulfills the important functions of connection, support, and protection; includes connective tissue proper and bone, cartilage, and blood

connective tissue proper a category of connective tissue that includes loose and dense connective tissue

Recall Activity

1. List the three functions of connective tissue. _____

   _____

2. Connective tissue underlies and supports _____ tissue.

3. What are the two main categories of connective tissue? _____

   _____

Concept 2: Extracellular Matrix

Most types of connective tissue are made of cells dispersed in an extracellular matrix. The *extracellular matrix* is a collection of material and fibers existing outside connective tissue cells; it provides support and structure. The material can be a liquid, semisolid gel, or solid and is also called the *ground substance*.

extracellular matrix a collection of material and fibers existing outside connective tissue cells; also called *ground substance*

Recall Activity

1. Most types of connective tissue are made of cells dispersed in a(n) _____ matrix.

2. The material of the extracellular matrix can be a(n) _____,

   _____, or _____.

Concept 3: Extracellular Fibers

Extracellular fibers are an important part of the extracellular matrix in connective tissue. There are three types of extracellular fibers: collagen fibers, elastic fibers, and reticular fibers. *Collagen fibers* are white and strong and contain the protein collagen. *Elastic fibers*, made of the protein elastin, are yellow and thin. Elastic fibers can branch off and stretch up to one and one-half times

collagen fiber an extracellular fiber that is white and strong and contains the protein collagen; is especially strong

elastic fiber an extracellular fiber that is made of the protein elastin and is yellow and thin; can stretch up to one and one-half times its resting length

reticular fiber an extracellular fiber that is thin and white and is made of the protein collagen; forms a network in the extracellular matrix

their resting length. *Reticular fibers* are thin and white and are made of the protein collagen. Reticular fibers form a network in the extracellular matrix (**Figure 8.10**).

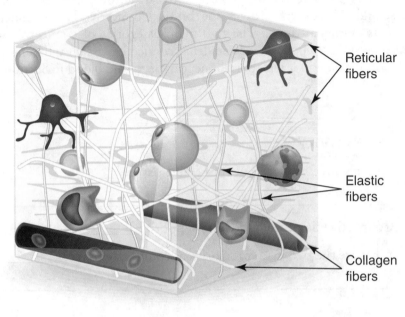

Reticular fibers

Elastic fibers

Collagen fibers

Figure 8.10   The extracellular fibers in connective tissue provide support for connective tissue cells.

Recall Activity

1. Which two types of extracellular fibers are made of collagen? _____

2. _____ fibers are thin and yellow.

Concept 4: Fibroblasts

fibroblast a cell that secretes collagen and elastin

Most connective tissue is made by fibroblasts. *Fibroblasts* are cells that secrete collagen and elastin. As they divide, they help form the extracellular fibers and extracellular matrix of connective tissue.

Recall Activity

1. Fibroblasts are cells that secrete _____ and _____.

2. As _____ divide, they help form the extracellular fibers and extracellular matrix of connective tissue.

Concept 5: Adipose Connective Tissue

Connective tissue proper includes types of loose and dense connective tissue. *Loose connective tissue* is composed of many cells with extracellular fibers winding through them. There are three types of loose connective tissue: adipose connective tissue, areolar connective tissue, and reticular connective tissue. *Adipose connective tissue* underlies the skin, where it insulates the body and acts as a shock absorber. The cells of adipose connective tissue are called *adipocytes*. Adipocytes store triglycerides (fat molecules), and the extracellular matrix around adipocytes is sparse. The purpose of adipocytes is to store energy (**Figure 8.11**).

loose connective tissue a type of connective tissue composed of many cells with extracellular fibers winding through them; includes adipose connective tissue, areolar connective tissue, and reticular connective tissue

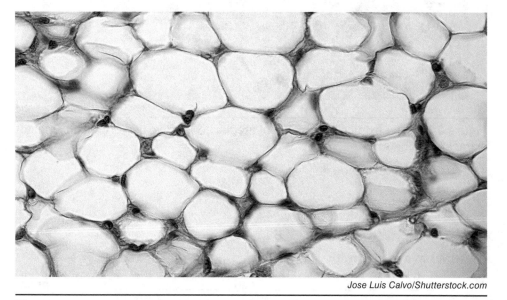

Jose Luis Calvo/Shutterstock.com

Figure 8.11 Adipose connective tissue insulates the body, acts as a shock absorber, and stores energy.

Recall Activity

1. Adipose connective tissue underlies the skin, where it _____ the body and acts as a(n) _____.

2. The cells of adipose connective tissue are called _____.

3. The purpose of adipocytes is to store _____.

Concept 6: Areolar Connective Tissue

The second type of loose connective tissue is areolar connective tissue. *Areolar connective tissue* is the most common type of connective tissue. It is located under the skin, where it serves as a reservoir for water and wraps, binds, and cushions most organs. The extracellular matrix of areolar connective tissue is a semisolid gel. The gel contains a loose arrangement of all three types of extracellular fibers (**Figure 8.12**).

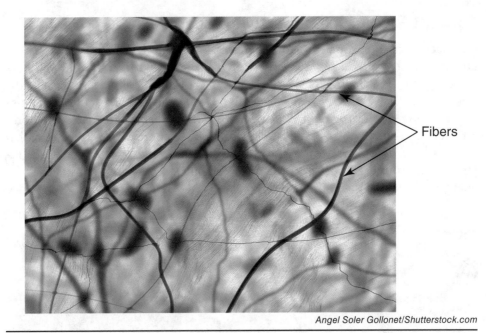

Angel Soler Gollonet/Shutterstock.com

Figure 8.12 The extracellular matrix of areolar connective tissue contains many extracellular fibers.

Recall Activity

1. Areolar connective tissue serves as a reservoir for _____ and _____, _____, and _____ most organs.

2. Which extracellular fibers are contained in the extracellular matrix for areolar connective tissue?

_____

Concept 7: Reticular Connective Tissue

Reticular connective tissue is the third type of loose connective tissue. The extracellular matrix of reticular connective tissue contains many reticular fibers. These fibers form a delicate network that supports the spleen, bone marrow, and lymph nodes.

Recall Activity

1. The extracellular matrix of reticular connective tissue contains many _____ fibers.

2. List the three organs containing reticular connective tissue. _____

_____

Concept 8: Irregular Dense Connective Tissue

While loose connective tissue contains many cells, *dense connective tissue* is composed mostly of extracellular fibers with few cells. There are three types of dense connective tissue: irregular dense connective tissue, regular dense connective tissue, and elastic connective tissue. *Irregular dense connective tissue* is a sheet of randomly positioned extracellular fibers with few fibroblasts. Collagen fibers make up most of the extracellular matrix. This sheet (as found in the lower layer of skin) exerts strength when pulled in any direction.

dense connective tissue a type of connective tissue composed mostly of extracellular fibers with few cells; includes irregular dense connective tissue, regular dense connective tissue, and elastic connective tissue

Recall Activity

1. The lower layer of skin is made of _____ connective tissue.

2. Irregular dense connective tissue is a sheet of randomly positioned _____ fibers with few _____.

Concept 9: Regular Dense Connective Tissue

Regular dense connective tissue is made of bundles of collagen fibers arranged in straight rows with few fibroblasts. This arrangement of fibers is very strong when pulled parallel to the rows of fibers. Examples of regular dense connective tissue are *tendons* (which connect bone to muscle), *ligaments* (which connect bone to bone), and the coverings of muscles. Because collagen fibers are extracellular and nonliving, they do not repair quickly after damage.

tendon a band of regular dense connective tissue that connects bone to muscle

ligament a band of regular dense connective tissue that connects bone to bone

Recall Activity

1. Which structure connects bone to bone? _____

2. Straight rows of bundled collagen fibers make up _____ connective tissue.

Concept 10: Elastic Connective Tissue

Elastic connective tissue is composed mostly of elastic fibers. Elastic fibers allow elastic connective tissue to stretch and recoil (**Figure 8.13**). One example of elastic connective tissue is found in the cardiovascular system. When the heart beats, it forces blood into a blood vessel called the *aorta*. Because the aorta contains elastic connective tissue, it expands and stretches as blood moves through it.

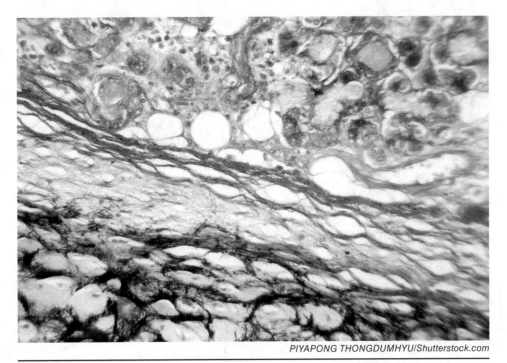

Figure 8.13 Elastic fibers make up elastic connective tissue.

Recall Activity

1. Elastic connective tissue contains _____ fibers.

2. One example of elastic connective tissue is found in the _____.

Section 8.3 Reinforcement

Answer the following questions using what you learned in this section.

1. *True or False.* All types of connective tissue connect body structures._____

2. Ligaments connect _____ to bone.

3. Which of the following extracellular fibers can stretch?
   A. collagen fiber   C. reticular fiber
   B. elastic fiber

4. Give an example of irregular dense connective tissue in the body._____

5. Unscramble the letters: rabbitflos. Define the word that is formed._____

   _____

6. Which of the following extracellular fibers forms a delicate network in the extracellular matrix?
   A. collagen fiber   C. reticular fiber
   B. elastic fiber

7. *True or False.* Irregular dense connective tissue has many fibroblasts. _____

8. Most types of _____ tissue are made of cells dispersed in an extracellular matrix.

9. What is the most common type of connective tissue? _____

10. The two types of connective tissue proper are _____ connective tissue and
_____ connective tissue.

11. *True or False.* Regular dense connective tissue is made of bundles of collagen fibers. _____

12. Connective tissue _____ and supports epithelial tissue.

13. List the types of extracellular fibers in alphabetical order. _____
_____

14. Describe the difference between loose connective tissue and dense connective tissue. _____
_____
_____

15. *True or False.* Adipocytes store biglycerides. _____

16. The _____ matrix, also called the _____ substance, is
a collection of material and fibers existing outside connective tissue cells.

17. *True or False.* Areolar connective tissue serves as a reservoir for water. _____

18. Tendons connect _____ to bone.

19. List the three types of loose connective tissue. _____
_____

20. Which of the following is *not* a type of dense connective tissue?
    A. irregular dense connective tissue   C. regular dense connective tissue
    B. elastic connective tissue   D. reticular connective tissue

21. The spleen, bone marrow, and lymph nodes are supported by _____ connective tissue.

Match the following terms with their definitions.

_____ 22. A cell that helps make extracellular fibers

_____ 23. The material and fibers existing outside connective
               tissue cells

_____ 24. Connective tissue that attaches bone to bone

_____ 25. An extracellular fiber that stretches

_____ 26. An extracellular fiber that is strong

_____ 27. An extracellular fiber that forms a network

_____ 28. Connective tissue that attaches muscle to bone

A. extracellular matrix
B. fibroblast
C. collagen fiber
D. elastic fiber
E. reticular fiber
F. tendon
G. ligament

Comprehensive Review (Chapters 1–8)

Answer the following questions using what you have learned so far in this book.

29. Which of the following is *not* an epithelial cell shape?

    A. stratified
    B. transitional
    C. cuboidal
    D. squamous

30. *True or False.* Your attitude is your way of feeling, thinking about, and viewing a situation. _____

31. Which of the following combining forms means "intestine"?

    A. oste/o
    B. gastr/o
    C. hepat/o
    D. enter/o

32. If the radius of a circle is 20 cm, what is the diameter of the circle? _____

33. Within the cell nucleus, DNA packages itself by wrapping around proteins called _____.

34. Constants are _____ factors that could affect the dependent variable.

35. List the two types of cell division. _____

36. Which of the following atoms has the highest atomic number?

    A. aluminum
    B. carbon
    C. lithium
    D. neon

Section 8.4 Bone, Cartilage, and Blood

Bone, cartilage, and blood—while not connective tissue proper—are also types of connective tissue. In this section, you will learn about bone, cartilage, and blood and their extracellular matrices.

The terms below are some of those that will be introduced in Section 8.4. To become familiar with these terms, reproduce each word on the line beside it. Pronounce each term as you write it. You will learn the definitions of these words as you complete this section.

1. bone _____

2. osteocyte _____

3. osteoblast _____

4. osteoclast _____

5. lacuna _____

6. compact bone _____

7. spongy bone _____

8. cartilage _____

9. chondrocyte _____

10. plasma _____

Concept 1: Bone

Bone is a type of connective tissue that is hard like rock. The extracellular matrix of bone is sturdy and solid, made of calcium salts reinforced with collagen fibers. Unlike rock, bone contains cells and is well supplied with blood. Bone tissue supports and protects the organs of the body.

bone a type of connective tissue made of cells and calcium salts reinforced with collagen fibers; is well supplied with blood

Recall Activity

1. List the two components of bone's extracellular matrix. _____

_____

2. *True or False.* Bone tissue is not well supplied with blood. _____

Concept 2: Bone Cells

Bone contains cells known as *osteocytes*. There are two types of osteocytes: osteoblasts and osteoclasts. *Osteoblasts* construct the bone matrix, and *osteoclasts* break down the bone matrix. Osteocytes live in *lacunae* (singular *lacuna*), which are cavities in the bone matrix (**Figure 8.14**). Nutrients and waste move through tiny tunnels that connect lacunae.

osteocyte a bone cell

osteoblast a bone cell that constructs the bone matrix

osteoclast a bone cell that breaks down the bone matrix

lacuna a cavity in the bone matrix

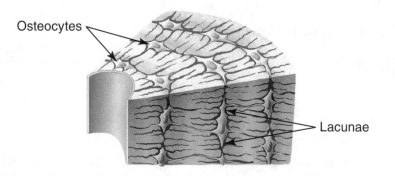

Osteocytes

Lacunae

© Body Scientific International

Figure 8.14   Osteocytes live in lacunae.

Recall Activity

1. Cavities in the bone matrix are called _____.

2. What are osteocytes?_____

3. List the two types of bone cells. _____

Concept 3: Types of Bone

compact bone a type of bone that looks solid

spongy bone a type of bone that looks like a honeycomb

There are two types of bone tissue: compact bone and spongy bone. *Compact bone* looks solid, whereas *spongy bone* looks like a honeycomb. The honeycomb of spongy bone is composed of spiked trabeculae. If an area of bone consists of compact bone and spongy bone, compact bone will form the border of the bone, and spongy bone will be on the inside (**Figure 8.15**).

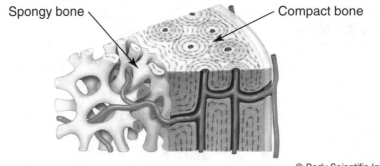

Spongy bone   Compact bone

© Body Scientific International

Figure 8.15 Compact bone forms the border of this bone, and spongy bone forms the inside.

Recall Activity

1. List the two types of bone tissue._____

2. If an area of bone consists of compact bone and spongy bone, _____ bone will form the border of the bone, and _____ bone will be on the inside.

Concept 4: Cartilage

cartilage an avascular connective tissue with an extracellular matrix made of extracellular fibers, carbohydrates, and water

chondrocyte a cartilage cell

Another type of connective tissue is cartilage. *Cartilage* is an avascular tissue with an extracellular matrix made of extracellular fibers, carbohydrates, and water. In cartilage, water binds to the collagen fibers of the extracellular matrix, making cartilage rubbery and flexible. Cartilage cells, called *chondrocytes*, are dispersed in a solid matrix within lacunae. Nutrients must move through the solid matrix to reach the lacunae, and there are no tunnels. Cartilage is not easily repaired when damaged. There are three types of cartilage: hyaline cartilage, elastic cartilage, and fibrocartilage.

Recall Activity

1. List the three components of cartilage's extracellular matrix. _____

_____

2. Is cartilage vascular or avascular? _____

3. In cartilage, _____ binds to _____ fibers, making cartilage rubbery and flexible.

Concept 5: Hyaline Cartilage

The first type of cartilage is hyaline cartilage. *Hyaline cartilage* is glassy and slick. It contains fine collagen fibers and covers the ends of bones, allowing frictionless motion at joints. Hyaline cartilage can also be found in your nose and in the cartilage rings in your trachea (**Figure 8.16**).

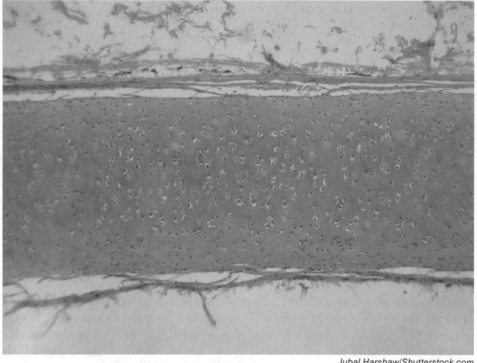

Jubal Harshaw/Shutterstock.com

Figure 8.16 Hyaline cartilage covers the ends of bones and is found in the nose and trachea.

Recall Activity

1. _____ cartilage is glassy and slick.

2. Hyaline cartilage covers the _____ of bones, allowing frictionless motion at

_____ .

Concept 6: Elastic Cartilage

Another type of cartilage is elastic cartilage. *Elastic cartilage* is a network of elastic fibers. Your ears are made of elastic cartilage. The flap that protects your trachea when you swallow, called the *epiglottis*, is also made of elastic cartilage.

Recall Activity

1. The _____ protects your trachea when you swallow.
2. _____ cartilage is a network of _____ fibers.

Concept 7: Fibrocartilage

A large number of thick collagen fibers make *fibrocartilage*, the strongest type of cartilage. Fibrocartilage is also flexible. The discs between your vertebrae (the bone segments that make up your spine), called *intervertebral discs*, are made of fibrocartilage.

Recall Activity

1. The strongest type of cartilage is _____.
2. The discs between your _____ are made of fibrocartilage.

Concept 8: Blood

Blood is a connective tissue that transports nutrients and waste. Blood is a connective tissue because it contains an extracellular matrix. The extracellular matrix of blood is called *plasma*. Plasma is primarily water, but also contains proteins such as *fibrinogen* (which is involved in forming blood clots). Blood is about 55% plasma and 45% formed elements (**Figure 8.17**). The formed elements include red blood cells (which carry oxygen), white blood cells (which fight infections), and platelets (which also help form blood clots).

plasma the extracellular matrix of blood; is primarily water, but also contains proteins

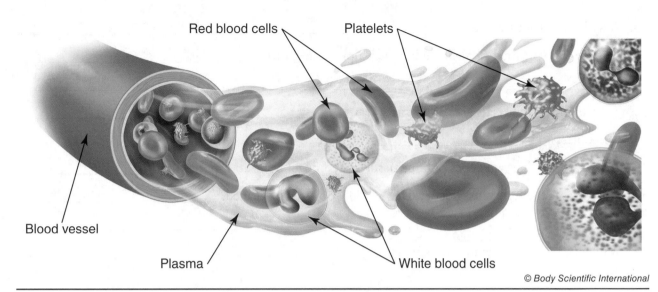

Figure 8.17 Blood is composed of plasma and formed elements.

© Body Scientific International

Recall Activity

1. Blood is about 55% _____ and 45% formed _____.

2. The extracellular matrix of blood is called _____.

3. Blood transports _____ and _____.

Section 8.4 Reinforcement

Answer the following questions using what you learned in this section.

1. Which of the following tissues makes up the nose?
   A. hyaline cartilage   C. bone
   B. elastic cartilage   D. fibrocartilage

2. The extracellular matrix of blood is called _____.

3. Osteocytes live in cavities in the bone matrix called _____.

4. List the types of cartilage in alphabetical order._____

   _____

5. Hyaline cartilage covers the ends of _____, allowing frictionless motion at

   _____.

6. Which of the following words are misspelled?
   A. mattrix   C. hyline cartilage   E. compact bone
   B. intervertebral disc D. spongi bone

7. *True or False.* Intervertebral discs cover the outsides of the vertebrae. _____

8. Why is blood considered a connective tissue?_____

9. List the three formed elements in blood in alphabetical order._____

_____

10. *True or False.* Bone cells are called *osteocytes.*_____

11. Osteoblasts _____ the bone matrix.

12. *True or False.* The two types of bone tissue are compact bone and spongy bone. _____

13. Unscramble the letters: tssalocoet. Define the word that is formed. _____

_____

14. Which of the following tissues is avascular?
   A. blood   C. bone
   B. cartilage

15. Which of the following are made of elastic cartilage?
   A. ears   C. epiglottis   D. intervertebral
   B. nose   discs

16. Unscramble the letters: ratibrolifecag. Define the word that is formed. _____

_____

17. Which of the following tissues is vascular?
   A. fibrocartilage   C. bone
   B. elastic cartilage   D. hyaline cartilage

18. The extracellular matrix of bone is made of _____ salts reinforced with
   _____ fibers.

19. What is the strongest type of cartilage?_____

20. *True or False.* Elastic cartilage is glassy and slick. _____

Match the following terms with their definitions.

_____ 21. A bone cell that constructs the bone matrix
                                                          A. osteoblast
_____ 22. Solid bone   B. osteoclast
                                                          C. lacuna
_____ 23. A cartilage cell
                                                          D. compact bone
_____ 24. A bone cell that breaks down the bone matrix
                                                          E. spongy bone
_____ 25. Bone that resembles a honeycomb
                                                          F. chondrocyte
_____ 26. The extracellular matrix of blood   G. plasma

_____ 27. A cavity in the bone matrix

Comprehensive Review (Chapters 1–8)

Answer the following questions using what you have learned so far in this book.

28. Protein buffers maintain the _____ of pH inside the cell.

29. *True or False.* You can concentrate on four or more tasks at one time. _____

30. List the types of extracellular fibers in connective tissue. _____

_____

31. List the steps of the diagnostic scientific method. _____

_____

32. *True or False.* One inch is the same length as 1.54 cm. _____

33. In a double covalent bond, how many electrons are shared? _____

34. What does a gastroenterologist study? _____

35. What type of endoplasmic reticulum contains no ribosomes? _____

Section 8.5 Muscle and Nerve Tissue

Muscle and nerve tissue are excitable tissues that perform important functions in the body. These tissues conduct electrical charges and are involved in the body's movement. In this section, you will learn about the properties of muscle and nerve tissue.

The terms below are some of those that will be introduced in Section 8.5. To become familiar with these terms, reproduce each word on the line beside it. Pronounce each term as you write it. You will learn the definitions of these words as you complete this section.

1. excitable tissue _____

2. action potential _____

3. neurotransmitter _____

4. muscle tissue _____

5. myocyte _____

6. voluntary muscle _____

7. involuntary muscle _____

8. nerve tissue _____

9. neuron _____

10. neuroglia _____

Concept 1: Excitable Tissue

Muscle and nerve tissue are types of excitable tissue. *Excitable tissue* produces an electrical charge when stimulated. For example, in muscle cells, an electrical charge known as *action potential* moves along the membranes of muscle cells and causes them to shorten. In nerve cells, action potential also moves along cell surfaces. When the action potential reaches the end of a nerve cell, it can cause a

excitable tissue a type of tissue that produces an electrical charge when stimulated; includes muscle and nerve tissue

action potential an electrical charge that moves along the membranes of cells; causes muscle cells to shorten and nerve cells to release neurotransmitters

neurotransmitter a chemical released from the end of a nerve cell that causes a new action potential to start in an adjacent cell

chemical called a *neurotransmitter* to be released (**Figure 8.18**). The neurotransmitter causes a new action potential to start in an adjacent nerve or muscle cell.

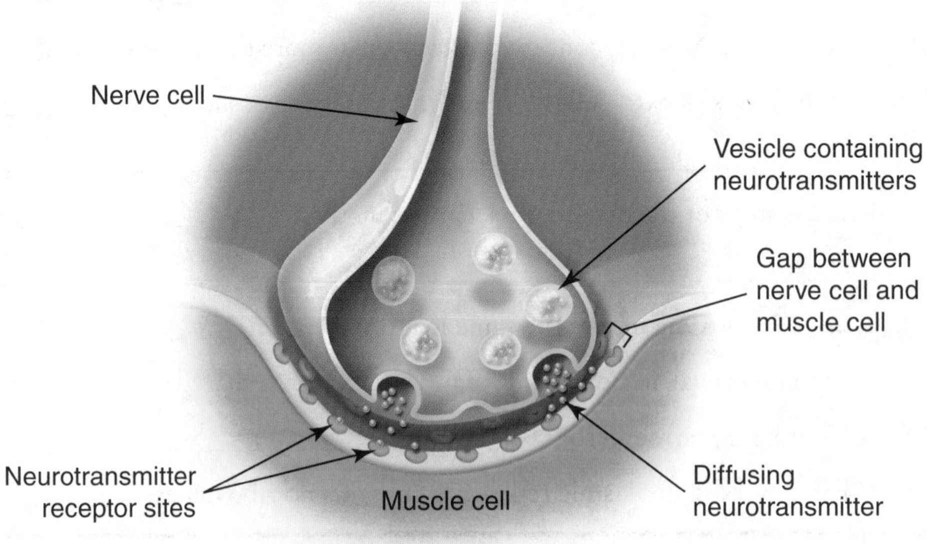

Nerve cell

Vesicle containing neurotransmitters

Gap between nerve cell and muscle cell

Neurotransmitter receptor sites

Muscle cell

Diffusing neurotransmitter

© Body Scientific International

Figure 8.18 Neurotransmitters are released at the end of this nerve cell to stimulate a muscle cell.

Recall Activity

1. _____ and _____ tissue are types of excitable tissue.

2. In muscle cells, an electrical charge known as _____ moves along the membranes of muscle cells.

3. *True or False*. Action potential causes muscle cells to shorten._____

4. When action potential reaches the end of a nerve cell, it can cause a(n) _____ to be released.

Concept 2: Muscle Tissue

muscle tissue an excitable tissue composed of muscle cells; contracts when stimulated

myocyte a muscle cell; also called a *muscle fiber*

Muscle tissue is an excitable tissue composed of muscle cells. When muscle cells are stimulated, they *contract* or shorten. After contracting, they return to normal length. Muscle cells are called *myocytes* or *muscle fibers*. There are three types of muscle tissue: skeletal muscle, smooth muscle, and cardiac muscle.

Recall Activity

1. When muscle cells are stimulated, they _____ or shorten.

2. List the three types of muscle tissue. _____

_____

3. Muscle cells are called _____ or _____ .

Concept 3: Skeletal Muscle

Skeletal muscle, as its name implies, is attached to bone. When skeletal muscles contract, the bones they are attached to move. Skeletal muscles are *voluntary muscles*, meaning you have conscious control of them, and skeletal muscle cells are long, rectangular, and multinucleate with visible bands called *striations* (**Figure 8.19**). Because muscles can only contract, skeletal muscles operate in pairs. In a pair of muscles, one muscle moves a bone one way, and the other muscle moves the bone back to its original position.

voluntary muscle muscle tissue that is consciously controlled

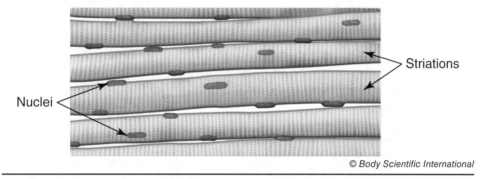

© Body Scientific International

Figure 8.19 Notice the striations of skeletal muscle.

Recall Activity

1. Skeletal muscle is attached to _____ .

2. *True or False.* A skeletal muscle cell has one nucleus._____

3. Visible bands in skeletal muscle cells are called _____ .

4. Skeletal muscles are _____ muscles, meaning you have

_____ control of them.

Concept 4: Smooth Muscle

Unlike skeletal muscle cells, the cells of *smooth muscle* do not have striations. Smooth muscle cells are shaped like spindles and tapered at both ends (**Figure 8.20**). Smooth muscles are *involuntary muscles*, meaning you do *not* have conscious control of them. Rather, the unconscious portion of your brain controls the contraction of smooth muscle. Hollow, tubelike organs, such as the small intestine, are circled by smooth muscle. When the smooth muscle of the small intestine contracts, the small intestine's diameter becomes smaller. This squeezing action moves food through the small intestine. Smooth muscle is also found in blood vessels.

involuntary muscle muscle tissue that is not consciously controlled

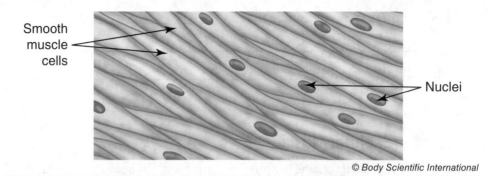

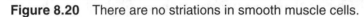

Figure 8.20   There are no striations in smooth muscle cells.

Recall Activity

1. How are smooth muscle cells different from skeletal muscle cells? _____

   _____

2. Where is smooth muscle found in the body? _____

3. Smooth muscles are _____ muscles, meaning you

   _____ have conscious control of them.

4. *True or False.* Smooth muscle cells do not have striations. _____

Concept 5: Cardiac Muscle

Cardiac muscle is a type of muscle tissue found only in the heart; it looks different from other types of muscle tissue. Cardiac muscle cells are involuntary and have branches. They are not as long as skeletal muscle cells and are *uninucleate* (having one nucleus). Cardiac muscle cells have striations as well as *intercalated discs* (where cardiac muscle cell branches meet), and they are bound together by desmosomes (**Figure 8.21**). The coordinated contraction of cardiac muscle cells is your heartbeat.

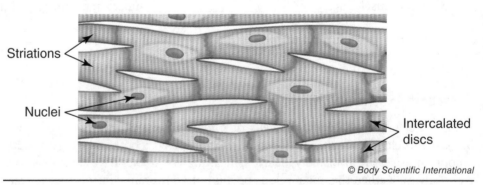

Figure 8.21   Cardiac muscle cells have striations and intercalated discs.

Recall Activity

1. Where in the body is cardiac muscle found? _____

2. Cardiac muscle is _____, meaning you _____ have conscious control of it.

3. Cardiac muscle branches meet at _____ discs.

4. The coordinated contraction of cardiac muscle cells is your _____.

Concept 6: Nerve Tissue

Nerve tissue is an excitable tissue composed of *neurons* (nerve cells that conduct electrical charges). A neuron consists of a *cell body* and two types of processes. The first process, known as a *dendrite*, receives electrical charges and then transmits them toward the cell body. The second process, known as an *axon*, transmits electrical charges away from the cell body (**Figure 8.22**). Neurons are responsible for communicating signals, such as movement and pain, all throughout the body. Nerve tissue also contains *neuroglia*, which are nonexcitable cells. Neuroglia support, insulate, and protect neurons.

nerve tissue an excitable tissue composed of neurons; is responsible for communicating signals, such as movement and pain, all throughout the body

neuron a nerve cell that conducts an electrical charge; has a cell body, dendrites, and an axon

neuroglia a nonexcitable nerve cell that supports, insulates, and protects neurons

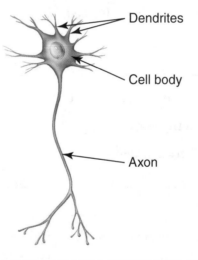

Dendrites

Cell body

Axon

© Body Scientific International

Figure 8.22 A neuron consists of a cell body, an axon, and dendrites.

Recall Activity

1. A neuron consists of a(n) _____ and _____ type(s) of process(es).

2. What is the purpose of neurons? _____

3. _____ support, insulate, and protect neurons.

Section 8.5 Reinforcement

Answer the following questions using what you learned in this section.

1. Which of the following types of muscle tissue is voluntary?

   A. cardiac muscle   C. smooth muscle

   B. skeletal muscle

2. Cardiac muscle cells are bound together by _____.

3. *True or False.* Neuroglia are excitable cells. _____

4. When _____ cells are stimulated, they contract or shorten.

5. Which of the following muscle cells have striations?

   A. smooth muscle cells   C. skeletal muscle cells

   B. cardiac muscle cells

6. A neuron consists of a(n) _____, dendrites, and a(n)

   _____.

7. Excitable tissue produces a(n) _____ charge when

   _____.

8. Unscramble the letters: lynovratu. Define the word that is formed. _____

   _____

9. Which type of muscle cell is tapered?_____

10. _____ support, insulate, and protect neurons.

11. *True or False.* Cardiac muscle is found only in the heart._____

12. List the three types of muscle tissue in alphabetical order. _____

    _____

13. Which type of muscle cell has intercalated discs? _____

14. *True or False.* Hollow, tubelike organs in the body are circled by smooth muscle. _____

15. Unscramble the letters: licbeetax. Define the word that is formed. _____

    _____

16. *True or False.* Muscle cells are also called *muscle fibers.* _____

17. Because muscles can only contract, skeletal muscles operate in _____.

18. Which type of muscle cell has branches?_____

19. Explain the difference between voluntary and involuntary muscles. _____

    _____

20. Which of the following types of muscle tissue are involuntary?
   A. smooth muscle   C. skeletal muscle
   B. cardiac muscle

21. _____ tissue produces an electrical charge when stimulated.

Match the following terms with their definitions.

_____ 22. An electrical charge that moves along the membranes of muscle and nerve cells

_____ 23. Muscle cell

_____ 24. Muscle that is consciously controlled

_____ 25. A chemical released from a neuron that causes a new action potential to start in an adjacent cell

_____ 26. Tissue that produces an electrical charge when stimulated

_____ 27. Nonexcitable cells that support, protect, and insulate neurons

_____ 28. Muscle that is not consciously controlled

_____ 29. A nerve cell that conducts an electrical charge

A. excitable tissue
B. action potential
C. neurotransmitter
D. myocyte
E. involuntary muscle
F. voluntary muscle
G. neuron
H. neuroglia

Comprehensive Review (Chapters 1–8)

Answer the following questions using what you have learned so far in this book.

30. Which of the following is *not* a type of endocytosis?
   A. pinocytosis   C. phagocytosis   D. receptor-mediated endocytosis
   B. diffusion

31. List the three parts of a nucleotide. _____

32. *True or False.* Your study sessions should last at least 80 minutes with no breaks. _____

33. *True or False.* All constants are the same for the experimental and control groups. _____

34. Both cytosol and interstitial fluid are primarily _____.

35. Which of the following represents the smallest mass?
   A. 0.2 kg   B. 20 g   C. 2 g   D. 200 g

36. Describe the composition of bone's extracellular matrix. _____

_____

37. Identify and define the combining form in the term *hepatocyte*. _____

Chapter 8 Review

Answer the following questions using what you learned in this chapter.

1. Epithelial tissue covers the _____ of the body and lines internal hollow _____ and _____.

2. Which type of tissue fulfills the important functions of connection, support, and protection?
   _____

3. The basal surface of epithelial tissue is attached to an acellular _____ membrane.

4. The _____ matrix is a collection of material and fibers existing outside connective tissue cells.

5. Which epithelial surface has contact with open space? _____

6. How does epithelial tissue receive nutrients and oxygen and dispose of waste? _____

   _____

   _____

   _____

7. List the two types of bone cells. _____

8. Which type of epithelial tissue lines the stomach? _____

9. *True or False.* Squamous cells are flat. _____

10. Which type of muscle tissue has intercalated discs? _____

11. _____ connective tissue is composed mostly of extracellular fibers with few cells.

12. Which of the following is *not* a part of a neuron?
    A. axon   C. striation
    B. dendrite   D. cell body

13. In _____ epithelium, the epithelial cells of the basal layer continually reproduce, and the epithelial cells of the apical layer are shed by abrasion.

14. Unscramble the letters: nattlionasir. Define the word that is formed. _____

    _____

15. Osteocytes live in _____, which are cavities in the bone matrix.

16. In muscle cells, an electrical charge known as _____ moves along the membranes of muscle cells and causes them to shorten.

17. *True or False.* Endocrine glands release products through a duct. _____

18. Describe the difference between voluntary and involuntary muscle. _____

    _____

19. Which of the following is *not* an extracellular fiber?
    A. elastic fiber   C. collagen fiber
    B. reticular fiber   D. hyaline fiber

20. Elastic fibers allow _____ connective tissue to stretch and recoil.

21. *True or False.* Neuroglia are excitable cells that conduct electrical charges. _____

22. A(n) _____ is made of different types of tissues working together to do a job.

23. Straight rows of bundled collagen fibers make up _____ connective tissue.

24. _____ connective tissue is composed of many cells with extracellular fibers winding through them.

25. Which type of tissue has direct access to a blood supply? _____

26. Which part of the neuron receives electrical charges and then transmits them toward the cell body?

27. *True or False.* In the simple arrangement, epithelial cells form a border that is only one cell thick. _____

28. Simple cuboidal epithelium is an epithelial tissue consisting of _____ layer(s) of _____ cells.

29. The extracellular matrix of bone is made of _____ salts reinforced with _____ fibers.

30. Which three organs contain reticular connective tissue? _____
   _____

Comprehensive Review (Chapters 1–8)

Using what you have learned so far in this book, match the following terms with their definitions.

_____ 31. Not attracted to water	A. fraction
_____ 32. Not having access to a blood supply	B. hydrophobic
_____ 33. The first stage of protein synthesis in which the sense strand of DNA is copied to make mRNA in a cell's nucleus	C. avascular
	D. scientific theory
	E. transcription
_____ 34. A protein catalyst	F. cortic/o
_____ 35. A part of a whole number	G. enzyme
_____ 36. A confirmed observation	H. cytoskeleton
_____ 37. The structure that supports the cell; includes microfilaments, intermediate filaments, and microtubules	I. fact
	J. -plasm
_____ 38. A combining form that means "outer region"	
_____ 39. A suffix that means "formation"	
_____ 40. The best explanation today of why a phenomenon occurs	

Chapter 9
Human Body Orientation

Introduction

Having a solid foundation in the knowledge of cells and tissues, you are now ready to study anatomy and physiology. As you have learned, *anatomy* is the study of body parts, and *physiology* is the study of how body parts function. This chapter will introduce you to the basic concepts that help students and healthcare professionals understand the human body. You will learn about body planes, cavities, and regions. You will also learn about terms related to anatomical location, the body's structural organization, and homeostasis in the body.

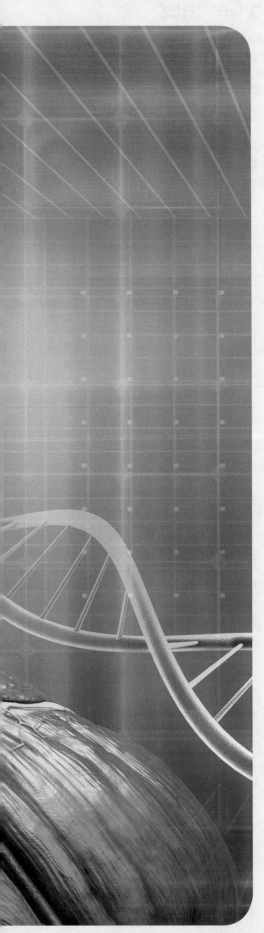

Objectives

After completing this chapter, you will be able to

- describe anatomical position
- identify and understand the body planes
- list the major dorsal and ventral cavities of the body
- know the regions of the body, including regions of the head and neck, trunk, and appendages
- identify the abdominopelvic regions
- use anatomical terms related to location and position
- understand the five levels of organization in the body
- explain how homeostatic body temperature, blood glucose concentration, and blood pH are maintained in the body

Key Terms

The following terms and phrases will be introduced and explained in Chapter 9. Read through the list to become familiar with the words.

abdominal cavity	intermediate
abdominal region	lateral
abdominopelvic cavity	lower limb
abdominopelvic region	manus
anatomical position	medial
appendicular region	midsagittal plane
axial region	negative feedback
blood glucose concentration	organism
body cavity	pedal
body plane	pelvic cavity
body system	pelvic region
body temperature	proximal
cephalic region	pubic region
cervical region	sagittal plane
cranial cavity	spinal cavity
deep	superficial
distal	superior
dorsal	thoracic cavity
frontal plane	thoracic region
glucagon	transverse plane
inferior	upper limb
insulin	ventral

Section 9.1 Body Planes and Cavities

The study of anatomy and physiology is the study of body parts and their functions. In the fields of anatomy and physiology, healthcare professionals and students use body planes to describe locations and positions on the body. Body cavities also help divide the human body into sections that can be studied. In this section, you will learn about anatomical position and about body planes and cavities.

The terms below are some of those that will be introduced in Section 9.1. To become familiar with these terms, reproduce each word on the line beside it. Pronounce each term as you write it. You will learn the definitions of these words as you complete this section.

1. anatomical position _____

2. body plane _____

3. midsagittal plane _____

4. sagittal plane _____

5. frontal plane _____

6. transverse plane _____

7. body cavity _____

8. cranial cavity _____

9. spinal cavity _____

10. thoracic cavity _____

11. abdominal cavity _____

12. pelvic cavity _____

13. abdominopelvic cavity _____

Concept 1: Anatomical Position

anatomical position a body position in which a person stands upright with feet apart, arms at the sides, feet and palms facing forward, and thumbs pointing away from the body

Anatomy and physiology describe the locations and positions of body structures and body movements. *Anatomy* is the study of body parts, and *physiology* is the study of how body parts function. In anatomy and physiology, body locations are described in reference to *anatomical position*. *Anatomical position* is a body position in which a person stands upright with feet apart, arms at the sides, feet and palms facing forward, and thumbs pointing away from the body (**Figure 9.1**).

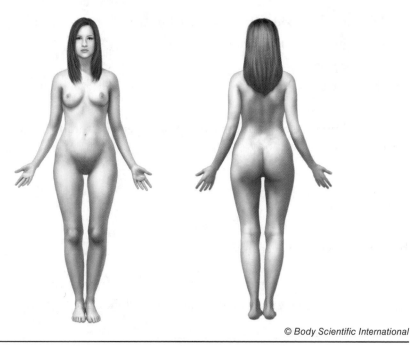
© Body Scientific International

Figure 9.1 Anatomy and physiology describe locations on the body in reference to anatomical position.

Recall Activity

1. In anatomy and physiology, body locations are described in reference to _____.

2. In anatomical position, the palms and feet face _____.

3. In anatomical position, the _____ point away from the body.

Concept 2: Body Planes

When describing locations, positions, and directions on the body, *body planes* serve as reference points. *Body planes* are imaginary, flat surfaces that divide the body into sections. They are also known as *anatomical planes*. Body planes divide the body in reference to anatomical position and divide the body into the same sections from any viewing angle (**Figure 9.2**).

body plane an imaginary, flat surface that divides the body into sections; also called an *anatomical plane*

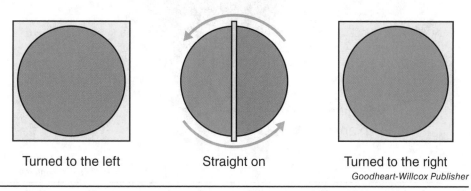

Turned to the left   Straight on   Turned to the right
Goodheart-Willcox Publisher

Figure 9.2 A plane divides this ball into left and right sections. The plane divides the ball into the same sections from all three viewing angles.

Four standard body planes are used in anatomy and physiology:

- midsagittal (median) plane
- sagittal plane
- frontal (coronal) plane
- transverse plane

By dividing the body into parts, you can get a better idea of how organs are positioned inside the body.

Recall Activity

1. List the four standard body planes used in anatomy and physiology._____

_____

2. Body _____ are imaginary, flat surfaces that divide the body into sections.

3. Body planes divide the body in reference to _____.

Concept 3: Midsagittal and Sagittal Planes

The *midsagittal* and *sagittal planes* divide the body into left and right sections. Both planes start at the top of the head and continue down through the body. The *midsagittal plane*, also known as the *median plane*, divides the body down the middle into equal left and right halves. The *sagittal plane* also divides the body into left and right sections, but not down the middle (**Figure 9.3**).

midsagittal plane a body plane that divides the body into equal left and right halves; also called the *median plane*

sagittal plane a body plane that divides the body into unequal left and right sections

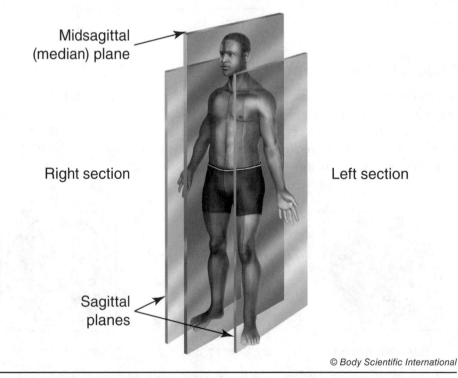

Midsagittal (median) plane

Right section

Left section

Sagittal planes

© Body Scientific International

Figure 9.3 The midsagittal plane divides the body into equal left and right halves. The sagittal plane divides the body into unequal left and right sections.

Recall Activity

1. Which body plane divides the body into equal left and right halves? _____

2. Which body plane divides the body into unequal left and right sections? _____

Concept 4: Frontal Plane

The *frontal plane* divides the body into front (ventral) and back (dorsal) sections. The frontal plane starts at the top of the head and continues down through the body (**Figure 9.4**). The sections on either side of the plane are not equal. The frontal plane is also called the *coronal plane*.

frontal plane a body plane that divides the body into front (ventral) and back (dorsal) sections; also called the *coronal plane*

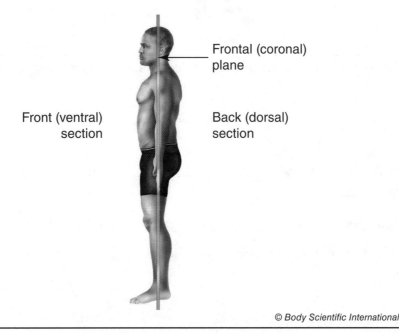

Frontal (coronal) plane

Front (ventral) section

Back (dorsal) section

© Body Scientific International

Figure 9.4 The frontal plane divides the body into front and back sections.

Recall Activity

1. The _____ plane divides the body into front and back sections.

2. *True or False.* The sections on either side of the frontal plane are not equal. _____

Concept 5: Transverse Plane

The *transverse plane* divides the body into top and bottom sections. The transverse plane passes through the middle of the body, starting at one arm and continuing through the body to the opposite arm (**Figure 9.5**). Sections of the body divided by the transverse plane are called *cross-sections*.

transverse plane a body plane that divides the body into top and bottom sections

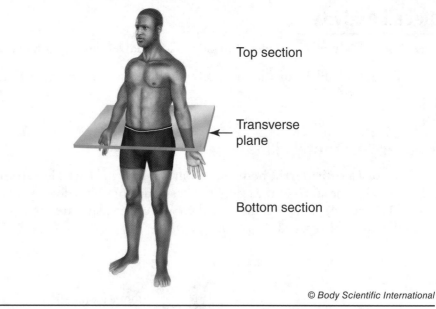

Top section

Transverse
plane

Bottom section

© Body Scientific International

Figure 9.5 The transverse plane divides the body into top and bottom sections.

Recall Activity

1. The transverse plane divides the body into _____ and

   _____ sections.

2. The transverse plane passes through the _____ of the body.

3. Sections of the body divided by the transverse plane are called _____.

Concept 6: Body Cavities

body cavity a space within the body that contains organs

A *body cavity* is a space within the body that contains organs. If you took the organs out of the body, the remaining body cavities would be empty. Some body cavities are surrounded by bone, and others are surrounded by muscle, connective tissue, or epithelial tissue. The body contains dorsal and ventral cavities.

Recall Activity

1. A body cavity is a space within the body that contains _____.

2. Some body cavities are surrounded by _____, and others are surrounded by

   muscle, _____ tissue, or _____ tissue.

Concept 7: Dorsal Cavities

The frontal plane divides the body into back (dorsal) and front (ventral) sections. The *dorsal* surface of the body is the back. There are two body cavities in the dorsal section: the cranial cavity and the spinal cavity. The skull forms the *cranial cavity*, which contains the brain. The hollow spaces inside vertebrae (bone segments of the spine) form the *spinal cavity*, which protects the spinal cord (**Figure 9.6**).

cranial cavity the dorsal body cavity that contains the brain

spinal cavity the dorsal body cavity that contains the spinal cord

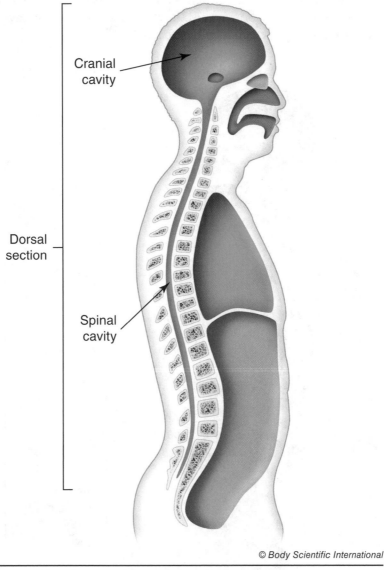

Cranial cavity

Dorsal section

Spinal cavity

© Body Scientific International

Figure 9.6 The dorsal cavities are the cranial and spinal cavities.

Recall Activity

1. Name the two body cavities in the dorsal section. _____

2. Which body cavity protects the brain? _____

Concept 8: Ventral Cavities

The *ventral* surface of the body is the front. There are three cavities in the ventral section: the thoracic cavity, the abdominal cavity, and the pelvic cavity.

thoracic cavity the ventral body cavity that contains the heart and lungs

abdominal cavity the ventral body cavity that contains the stomach, liver, spleen, and intestines

pelvic cavity the ventral body cavity that contains the urinary bladder and some reproductive organs

abdominopelvic cavity the abdominal and pelvic cavities; contains the stomach, liver, spleen, intestines, urinary bladder, and some reproductive organs

The *thoracic cavity* is formed by the rib cage and protects the heart and lungs. A portion of the rib cage forms the upper *abdominal cavity*; the rest of the abdominal cavity is surrounded with soft tissue. The major organs of the abdominal cavity are the stomach, liver, spleen, and intestines. The *pelvic cavity* is surrounded by the bones of the pelvis and contains the urinary bladder and some reproductive organs. Sometimes the abdominal and pelvic cavities are referred to collectively as the *abdominopelvic cavity* (**Figure 9.7**).

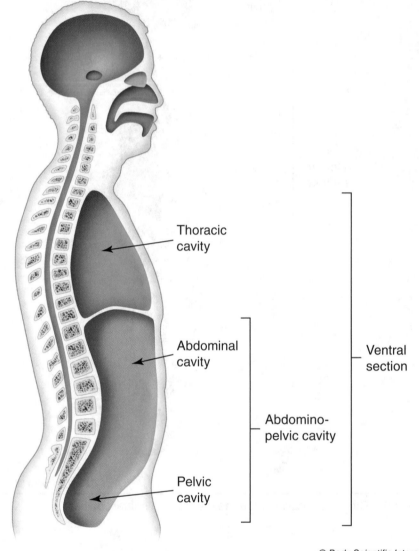

Thoracic cavity

Abdominal cavity

Pelvic cavity

Abdomino-pelvic cavity

Ventral section

© *Body Scientific International*

Figure 9.7 The ventral cavities are the thoracic, abdominal, and pelvic cavities.

Recall Activity

1. The _____ cavity protects the heart and lungs.

2. The abdominal and pelvic cavities are referred to collectively as the _____ cavity.

3. The urinary bladder and some reproductive organs are housed in the _____ cavity.

Section 9.1 Reinforcement

Answer the following questions using what you learned in this section.

1. In anatomical position, the _____ and _____ face forward.

2. Which of the following body planes divides the body into equal left and right halves?
   A. sagittal plane   C. frontal plane
   B. midsagittal plane   D. transverse plane

3. A(n) _____ is a space within the body that contains organs.

4. *True or False.* The frontal plane is also called the *coronal plane.* _____

5. Unscramble the letters: nertlav. Define the word that is formed. _____

   _____

6. Which of the following words are misspelled?
   A. dorsal   C. saggital
   B. ventrile   D. median

7. Which of the following is *not* a ventral cavity?
   A. thoracic cavity   C. pelvic cavity
   B. spinal cavity   D. abdominal cavity

8. The two body cavities of the dorsal section are the _____ cavity and the
   _____ cavity.

9. *True or False.* The stomach, liver, and intestines are housed in the pelvic cavity. _____

10. Describe the difference between the midsagittal plane and the sagittal plane. _____

    _____

    _____

11. Which of the following are ventral body cavities?
    A. thoracic cavity   C. pelvic cavity
    B. spinal cavity   D. abdominal cavity

12. The _____ plane divides the body into front and back sections.

13. Sections of the body divided by the _____ plane are called cross-sections.

14. *True or False.* All body cavities are surrounded by bone. _____

15. Which body cavity contains the heart and lungs? _____

16. *True or False.* The term *ventral* refers to the back section of the body. _____

17. The skull forms the _____ cavity.

18. In anatomical position, which direction do the thumbs point? _____

19. Unscramble the letters: haccroti. Define the word that is formed. _____

    _____

20. Which of the following are dorsal body cavities?

    A. thoracic cavity   C. pelvic cavity

    B. spinal cavity   D. cranial cavity

21. Which body plane divides the body into top and bottom sections?_____

Match the following terms with their definitions.

_____ 22. A body plane that divides the body into unequal left and right sections

_____ 23. A body plane that divides the body into equal left and right halves

_____ 24. A body plane that divides the body into front and back sections

_____ 25. A body plane that divides the body into top and bottom sections

_____ 26. An imaginary, flat surface that divides the body into sections

_____ 27. A body position in which a person stands upright with feet apart, arms at the sides, feet and palms facing forward, and thumbs pointing away from the body

A. anatomical position
B. body plane
C. midsagittal plane
D. sagittal plane
E. frontal plane
F. transverse plane

Comprehensive Review (Chapters 1–9)

Answer the following questions using what you have learned so far in this book.

28. Which body plane divides the body into equal left and right halves? _____

29. The "then" portion of a hypothesis is the _____ variable.

30. Why are hydrogen bonds the weakest type of atomic bond? _____

    _____

31. Science's body of knowledge is the _____ that scientists have accumulated about the natural world.

32. *True or False.* Cytoplasm is all the material found inside a cell except for the nucleus. _____

33. Which of the following word parts means "layer"?

    A. alb/o   C. rect/o   E. strat/o

    B. sten/o   D. lat/o   F. rubr/o

34. When atoms move from areas of high concentration to areas of low concentration, this is called a(n) _____ reaction.

35. The volume measurement of 1000 mL is the same as _____ L.

36. Which type of muscle tissue is voluntary? _____

Section 9.2 Regions of the Body

In anatomy and physiology, healthcare professionals and students use an array of terms to refer to specific regions of the body. In this section, you will learn about abdominopelvic regions and about anatomical terms related to the head and neck, trunk, and limbs.

The terms below are some of those that will be introduced in Section 9.2. To become familiar with these terms, reproduce each word on the line beside it. Pronounce each term as you write it. You will learn the definitions of these words as you complete this section.

1. axial region _____

2. appendicular region _____

3. cephalic region _____

4. cervical region _____

5. thoracic region _____

6. abdominal region _____

7. pelvic region _____

8. pubic region _____

9. abdominopelvic region _____

10. upper limb _____

11. manus _____

12. lower limb _____

13. pedal _____

Concept 1: Axial Versus Appendicular Regions

The body can be divided into axial and appendicular regions. The *axial region* of the body is the body's core: the head, neck, and trunk. The *appendicular region* includes the *appendages*, or limbs (arms and legs). The appendicular region is attached to the axial region, and regional terms identify specific surfaces of axial and appendicular parts (**Figure 9.8**).

axial region the head, neck, and trunk of the body

appendicular region the limbs (arms and legs) of the body

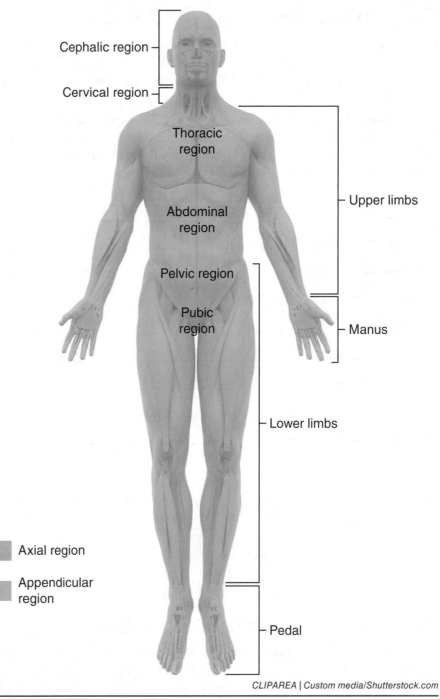

Cephalic region

Cervical region

Thoracic region

Abdominal region

Pelvic region

Pubic region

Upper limbs

Manus

Lower limbs

Axial region

Appendicular region

Pedal

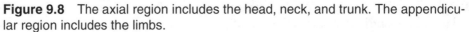
CLIPAREA | Custom media/Shutterstock.com

Figure 9.8 The axial region includes the head, neck, and trunk. The appendicular region includes the limbs.

Recall Activity

1. The limbs are part of the _____ region of the body.

2. *True or False.* The axial region and the appendicular region are attached. _____

3. The _____ region of the body includes the head, neck, and trunk.

Concept 2: Head and Neck

At the top of the body, the head and neck are part of the axial region. The head area is called the *cephalic region*. Some surface parts of the cephalic region include the forehead, scalp, eyes, nose, mouth, cheeks, lips, and ears. The neck area is called the *cervical region* and includes the cervical vertebrae (bone segments of the spine that make up the neck).

cephalic region the head area of the body

cervical region the neck area of the body

Recall Activity

1. The head area is called the _____ region.

2. The cervical region makes up the _____ area and includes the cervical vertebrae.

3. List three surface parts of the cephalic region. _____

Concept 3: Trunk

The *trunk* of the body encompasses the chest, thorax, and hips. The body's trunk can be divided into four regions: the thoracic region, the abdominal region, the pelvic region, and the pubic region. The *thoracic region* includes the chest or breast. The *abdominal region* encompasses the belly and navel (belly button). The *pelvic region* includes the hips, and the *pubic region* refers to the groin and genitals.

thoracic region the chest or breast area of the body

abdominal region the belly area of the body

pelvic region the hip area of the body

pubic region the groin and genital area of the body

Recall Activity

1. Which region refers to the groin and genitals? _____

2. The _____ region includes the chest or breast.

3. The abdominal region encompasses the _____ and
_____.

Concept 4: Abdominopelvic Regions

The abdominal and pelvic regions encompass the *abdominal cavity* and the *pelvic cavity*, known collectively as the *abdominopelvic cavity*. The abdominopelvic cavity can be divided into nine regions, much like a tic-tac-toe box. When referring to the *abdominopelvic regions*, envision the body in anatomical position. In anatomy, *left* always refers to the body's left (not your left), and *right* always refers to the body's right (not your right). The abdominopelvic regions are organized into three rows and three columns (**Figure 9.9**).

abdominopelvic region an area of the abdominopelvic cavity

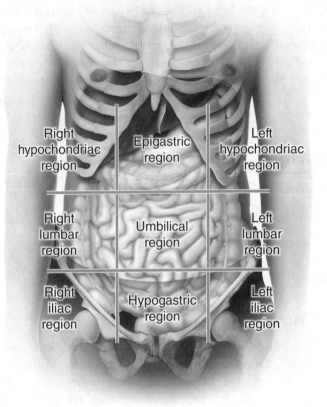

© Body Scientific International

Figure 9.9 There are nine abdominopelvic regions.

Recall Activity

1. The abdominopelvic regions are organized into three _____ and three _____.

2. In anatomy, *left* always refers to _____ left, and *right* always refers to _____ right.

3. The abdominopelvic cavity is divided into _____ region(s).

Concept 5: First Row

In the first row of abdominopelvic regions are the right hypochondriac region, the epigastric region, and the left hypochondriac region. The prefix *hypo-* means "below," and the root word *chondr* (meaning "cartilage") refers to the cartilage of the rib cage. Thus, the *right hypochondriac region* and the *left hypochondriac region* refer to the abdominopelvic areas just below the rib cage. The prefix *epi-* means "upon," and the root word *gastr* refers to the stomach. Thus, the *epigastric region* encompasses the area above the stomach.

Recall Activity

1. List the three abdominopelvic regions in the first row. _____

   _____

2. Disassemble and define the word *epigastric*. _____

3. Which of the following word parts means "below"?
   A. hypo-   C. chondr
   B. epi-   D. gastr

Concept 6: Second Row

The second row of abdominopelvic regions contains the right lumbar region, the umbilical region, and the left lumbar region. The word *lumbar* is formed from the root word *lumb* (meaning "lower back") and the suffix *-ar* (meaning "pertaining to"). Thus, the *right lumbar region* and the *left lumbar region* refer to abdominopelvic areas of the lower back. The *umbilical region* identifies the area where the navel (the remnant of the *umbilical* cord) is located.

Recall Activity

1. The navel is the remnant of the _____ cord.

2. The second row of abdominopelvic regions contains the right _____ region, the _____ region, and the left _____ region.

3. The right lumbar region and the left lumbar region refer to abdominopelvic areas of the _____.

Concept 7: Third Row

In the third row of abdominopelvic regions are the right iliac region, the hypogastric region, and the left iliac region. The word *iliac* is formed from the root word *ili* (meaning "ilium") and the suffix *-ac* (meaning "pertaining to") and refers to the portion of the pelvis called the *ilium* (**Figure 9.10**). The *right iliac region* and the *left iliac region* encompass the area around the ilium. The prefix *hypo-* means "below," and the root word *gastr* refers to the stomach; therefore, the *hypogastric region* is the area below the stomach.

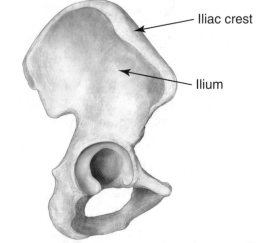

Iliac crest

Ilium

© Body Scientific International

Figure 9.10   The ilium is a portion of the pelvis.

Recall Activity

1. The hypogastric region is the area below the _____.

2. The word *iliac* refers to a portion of the pelvis called the _____.

3. List the three abdominopelvic regions in the third row. _____

_____

Concept 8: Limbs

upper limb the arm and shoulder area of the body

manus the hand area of the body

lower limb the leg and hip area of the body

pedal the foot area of the body

The limbs, or *appendages*, make up the appendicular region of the body and include the arms, hands, legs, and feet. The arms are called the *upper limbs*, and the surfaces of the upper limbs include the shoulder, upper arm, elbow (front and back), forearm, and wrist. The hands are referred to as *manus* and include the surfaces of your thumbs, palms, and digits (fingers). The *lower limbs* are the legs. The surfaces of the lower limbs are the hip, thigh, knee (front and back), calf, shin, and ankle. The feet are called *pedal* and include the surfaces of the sole, heel, and digits (toes). An easy way to distinguish between manus and pedal is that *manicures* are for your hands, and *pedicures* are for your feet.

Recall Activity

1. The hands are referred to as _____.

2. The _____ are called pedal.

3. Explain the difference between the upper and lower limbs. _____

_____

Section 9.2 Reinforcement

Answer the following questions using what you learned in this section.

1. The _____ area is called the *cephalic region*.

2. *True or False.* The navel is also known as the *belly button*. _____

3. The pubic region refers to the _____ and genitals.

4. Name the abdominopelvic regions in the second row. _____

   _____

5. In which region is the chest found?
   - A. pelvic region
   - B. thoracic region
   - C. abdominal region
   - D. pubic region

6. Which body cavity is divided into nine regions? _____

7. *True or False.* The pelvic region encompasses the belly and navel. _____

8. Which of the following words are misspelled?
   - A. epigastric
   - B. hypochondric
   - C. lumbar
   - D. umbiblical

9. Name the abdominopelvic regions in the third row. _____

   _____

10. *True or False.* The term *pedal* refers to the hand. _____

11. Which region of the body encompasses the head, neck, and trunk? _____

12. The _____ region of the body includes the limbs (arms and legs).

13. Which of the following is *not* an abdominopelvic region of the first row?
    - A. epigastric region
    - B. left hypochondriac region
    - C. umbilical region
    - D. right hypochondriac region

14. Unscramble the letters: schryogipta. Define the word that is formed. _____

   _____

15. The _____ area is called the *cervical region*.

16. *True or False.* The surfaces of the upper limbs include the shoulder, upper arm, elbow (front and back), forearm, and wrist. _____

17. List the four regions of the trunk. _____

   _____

18. Unscramble the letters: enaclapdipru. Define the word that is formed. _____

   _____

19. *True or False.* The prefix *hypo-* means "below." _____

20. Which of the following word parts means "stomach"?

    A. chondr   C. hypo-

    B. gastr   D. epi-

21. The feet are called _____ and include the surfaces of the sole, heel, and digits (toes).

Match the following terms with their definitions.

_____ 22. The hands

_____ 23. The neck area

_____ 24. The feet

_____ 25. The area containing the chest

_____ 26. The area containing the groin

_____ 27. The arms

_____ 28. The legs

_____ 29. The head, neck, and trunk

_____ 30. The head area

_____ 31. The abdominal and pelvic cavities

_____ 32. The area containing the hips

_____ 33. The area containing the belly

_____ 34. The limbs (arms and legs)

A. abdominopelvic cavity
B. axial region
C. appendicular region
D. cephalic region
E. cervical region
F. thoracic region
G. abdominal region
H. pelvic region
I. pubic region
J. upper limbs
K. manus
L. lower limbs
M. pedal

Comprehensive Review (Chapters 1–9)

Answer the following questions using what you have learned so far in this book.

35. The prefix *meso-* means "_____."

36. An explanation is supernatural if it cannot be _____.

37. Arrange the following phases of mitosis from first to last: anaphase, prophase, telophase, and metaphase.

    _____

38. A scientific law is a general statement of _____.

39. Describe anatomical position. _____

    _____

40. What is the complementary base of guanine? _____

41. Water freezes at _____°C.

42. *True or False.* A cell's plasma membrane is selectively permeable. _____

43. Which of the following body parts are made of elastic cartilage?

    A. nose   C. ear

    B. mouth   D. epiglottis

Section 9.3 Terms of Location

Anatomy and physiology includes many terms related to the locations of body parts. All of these terms apply only when the body is in anatomical position. Some of the terms you will learn about in this section include *superior, inferior, ventral, dorsal, medial, lateral, intermediate, proximal, distal, superficial,* and *deep.* By the end of this section, you will know how to use all of these terms correctly.

The terms below are some of those that will be introduced in Section 9.3. To become familiar with these terms, reproduce each word on the line beside it. Pronounce each term as you write it. You will learn the definitions of these words as you complete this section.

1. superior _____

2. inferior _____

3. ventral _____

4. dorsal _____

5. medial _____

6. lateral _____

7. intermediate _____

8. proximal _____

9. distal _____

10. superficial _____

11. deep _____

Concept 1: Describing Location

In anatomy and physiology, healthcare professionals and students often describe the locations of body parts in comparison to other body parts. Comparing the locations of body parts in relation to each other makes it easier to envision positions on the body. Note that the terms of location introduced in this section only apply to body parts when the body is in anatomical position.

Recall Activity

1. Healthcare professionals and students often describe the locations of body parts in comparison to _____.

2. Terms of location only apply to body parts when the body is in _____.

3. *True or False.* Terms of location apply to body parts when the body is in any position. _____

Concept 2: Superior and Inferior

The terms *superior* and *inferior* indicate whether a body part is closer to the head or closer to the feet. If a body part is *superior*, it is closer to the head. If a body part is *inferior*, it is closer to the feet. For example, your head is superior to your neck, and your neck is inferior to your head. Your neck is superior to your shoulder, and your shoulder is inferior to your neck (**Figure 9.11**).

superior closer to the head of the body

inferior closer to the feet of the body

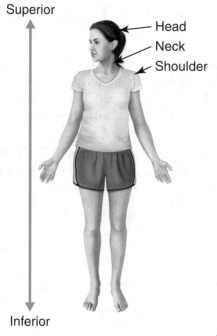

Superior

Head
Neck
Shoulder

Inferior

© Body Scientific International

Figure 9.11 If a body part is superior, it is closer to the head. If it is inferior, it is closer to the feet.

Recall Activity

1. Which of the following body parts is most superior?

   A. hip   C. ankle

   B. chest   D. knee

2. Your navel is _____ to your neck.

3. Which of the following body parts is most inferior?

   A. eye   C. neck

   B. nose   D. shoulder

4. Your elbow is _____ to your knee.

Concept 3: Ventral and Dorsal

ventral closer to the front of the body; also called *anterior*

dorsal closer to the back of the body; also called *posterior*

Ventral and *dorsal* describe locations in relation to the front and back of the body. If a body part is *ventral*, it is closer to the front of the body. Another word for ventral is *anterior*. If a body part is *dorsal*, it is closer to the back of the body. Another word for dorsal is *posterior*. Your heart is ventral (anterior) to your spine, and your spine is dorsal (posterior) to your heart. Your sternum is ventral (anterior) to your heart, and your heart is dorsal (posterior) to your sternum (**Figure 9.12**).

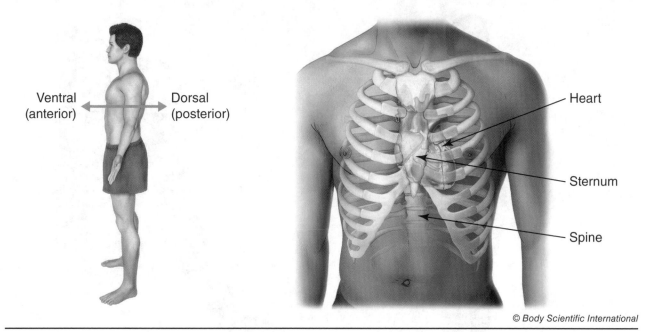

Ventral
(anterior)

Dorsal
(posterior)

Heart

Sternum

Spine

© Body Scientific International

Figure 9.12 *Ventral* refers to the front of the body, and *dorsal* refers to the back.

Recall Activity

1. Ventral is to _____ as dorsal is to posterior.

2. Which body part is more ventral: the toes or the heel? _____

3. If a body part is dorsal, it is closer to the _____ of the body.

4. Which body part is more dorsal: the fingernails or the palms? _____

5. If a body part is ventral, it is closer to the _____ of the body.

6. Which body part is more anterior: the tip of the nose or the eyes? _____

Concept 4: Medial, Lateral, and Intermediate

The terms *medial*, *lateral*, and *intermediate* describe locations in reference to the middle (midsagittal plane) of the body. If a body part is *medial*, it is closer to the middle (midsagittal plane). If a body part is *lateral*, it is farther from the middle. A body part that is between one medial and one lateral body part is called *intermediate*. For example, the radial nerve of your arm is lateral to your sternum. Your sternum is medial to your arm's ulnar nerve. The ulnar nerve is intermediate to the radial nerve and the sternum (**Figure 9.13**).

medial closer to the middle (midsagittal plane) of the body

lateral farther from the middle (midsagittal plane) of the body

intermediate between one medial and one lateral body part

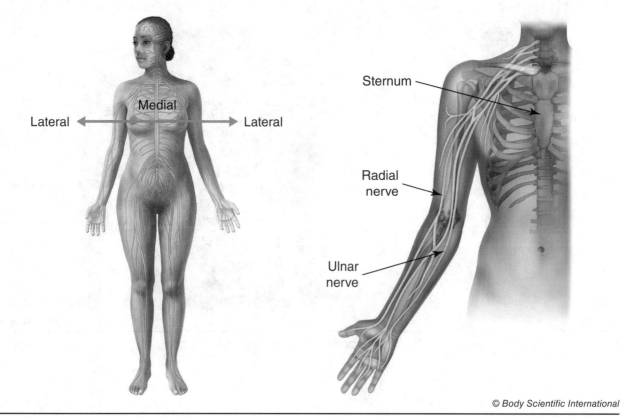

© Body Scientific International

Figure 9.13 A body part is lateral if it is farther from the middle of the body. It is medial if it is closer to the middle of the body.

Recall Activity

1. Which of the following body parts is most lateral?
   A. nose
   B. eye
   C. ear
   D. neck

2. *Medial*, *lateral*, and *intermediate* describe locations in reference to the _____ plane.

3. Compared to the nose and ears, the eyes are _____ .

4. Which of the following body parts is most medial?
   A. thumb
   B. index finger
   C. middle finger
   D. little finger

5. Compared to the ears and nose, the arms are _____ .

Concept 5: Proximal and Distal

The terms *proximal* and *distal* only apply to limbs. If a body part is *proximal*, it is closer to the place where a limb is attached to the body's trunk. If a body part is *distal*, it is farther from the place where a limb is attached to the body's trunk. For example, the muscles of the forearm are distal to the muscles of the upper arm, and the muscles of the upper arm are proximal to the muscles of the forearm. The calf muscles are distal to the muscles of the thigh, and the muscles of the thigh are proximal to the calf muscles (**Figure 9.14**).

proximal closer to the place where a limb is attached to the body's trunk

distal farther from the place where a limb is attached to the body's trunk

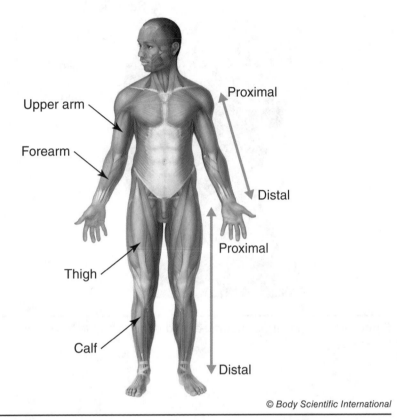

Figure 9.14 The terms *proximal* and *distal* apply to the arms and legs.

Recall Activity

1. If a body part is _____, it is closer to the place where a limb is attached to the body's trunk.

2. The hand is _____ to the elbow.

3. If a body part is _____, it is farther from the place where a limb is attached to the body's trunk.

4. The terms *proximal* and *distal* only apply to _____.

5. The ankle is _____ to the knee.

Concept 6: Superficial and Deep

The terms *superficial* and *deep* describe locations in relation to the surface of the body. If a body part is *superficial*, it is closer to the surface of the body. If a body part is *deep*, it is farther from the surface of the body. For example, the muscles of the face are superficial to the brain. The brain is deep to the muscles of the face. The skull is deep to the muscles of the face, but superficial to the brain (**Figure 9.15**).

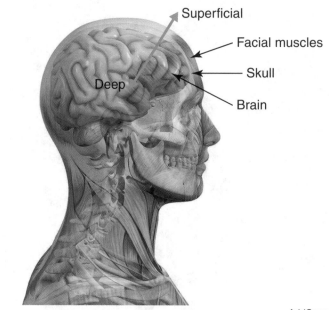

AridOcean/Shutterstock.com

Figure 9.15   The terms *superficial* and *deep* describe how close a body part is to the surface.

Recall Activity

1. Which body part is deeper: the heart or the ribs? _____

2. If a body part is superficial, it is _____ to the surface of the body.

3. The terms *superficial* and *deep* describe location in relation to the _____ of the body.

4. Which body part is more superficial: the stomach or the skin? _____

5. If a body part is deep, it is _____ from the surface of the body.

Section 9.3 Reinforcement

Answer the following questions using what you learned in this section.

1. Compared to the nose and ears, the eyes are _____.

2. Which of the following terms indicates that a body part is closer to the surface?
   A. deep
   B. medial
   C. superficial
   D. dorsal

3. If a body part is _____, it is closer to the head; if a body part is _____, it is closer to the feet.

4. Which of the following body parts is most lateral?
   A. hip
   B. finger
   C. nose
   D. left eye

5. *True or False.* The term *medial* describes location in reference to the frontal plane. _____

6. *Superficial* and *deep* describe locations in relation to the _____ of the body.

7. If a body part is ventral, it is closer to the _____ of the body; if a body part is dorsal, it is closer to the _____ of the body.

8. Which of the following body parts is most medial?
   A. right hand
   B. navel
   C. left cheek
   D. left knee

9. Compared to the skin, is the brain superficial or deep? _____

10. *True or False.* The terms *proximal* and *distal* apply only to the trunk of the body. _____

11. Which of the following body parts is most superior?
    A. knee
    B. hip
    C. foot
    D. ankle

12. *Medial*, *lateral*, and *intermediate* describe locations in reference to the _____ plane.

13. Which of the following body parts is most proximal?
    A. knee
    B. hip
    C. foot
    D. ankle

14. The terms *ventral* and _____ mean that a body part is closer to the front of the body.

15. *True or False.* The term *lateral* describes location in reference to the sagittal plane. _____

16. If a body part is superior, it is closer to the _____.

17. Which of the following body parts is intermediate to the others?
    A. right thumb
    B. right forearm
    C. right collarbone

18. *True or False.* The brain is deep to the skin._____

19. Terms of location only apply to body parts when the body is in _____.

20. Which body part is deeper: the stomach or the skin?_____

21. If a body part is _____, it is farther from the middle of the body.

22. The terms *dorsal* and _____ mean that a body part is closer to the back of the body.

Match the following terms with their definitions.

_____ 23. Closer to the front of the body

_____ 24. Closer to the back of the body

_____ 25. Between medial and lateral body parts

_____ 26. Closer to the point of limb attachment

_____ 27. Farther from the point of limb attachment

_____ 28. Closer to the middle of the body

_____ 29. Farther from the middle of the body

_____ 30. Closer to the head

_____ 31. Closer to the feet

_____ 32. Closer to the surface of the body

_____ 33. Farther from the surface of the body

A. superior
B. inferior
C. ventral
D. dorsal
E. medial
F. lateral
G. intermediate
H. proximal
I. distal
J. superficial
K. deep

Comprehensive Review (Chapters 1–9)

Answer the following questions using what you have learned so far in this book.

34. Which connective tissue structure connects bone to bone?_____

35. A hemisphere is _____ of a sphere.

36. Convert 2376 g into kg. _____

37. A macromolecule made of repeating subunits is called a(n) _____.

38. *True or False.* There is always some degree of uncertainty in science._____

39. Which of the following structures make up a cell's plasma membrane?
    A. ribosomes   C. proteins
    B. phospholipids   D. lysosomes

40. Facts are _____ of people and opinions.

41. Describe the difference between diffusion and facilitated diffusion._____
    _____

42. Which region of the body encompasses the head, neck, and trunk? _____

Section 9.4 Body Organization

In anatomy and physiology, the body is organized into five different levels. These levels differ in complexity, from the most basic cell level to the organism level that considers cells, tissues, organs, and body systems. In this section, you will learn about body organization and about the characteristics of each organizational level.

The terms below are some of those that will be introduced in Section 9.4. To become familiar with these terms, reproduce each word on the line beside it. Pronounce each term as you write it. You will learn the definitions of these words as you complete this section.

1. body system _____

2. organism_____

Concept 1: Five Levels of Organization

The human body is organized into five levels that progress from simple to more complex. The five levels of organization are

- cells
- tissues
- organs
- body systems
- organisms

For example, *cells* make up *tissue*. Different types of tissue compose the *organs* involved in digestion, including the organs of the alimentary canal (mouth, pharynx, esophagus, stomach, small intestine, colon, rectum, and anus). The organs involved in digestion make up the body system known as the *digestive system*. Together, all of the body systems make up the human *organism* (**Figure 9.16**).

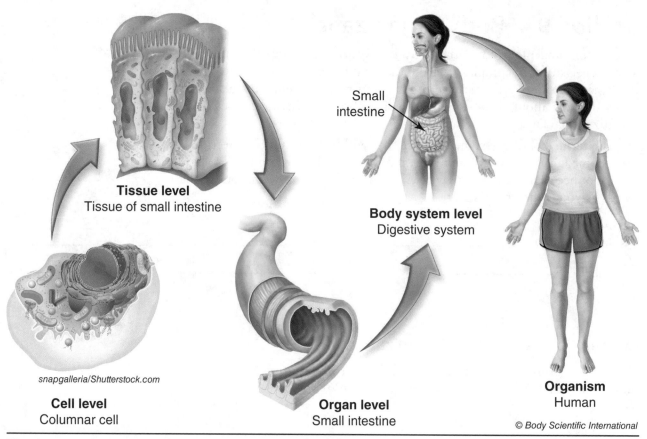

Small intestine

Tissue level
Tissue of small intestine

Body system level
Digestive system

Organism
Human

snapgalleria/Shutterstock.com

Cell level
Columnar cell

Organ level
Small intestine

© Body Scientific International

Figure 9.16   The body is organized into five different levels.

Recall Activity

1. List the five levels of organization in order of complexity from complex to simple. _____

_____

2. Together, all of the _____ make up the human organism.

Concept 2: Cell Level

As you have learned, the *cell* is the basic unit of life. Human body cells are specialized to perform specific functions in the body. If you were to look at the body's alimentary canal on a cellular level, you would study many types of cells and their functions. For example, in the stomach, *parietal cells* release hydrochloric acid to make the environment acidic. *Chief cells* in the stomach secrete pepsinogen, which aids in digestion, and *mucous neck cells* produce mucus to protect the cells lining the stomach. *Smooth muscle cells* move food through the alimentary canal, and *simple columnar epithelial cells* with microvilli absorb digested macromolecules.

Recall Activity

1. Simple columnar epithelial cells with _____ absorb digested macromolecules.

2. Which cells in the stomach release hydrochloric acid? _____

3. Mucous neck cells produce _____ to protect the cells lining the stomach.

Concept 3: Tissue Level

A *tissue* is a group of cells that work together to do a job. On a tissue level, you study groups of cells that work with one another. In the alimentary canal, for example, muscle tissue contracts to move food through the canal. Through most of the alimentary canal, muscle tissue is composed of two sheets of muscle cells. The first sheet of smooth muscle cells is arranged in a circle around the tubelike canal. When these muscle cells contract in unison, the tube becomes smaller in diameter. The second sheet of muscle cells is perpendicular to the circular muscle cells. In the second sheet, muscle cells are arranged lengthwise around the tube. When these muscle cells contract, the tube becomes shorter in length.

Recall Activity

1. Through most of the alimentary canal, muscle tissue is composed of _____ sheet(s) of muscle cells.

2. In the alimentary canal, muscle tissue _____ to move food through the canal.

3. A(n) _____ is a group of cells working together to do a job.

Concept 4: Organ Level

An *organ* is a group of tissues that work together to do a job. An organ is composed of different types of tissue. For example, the job of the small intestine is to move food, break down food into macromolecules, and absorb macromolecules into the blood. To achieve this, the small intestine contains several types of tissue. Lining the inside of the small intestine is a layer of epithelial tissue called *mucosa*. The cells of this tissue layer have microvilli and absorb macromolecules from digested food. The mucosa is supported by a layer of connective tissue called the *lamina propria*. Two layers of muscle tissue are next. Cells in these tissue layers contract to move food through the small intestine. Finally, another layer of epithelial tissue covers the outside of the small intestine. This layer of epithelial tissue is called *serosa* (**Figure 9.17**).

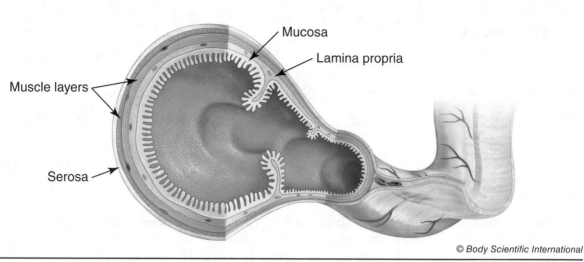

Muscle layers

Mucosa

Lamina propria

Serosa

© Body Scientific International

Figure 9.17 The small intestine has four layers of tissue.

Recall Activity

1. The two layers of epithelium in the small intestine are the _____ and the _____.

2. The layer of connective tissue in the small intestine is called the _____.

3. Which tissue layer lines the inside of the alimentary canal? _____

Concept 5: Body System Level

body system a group of organs that work together to perform several functions; also called an *organ system*

Organs that work together to perform a group of functions make up a *body system* (also known as an *organ system*). For example, the organs of the alimentary canal, as well as some other organs (such as the salivary glands, liver, pancreas, and gallbladder), make up the *digestive system*. Together, all of these organs perform the functions of moving food, *digesting* food (chewing food into small pieces and breaking pieces into macromolecules), and absorbing macromolecules for use throughout the body.

The human body has 11 systems (**Figure 9.18**):

- integumentary system
- skeletal system
- muscular system
- nervous system
- endocrine system
- respiratory system
- cardiovascular system
- lymphatic system
- digestive system
- urinary system
- reproductive systems (male and female)

You will learn about the basic organs and functions of these body systems in Chapter 10.

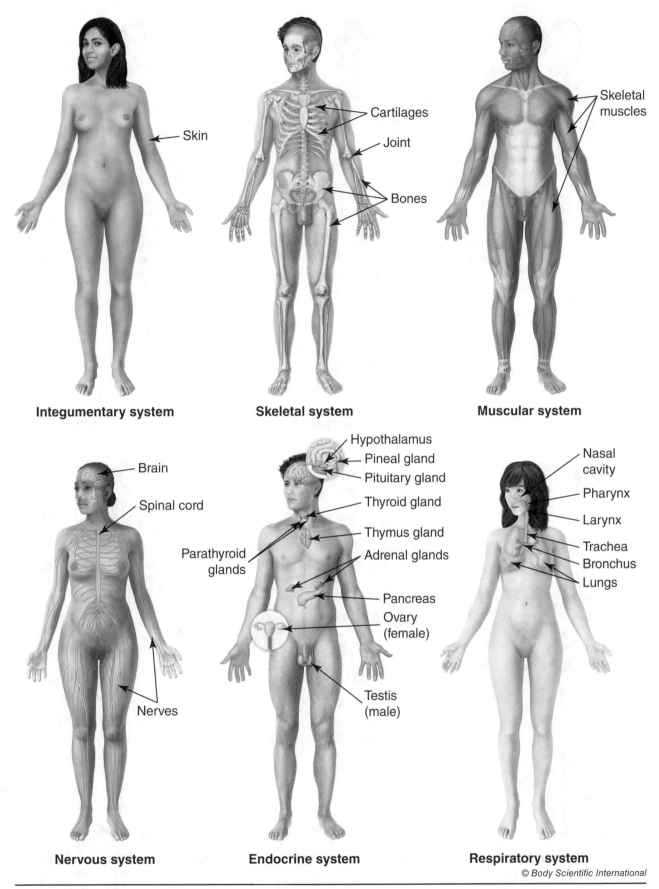

Skin

Cartilages
Joint
Bones

Skeletal muscles

Integumentary system

Skeletal system

Muscular system

Brain

Spinal cord

Nerves

Hypothalamus
Pineal gland
Pituitary gland

Thyroid gland

Thymus gland
Adrenal glands

Parathyroid glands

Pancreas
Ovary (female)

Testis (male)

Nasal cavity
Pharynx
Larynx
Trachea
Bronchus
Lungs

Nervous system

Endocrine system

Respiratory system

© Body Scientific International

Figure 9.18 Eleven body systems make up the human body.

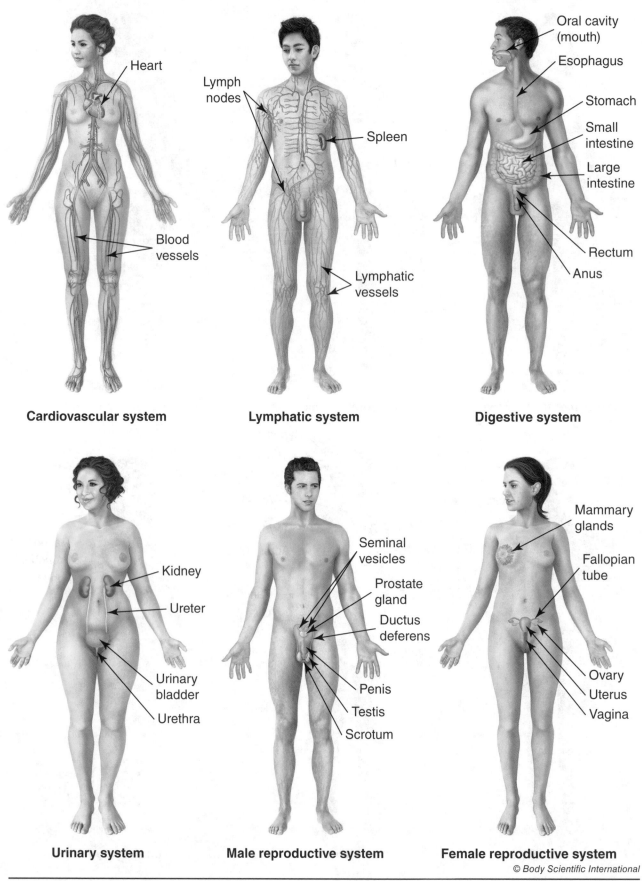

Cardiovascular system

Heart

Blood vessels

Lymphatic system

Lymph nodes

Spleen

Lymphatic vessels

Digestive system

Oral cavity (mouth)

Esophagus

Stomach

Small intestine

Large intestine

Rectum

Anus

Urinary system

Kidney

Ureter

Urinary bladder

Urethra

Male reproductive system

Seminal vesicles

Prostate gland

Ductus deferens

Penis

Testis

Scrotum

Female reproductive system

Mammary glands

Fallopian tube

Ovary

Uterus

Vagina

© *Body Scientific International*

Figure 9.18 *Continued.*

Recall Activity

1. A body system is a group of _____ working together to perform several functions.

2. _____ is chewing food into small pieces and breaking pieces into macromolecules.

3. How many systems does the human body have?_____

4. List the human body systems._____

_____

_____

Concept 6: Organism Level

The most complex level of body organization is the organism level. An *organism* is a complex life form made of many interdependent parts. The human organism is a cooperative community of the 11 body systems. All of the body systems work together to maintain life.

organism a complex life form made of many interdependent parts

Recall Activity

1. The human organism is a cooperative _____ of body systems.

2. An organism is a complex life form made of many _____ parts.

Section 9.4 Reinforcement

Answer the following questions using what you learned in this section.

1. Which of the following organs is *not* part of the alimentary canal?
   A. liver
   B. stomach
   C. esophagus
   D. mouth

2. *True or False.* An organ is a group of tissues working together to do a job. _____

3. The epithelial tissue layer lining the inside of the alimentary canal is called the

   _____.

4. List the five levels of body organization in order of complexity from simple to complex. _____

   _____

5. Which of the following cells makes pepsinogen?
   A. chief cell
   B. goblet cell
   C. smooth muscle cell
   D. parietal cell

6. The basic unit of life is the _____.

7. Organs that work together to perform a group of functions make up a(n) _____.

8. *True or False.* The colon is not part of the alimentary canal._____

9. Unscramble the letters: stusie. Define the word that is formed._____
   _____

10. *True or False.* The digestive system is composed only of organs that make up the alimentary canal.
    _____

11. The cells of the mucosa have _____ that help them absorb macromolecules from digested food.

12. A group of cells working together to do a job is a(n) _____.

13. List the five levels of body organization in alphabetical order. _____
    _____

14. How many body systems does the human body have?_____

15. *True or False.* The lamina propria is the muscle layer of the small intestine. _____

16. List the human body systems in alphabetical order._____
    _____

    _____

17. In the stomach, _____ cells release hydrochloric acid to make the environment acidic.

18. The human organism is a cooperative community of 11 _____.

19. Which of the following words are misspelled?
    A. organ   C. salivary
    B. alimatary   D. esophgous

20. A(n) _____ is a complex life form made of many interdependent parts.

21. Which level of body organization is concerned with several organs that work together to perform a group of functions? _____

Match the following terms with their definitions.

_____ 22. Organs working together to perform a group of functions

_____ 23. A group of cells working together to do a job

_____ 24. A group of tissues working together to do a job

_____ 25. The basic unit of life

_____ 26. A complex life form made of many interdependent parts

A. cell
B. tissue
C. organ
D. body system
E. organism

Comprehensive Review (Chapters 1–9)

Answer the following questions using what you have learned so far in this book.

27. What does the prefix *inter-* mean?_____

28. An explanation is natural if it is _____ and _____.

29. The first step in the diagnostic scientific method is _____.

30. What is the value of pi?_____

31. In a covalent bond, are electrons accepted, donated, or shared? _____

32. Which of the following body parts is most distal?
    A. knee   C. foot
    B. hip   D. ankle

33. *True or False.* Tight junctions prevent heart muscle cells from separating. _____

34. Which type of tissue is composed mostly of extracellular fibers with few cells? _____

35. *True or False.* Energy is required to move from low concentration to high concentration. _____

Section 9.5 Homeostasis in the Body

Homeostasis is a state of relative stability. In Section 7.7, you learned about how the cell maintains homeostasis for its continued survival. Homeostasis is also maintained in the body at large. In this section, you will learn about the body's functions for maintaining homeostasis. Understanding these functions will prepare you for anatomy and physiology.

The terms below are some of those that will be introduced in Section 9.5. To become familiar with these terms, reproduce each word on the line beside it. Pronounce each term as you write it. You will learn the definitions of these words as you complete this section.

1. negative feedback _____

2. body temperature _____

3. blood glucose concentration_____

4. insulin _____

5. glucagon _____

Concept 1: Reviewing Homeostasis

As you have learned, life can only exist within a narrow range of circumstances. For life to continue, the body and its cells must maintain *homeostasis* (a state of relative stability). The environment outside your body can constantly change. You can walk out of a warm house into the cold street outside. In the midst of this external temperature change, your body makes adjustments to maintain a stable internal body temperature. The environment inside your body can also change. For example, if you do not eat for several hours, your body will maintain a constant blood glucose concentration to supply your cells. In both of these examples, your body is maintaining homeostasis. In Section 7.7, you learned about homeostasis inside the cell. Now you will learn about homeostasis inside the body as a whole.

Recall Activity

1. For life to continue, the body and its cells must maintain _____.

2. If you do not eat for several hours, your body will maintain a constant blood _____ concentration to supply your cells.

Concept 2: Negative Feedback

negative feedback the cycle of taking action to correct a concentration or factor back to its set value within the body

Your body is constantly monitoring the concentrations of hundreds of molecules and other factors necessary for life. When a concentration or factor falls below or climbs above a set value, your body will take action to correct the concentration or factor back to the set value. Once the set value is reached, the body will stop this action. This cycle of taking action to correct concentrations and factors inside the body is called *negative feedback*. To maintain a set value, your body signals cells to make products and perform certain actions and then signals them to stop when the set value is reached.

Recall Activity

1. In _____, the body takes action to correct a concentration or factor back to its set value.

2. Once the set value of a concentration or factor is reached, the body will _____ its action.

Concept 3: Body Temperature

body temperature the temperature inside the body; in homeostasis, 37°C (98.6°F)

The process of negative feedback enables your body to maintain homeostasis when the environment outside the body changes. An example of this is *body temperature*. In homeostasis, the body's internal temperature is 37°C (98.6°F). If you are in a cold environment, your body will lose heat to the environment. In response to this change, your hypothalamus directs your body to adjust reactions inside cells to increase the amount of heat produced and make up for heat lost. If you are in a hot environment, your body will gain heat from the environment. In response, your hypothalamus directs your body to sweat, losing heat to the environment as sweat evaporates (**Figure 9.19**). As you might imagine, sweating upsets the homeostasis of water inside your body. This is why you need to drink water to replace water lost as sweat.

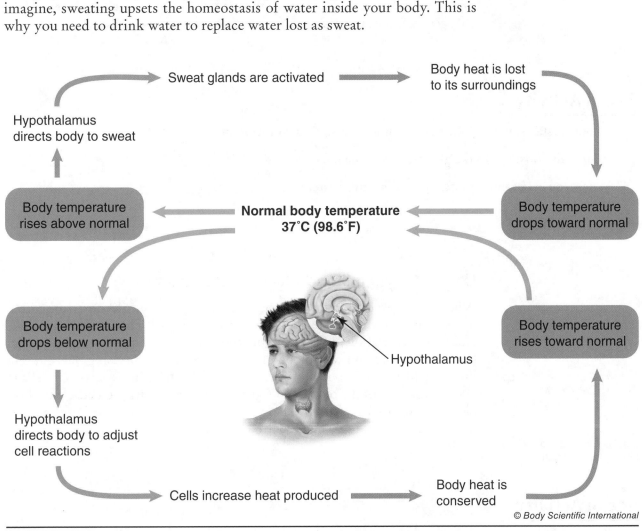

Figure 9.19   The hypothalamus maintains the homeostasis of body temperature.

Recall Activity

1. Sweating upsets the _____ of water inside your body.

2. Your body adjusts to cold by _____ the amount of heat produced by cellular reactions.

3. In homeostasis, the body's internal temperature is _____°C (_____°F).

Concept 4: Blood Glucose Concentration

Negative feedback also enables your body to maintain homeostasis when the environment *inside* the body changes. One factor that must remain stable inside the body is *blood glucose concentration*. In homeostasis, your blood maintains a glucose concentration of 90 mg/100 mL. However, the concentration of glucose in your blood is always changing. Your cells constantly take

blood glucose concentration the number of glucose molecules per a volume of blood; in homeostasis, 90 mg/100 mL

glucose out of the blood for use in cell respiration. When you eat carbohydrates, your digestive system puts glucose into the blood. In response to these changes, your body takes several actions to maintain homeostasis.

Recall Activity

1. In homeostasis, your blood maintains a glucose concentration of _____.

2. Your cells constantly take glucose out of the blood for use in cell _____.

3. When you eat carbohydrates, your digestive system puts _____ into the blood.

Concept 5: High Blood Glucose Concentration

insulin a hormone produced by the beta cells of the pancreas that signals cells to take glucose out of the blood and signals the liver to draw glucose out of the blood and store it as glycogen

When you digest carbohydrates, your digestive system breaks down the carbohydrates into glucose and puts glucose into your blood. This causes your blood glucose concentration to rise, climbing above 90 mg/100 mL. In response, your body takes action to lower blood glucose concentration, causing the beta cells in your pancreas to produce the hormone *insulin*. Insulin signals your cells to take glucose out of the blood and signals your liver to draw glucose out of the blood and store it as *glycogen*. These actions lower the concentration of glucose in your blood back to 90 mg/100 mL (**Figure 9.20**).

Recall Activity

1. When you digest carbohydrates, does your blood glucose concentration rise or fall? _____

2. Beta cells in your pancreas produce the hormone _____.

3. Insulin signals your _____ to take glucose out of the blood and signals your _____ to draw glucose out of the blood and store it as glycogen.

Concept 6: Low Blood Glucose Concentration

glucagon a hormone produced by the alpha cells of the pancreas that signals the liver to break down stored glycogen into glucose and release glucose into the blood

Because of cell respiration, your cells are constantly taking glucose out of the blood. This causes your blood glucose concentration to decrease, falling below 90 mg/100 mL. Digesting carbohydrates increases blood glucose concentration, but you are not constantly eating. Because of this, your liver stores a polysaccharide known as *glycogen* that can be broken into glucose and put into the blood if glucose concentration is low. When blood glucose concentration is too low, alpha cells in the pancreas produce the hormone *glucagon*. Glucagon signals the liver to break down stored glycogen into glucose and release glucose into the blood. These actions raise the concentration of glucose in your blood back to 90 mg/100 mL (Figure 9.20).

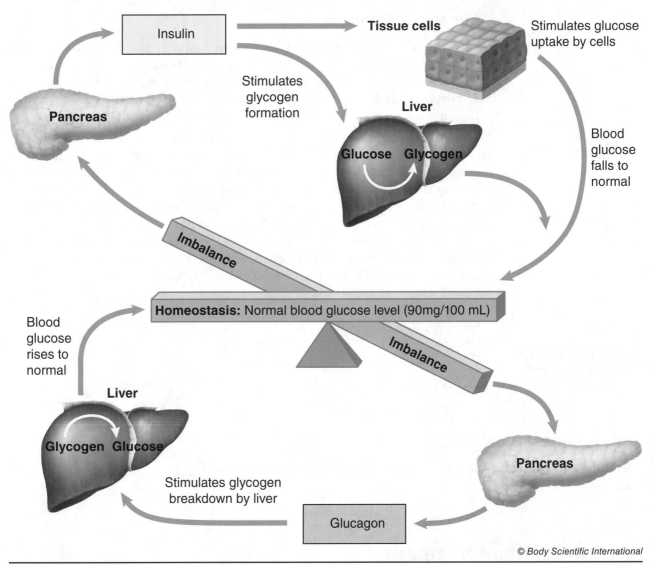

Figure 9.20 The hormones insulin and glucagon maintain homeostatic blood glucose concentration in the body.

Recall Activity

1. Alpha cells in the pancreas produce the hormone _____.

2. Glucagon signals the liver to break down stored _____ into glucose.

3. Does the action of glucagon cause blood glucose concentration to increase or decrease?

   _____

Concept 7: Blood pH

pH is another factor that must be kept in homeostasis. In Section 7.7, you learned about how cells regulate internal pH. pH must also be regulated in the blood. As you have learned, pH is the measurement of acid or base in a liquid and depends on the numbers of hydrogen ions (H^+) and hydroxide ions (OH^-). In homeostasis, the pH of blood is slightly basic, between 7.35 and 7.45.

The kidneys maintain the homeostasis of blood pH. Blood is constantly entering and leaving the kidneys. In fact, every four minutes, all the blood in your body will travel through a kidney. The kidneys sort through what to keep in the blood and what to remove from the blood, and molecules and ions that are removed from the blood become *urine*. The body's metabolism is constantly producing hydrogen ions (H^+). If blood pH is too low, the kidneys will remove hydrogen ions (H^+) from the blood, raising blood pH. If blood pH is too high, the kidneys will retain hydrogen ions (H^+), and as the body continues to produce hydrogen ions (H^+), blood pH will fall.

Recall Activity

1. Removing hydrogen ions (H^+) from the blood _____ blood pH.

2. In homeostasis, the pH of blood is between _____ and

   _____.

3. If the kidneys retain hydrogen ions (H^+) in the blood, blood pH will _____.

Section 9.5 Reinforcement

Answer the following questions using what you learned in this section.

1. Which hormone is produced by the alpha cells of the pancreas?_____

2. Glucagon signals the _____ to break down stored glycogen into glucose.

3. When the kidneys retain hydrogen ions (H^+) in the blood, does blood pH rise or fall?_____

4. *True or False.* The body's homeostatic internal temperature is 39°C. _____

5. Which organ maintains homeostatic blood pH by choosing what to keep in the blood and what to remove from the blood? _____

6. The hormone _____ signals your cells to take glucose out of the blood.

7. *True or False.* Molecules and ions that are removed from the blood become urine._____

8. Which hormone is produced by the beta cells of the pancreas?_____

9. Unscramble the letters: anoggclu. Define the word that is formed. _____

   _____

10. The hormone insulin signals the liver to take glucose out of the blood and store it as
    _____.

11. Does removing hydrogen ions (H^+) from the blood raise or lower blood pH? _____

12. The hormone _____ raises blood glucose concentration.

13. What happens in negative feedback? _____

    _____

14. *True or False.* The kidneys keep the pH of blood between 7.25 and 7.55. _____

15. To maintain a set value, your body signals cells to make _____ and perform
    certain _____ and then signals them to _____ when
    the set value is reached.

16. Which hormone causes the breakdown of glycogen in the liver? _____

17. In response to a hot environment, your body sweats, losing heat to the environment as sweat
    _____.

18. What is the body's homeostatic internal temperature? _____

19. Unscramble the letters: smashsootie. Define the word that is formed. _____

    _____

20. *True or False.* In homeostasis, blood glucose concentration is 90 mg/100 mL. _____

21. In homeostasis, the pH of blood is slightly _____, between
    _____ and _____.

Comprehensive Review (Chapters 1–9)

Answer the following questions using what you have learned so far in this book.

22. pH values range from _____ to _____.

23. Name the three types of extracellular fibers. _____

24. *True or False.* If additional evidence leads to a better explanation, science will change. _____

25. What is the second step of the experimental scientific method? _____

26. If the diameter of a circle is 100 cm, the radius is _____ mm.

27. List the three building blocks of the cytoskeleton. _____

28. The prefix _____ means "false."

29. Which will diffuse faster: a molecule containing few atoms or a molecule containing many atoms?

    _____

30. Organs that work together to perform a group of functions make up a(n) _____.

Chapter 9 Review

Answer the following questions using what you learned in this chapter.

1. List the four body planes used in anatomy and physiology. _____

   _____

2. In anatomical position, the thumbs point _____ the body.

3. *True or False.* The word *manus* refers to the hand. _____

4. Which of the following is *not* a region of the trunk?

   A. thoracic region   C. abdominal region

   B. pubic region   D. cervical region

5. Is your knee proximal or distal to your hip? _____

6. *True or False.* The nose is intermediate to the eyes and ears. _____

7. Which of the following body parts is most superficial?

   A. liver   C. skin

   B. kidney   D. heart

8. Is your ankle superior or inferior to your shin? _____

9. The _____ plane divides the body into front and back sections.

10. *True or False.* Both the midsagittal plane and the sagittal plane divide the body down the middle. _____

11. List the human body systems. _____

    _____

    _____

12. Which of the following body parts is most medial?

    A. hip   C. nose

    B. finger   D. left eye

13. When you digest carbohydrates, does your blood glucose concentration rise or fall? _____

14. *True or False.* The heart is deep to the rib cage. _____

15. A(n) _____ is a group of organs working together to perform a group of functions.

16. The cranial and _____ cavities are found in the dorsal section of the body.

17. When blood glucose concentration is too high, beta cells in the pancreas produce the hormone

    _____.

18. Is the sternum dorsal or ventral to the spine? _____

19. *True or False.* If a body part is inferior, it is closer to the head. _____

20. In homeostasis, what is the body's blood glucose concentration? _____

21. List the five levels of body organization in order of complexity from simple to complex. _____

    _____

22. List the three abdominopelvic regions in the first row. _____

_____

23. *True or False.* The head area is called the cephalic region. _____

24. Which of the following body planes divides the body into top and bottom sections?
    A. sagittal plane   C. frontal plane
    B. midsagittal plane   D. transverse plane

25. What is the body's homeostatic internal temperature? _____

26. The _____ region of the body includes the limbs (arms and legs).

27. In homeostasis, the pH of blood is between _____ and

    _____.

Comprehensive Review (Chapters 1–9)

Using what you have learned so far in this book, match the following terms with their definitions.

_____ 28. An area of biology that studies tissues

_____ 29. A combining form that means "belly side (of the body)"

_____ 30. Facts that relate to a possible cause

_____ 31. The movement of atoms from areas of low concentration to areas of high concentration using solute pumps

_____ 32. A type of connective tissue made of cells and calcium salts reinforced with collagen fibers

_____ 33. The speed of enzymatic reactions

_____ 34. An avascular connective tissue with an extracellular matrix made of extracellular fibers, carbohydrates, and water

_____ 35. A body plane that divides the body into front and back sections

_____ 36. A combining form that means "back (of the body)"

_____ 37. Finger-like projections of the plasma membrane that increase the surface area of the cell to allow for more absorption

_____ 38. A liquid that contains more H^+ ions than OH^- ions

_____ 39. The total area of the outer surface of an object

_____ 40. A body plane that divides the body into top and bottom sections

_____ 41. The spreading out of atoms from areas of high concentration into areas of low concentration

A. evidence
B. ventr/o
C. surface area
D. turnover rate
E. microvilli
F. histology
G. diffusion
H. bone
I. frontal plane
J. dors/o
K. acid
L. cartilage
M. active transport
N. transverse plane

Chapter 10
Human Body Systems

Introduction

This chapter is an introduction to what you will study in an anatomy and physiology class. In anatomy and physiology, healthcare professionals and students study human body systems. Body systems, also called *organ systems*, are groups of organs that work together to perform several functions. The human body is composed of 11 body systems: the integumentary system, the skeletal system, the muscular system, the nervous system, the endocrine system, the respiratory system, the cardiovascular system, the lymphatic system, the digestive system, the urinary system, and the reproductive systems. In this chapter, you will learn about the functions and structures of these body systems.

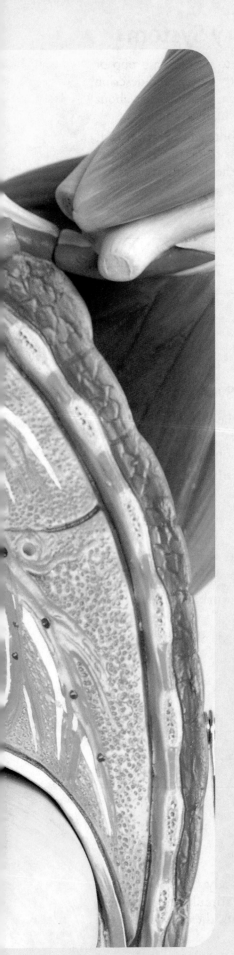

Objectives

After completing this chapter, you will be able to

- understand the function and structure of the integumentary system
- describe the skeletal system and its role in the body
- explain the components and movements of the muscular system
- outline the structure of the nervous system and explain its function
- name the organs of the endocrine system and explain the role of hormones
- identify the parts of the respiratory system
- describe how blood circulates through the cardiovascular system
- understand the structure and function of the lymphatic system
- identify how food travels through the digestive system
- explain the purpose of the urinary system and name its components
- distinguish among the organs of the male and female reproductive systems

Key Terms

The following terms and phrases will be introduced and explained in Chapter 10. Read through the list to become familiar with the words.

abduction
absorption
adduction
afferent nerve
alimentary canal
appendicular skeleton
artery
atrioventricular (AV) valve
atrium
axial skeleton
brain
capillary
cardiovascular system
central nervous system (CNS)
chemical digestion
defecation
dermis
diaphragm
digestive system
ductus deferens
efferent nerve
endocrine system
epidermis
epididymis
expiration
extension
external respiration
fallopian tube
filtration

flexion
hair
heart
hormone
hypodermis
ingestion
insertion
inspiration
integumentary system
internal respiration
joint
kidney
lung
lymph
lymph node
lymphatic system
lymphocyte
mammary gland
mechanical digestion
muscular system
nail
nephron
nervous system
nontropic hormone
origin
ovary
parathyroid gland
pectoral girdle
pelvic girdle
penis

peripheral nervous system (PNS)
peristalsis
pituitary gland
pulmonary circulation
reabsorption
reproductive system
respiratory system
rotation
secretion
semilunar (SL) valve
skeletal system
skin
skull
spinal cord
spine
spleen
systemic circulation
testis
thoracic cage
thymus
thyroid gland
tropic hormone
ureter
urethra
urinary bladder
urinary system
uterus
vagina
vein
ventricle

Section 10.1 The Integumentary System

A *body system* is made up of organs working together to perform a group of functions. Each section in this chapter will cover one body system and describe its functions and primary structures. The first body system you will learn about is the *integumentary system*, which is composed of the skin, hair, and nails.

The terms below are some of those that will be introduced in Section 10.1. To become familiar with these terms, reproduce each word on the line beside it. Pronounce each term as you write it. You will learn the definitions of these words as you complete this section.

1. integumentary system _____

   _____

2. skin _____

3. epidermis _____

4. dermis _____

5. hypodermis _____

6. hair _____

7. nail _____

Concept 1: Functions of the Integumentary System

integumentary system a body system consisting of the skin, hair, and nails; protects the body, helps maintain homeostasis, makes vitamin D, removes waste, and perceives sensations

The *integumentary system* is a body system that includes the skin, hair, and nails. The glands of the skin are also part of the integumentary system. The integumentary system performs the following important functions in the body:

- protects the body from infection, ultraviolet (UV) radiation, dehydration, physical harm (such as scrapes), and chemicals
- maintains the homeostasis of body temperature
- makes vitamin D
- removes waste from the body through perspiration (sweating)
- perceives pressure, touch, pain, and temperature

All of the structures in the integumentary system work together to perform this group of functions.

Recall Activity

1. What organs are included in the integumentary system? _____

2. List three functions of the integumentary system. _____

   _____

Concept 2: Skin

skin an organ that forms the covering of the body; protects the body and contains organs that perceive sensory stimuli and cause perspiration

The *skin* is the covering of the body. It protects the body from the outside environment and contains organs that perceive sensory stimuli and cause perspiration. The skin is made of three layers: the *epidermis*, the *dermis*, and the *hypodermis* (**Figure 10.1**). The dermis and hypodermis are much thicker than the epidermis. For example, when a blister forms, fluid separates the dermis and epidermis. The thin surface of the blister is the epidermis, and the skin beneath the blister is the dermis.

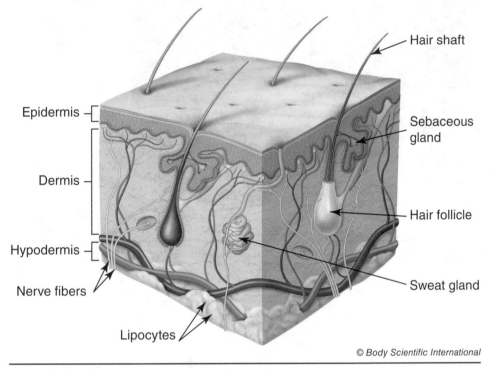

Figure 10.1   The skin is composed of three layers.

Recall Activity

1. Which layer of skin is most superficial? _____

2. *True or False*. The dermis is much thicker than the epidermis. _____

3. Which layer of skin is deepest? _____

Concept 3: Epidermis

The *epidermis* is the outermost, most superficial layer of skin. The epidermis is made of *stratified squamous epithelium*, and cell division takes place deep in the epidermis. Cells called *keratinocytes* are pushed up to the apical surface of the epidermis as superficial cells are shed. As they move toward the surface, keratinocytes die, flatten, and gradually fill with a tough, water-resistant protein called *keratin*. Because of this, keratinocytes at the surface of the epidermis form a waterproof barrier. The epidermis also contains *melanocytes*, which affect skin color. The epidermis contains four or five strata (layers), as illustrated in **Figure 10.2**. The stratum lucidum is found only in thick skin.

epidermis the outermost, most superficial layer of skin; is made of stratified squamous epithelium and contains keratinocytes and melanocytes

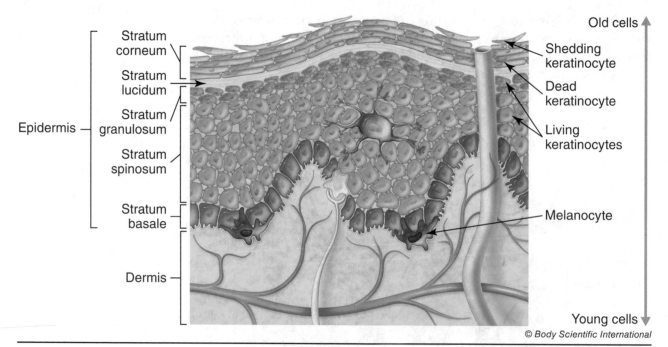

Figure 10.2 This portion of the epidermis has five layers. The stratum lucidum is found only in thick skin.

Recall Activity

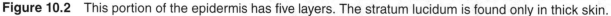

1. Which skin cells form a waterproof barrier at the surface of the epidermis? _____

2. *True or False*. The most superficial cells of the epidermis are dead. _____

3. The epidermis is made of _____ squamous epithelium.

4. List the layers of the epidermis in order from superficial to deep. _____

_____

5. In thin skin, how many strata does the epidermis have? _____

Concept 4: Dermis

dermis the middle layer of skin; contains connective tissue, blood vessels, sweat and sebaceous glands, hair follicles, and nerve endings

The *dermis* is the middle layer of skin. Connective tissue, blood vessels, glands, hair follicles, and nerve endings make up the dermis. Nerve endings perceive touch, pressure, temperature, and pain and communicate these signals back to the spinal cord and brain. *Sweat glands* cause *perspiration*, which helps lower body temperature. The dermis also contains *sebaceous glands*, which secrete *sebum*, a substance that coats the hair and skin.

Recall Activity

1. The dermis is the _____ layer of skin.

2. Name two glands that are found in the dermis. _____

Concept 5: Hypodermis

The deepest layer of skin is the *hypodermis*. The hypodermis is made of *lipocytes* (cells that produce and store fat) and connects the dermis to muscles beneath the skin. The hypodermis helps insulate the body and protects deeper tissues.

hypodermis the deepest layer of skin that connects the dermis to muscles beneath the skin; helps insulate the body and protects deeper tissues

Recall Activity

1. The deepest layer of skin is the _____.

2. Identify two functions of the hypodermis. _____

Concept 6: Hair and Nails

The integumentary system also includes the hair and nails. *Hair* is made of dead, protein-filled cells and grows from hair follicles in the dermis (Figure 10.1). It helps protect the body and regulate body temperature. *Nails* are made of keratin and protect the ends of the phalanges (fingers and toes).

hair a strand of dead, protein-filled cells that grows from a hair follicle in the dermis

nail a plate of keratin that protects the end of a phalanx (finger or toe)

Recall Activity

1. Hair is made of _____, protein-filled cells.

2. Which protein makes up the nails? _____

Section 10.1 Reinforcement

Answer the following questions using what you learned in this section.

1. List the three layers of the skin in order from superficial to deep. _____

2. *True or False.* The deepest cells of the epidermis are dead. _____

3. Which of the following layers of the epidermis is *not* found in thin skin?

   A. stratum basale   C. stratum corneum

   B. stratum lucidum   D. stratum spinosum

4. *True or False.* The dermis has four layers._____

5. Where in the epidermis does cell division take place? _____

6. Unscramble the letters: netarki. Define the word that is formed. _____

   _____

7. In thick skin, the epidermis contains _____ layer(s).

8. Which skin layer is made of lipocytes? _____

9. Nails are made of _____ and protect the ends of the fingers and toes.

10. As they move toward the surface, cells of the epidermis gradually fill with a tough, water-resistant protein called _____.

11. *True or False.* The epidermis contains melanocytes, which affect skin color. _____

12. Which layer of the skin contains hair follicles? _____

13. *True or False.* The epidermis has two layers. _____

14. Nerve endings in the dermis perceive _____, _____, _____, and _____.

15. Identify the five functions of the integumentary system. _____
_____
_____

16. Is the dermis deep or superficial to the epidermis? _____

17. Which two glands are found in the dermis? _____

18. *True or False.* The epidermis is thinner than the dermis. _____

Comprehensive Review (Chapters 1–10)

Answer the following questions using what you have learned so far in this book.

19. *True or False.* When a cell is dividing, DNA is packaged as chromatin. _____

20. A fact is a confirmed _____.

21. If all constants in an experiment are the same, any differences *must* be caused by the _____ variable.

22. Identify and define the prefix in the word *abduction.* _____

23. *True or False.* A volume of 0.1 L is the same as 100 mL. _____

24. List the layers of the epidermis in order from deep to superficial. _____
_____

25. Which of the following pH values represents the strongest base?
    A. 2   C. 8
    B. 6   D. 10

26. The two steps in protein synthesis are _____ and _____.

27. The extracellular matrix of bone is made of calcium salts reinforced with _____ fibers.

28. Which body plane divides the body into top and bottom sections? _____

Section 10.2 The Skeletal System

The skeletal system includes the bones and joints. This body system provides structure and support for the body and facilitates body movement. In this section, you will learn about the functions and structures of the skeletal system.

The terms below are some of those that will be introduced in Section 10.2. To become familiar with these terms, reproduce each word on the line beside it. Pronounce each term as you write it. You will learn the definitions of these words as you complete this section.

1. skeletal system _____

2. axial skeleton _____

3. appendicular skeleton _____

   _____

4. skull _____

5. thoracic cage _____

6. spine _____

7. pectoral girdle _____

8. pelvic girdle _____

9. joint _____

Concept 1: Functions of the Skeletal System

The *skeletal system* encompasses the *skeleton* (the bones and joints of the body). It is composed mostly of bone tissue and cartilage. The skeletal system performs the following functions in the body:

- protects the body by surrounding internal structures
- provides support, structure, and shape for the body
- produces red blood cells (bone marrow)
- facilitates body movement
- stores calcium

The structures of the skeletal system work in concert to perform these functions.

skeletal system a body system consisting of the bones and joints of the body; protects the body, provides support, produces red blood cells, facilitates movement, and stores calcium

Recall Activity

1. Which two tissues make up most of the skeletal system?_____

2. List four functions of the skeletal system. _____

   _____

3. The skeletal system includes the bones and _____.

Concept 2: Axial Versus Appendicular Skeleton

The skeletal system can be divided into two major parts: the axial skeleton and the appendicular skeleton (**Figure 10.3**). The *axial skeleton* consists of the skull, the thoracic cage, and the spine. The *appendicular skeleton* contains the pectoral girdle, the pelvic girdle, the upper limbs, and the lower limbs.

axial skeleton the portion of the skeleton containing the skull, thoracic cage, and spine

appendicular skeleton the portion of the skeleton containing the pectoral girdle, pelvic girdle, upper limbs, and lower limbs

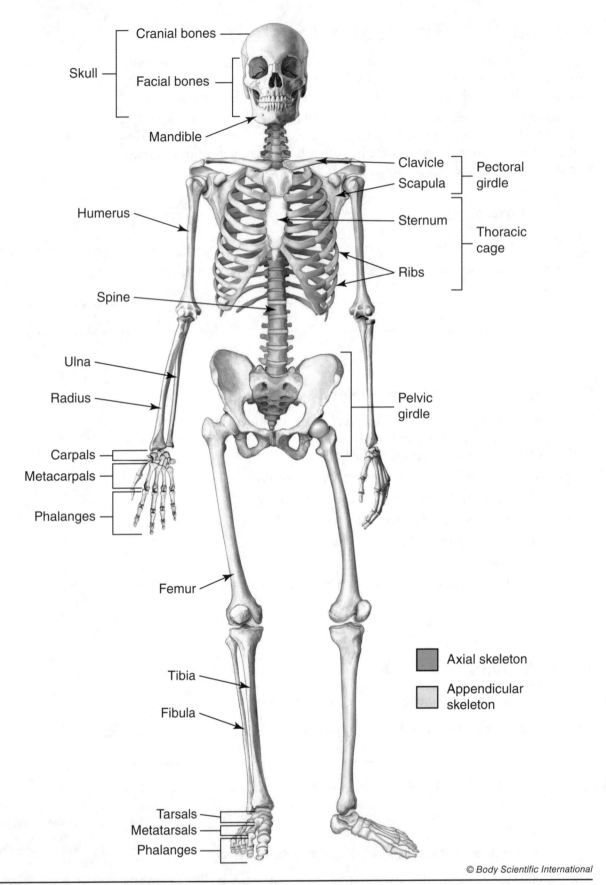

Skull
— Cranial bones
— Facial bones
— Mandible

Clavicle — Pectoral girdle
Scapula

Humerus

Sternum — Thoracic cage

Ribs

Spine

Ulna

Radius

Pelvic girdle

Carpals
Metacarpals

Phalanges

Femur

Tibia

Fibula

Axial skeleton

Appendicular skeleton

Tarsals
Metatarsals
Phalanges

© *Body Scientific International*

Figure 10.3 In this illustration, the appendicular skeleton is beige, and the axial skeleton is red.

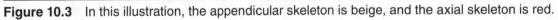

Recall Activity

1. The axial skeleton consists of the _____, the _____, and the _____.

2. The appendicular skeleton consists of the _____, the _____, the _____, and the _____.

Concept 3: Skull

The *skull* is a group of bones that make up the head. The skull contains *cranial bones* (which protect the brain) and *facial bones* (to which facial muscles attach). Most bones in the skull are fused together and thus are immovable. The one exception is the *mandible* (jawbone), which is capable of movement for chewing and speaking.

skull the cranial and facial bones that make up the head

Recall Activity

1. _____ bones protect the brain, and _____ bones attach to facial muscles.

2. Which bone of the skull is movable? _____

Concept 4: Thoracic Cage

The bones of the *thoracic cage* include the sternum (breastbone) and the 12 ribs (also called *costals*). There are three types of ribs: true ribs, false ribs, and floating ribs (**Figure 10.4**). *True ribs* attach directly to the sternum, *false ribs* attach indirectly to the sternum, and *floating ribs* are not connected to the sternum.

thoracic cage the sternum and ribs that surround the thoracic cavity

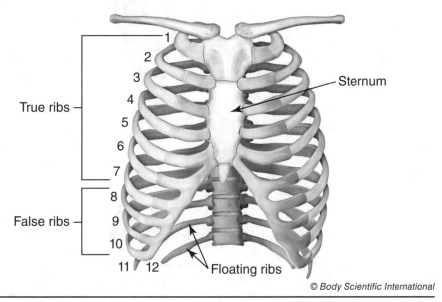

© Body Scientific International

Figure 10.4 Numbers 1–7 are true ribs, numbers 8–10 are false ribs, and numbers 11–12 are floating ribs.

Recall Activity

1. List the three types of ribs. _____

2. The bones of the _____ cage include the sternum and the 12 ribs.

Concept 5: Spine

spine a stack of block-like vertebrae that surround the spinal cord; also called the *vertebral column*

The *spine* is a stack of block-like *vertebrae* (bone segments) that surround the spinal cord. The spine is also called the *vertebral column*. The spine has four regions. From superior to inferior, these regions are the *cervical region*, the *thoracic region*, the *lumbar region*, and the *sacral region* (**Figure 10.5**). The vertebrae of the sacral region are fused together. Vertebrae that are not fused together are separated by *intervertebral discs* made of cartilage.

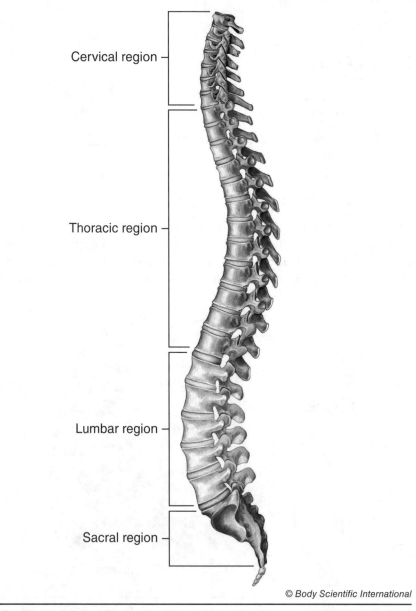

Cervical region

Thoracic region

Lumbar region

Sacral region

© Body Scientific International

Figure 10.5   The spine has four regions.

Recall Activity

1. List the regions of the spine. _____

   _____

2. Vertebrae that are not fused together are separated by _____ discs.

3. The spine is a stack of block-like vertebrae that surround the _____.

Concept 6: Pectoral Girdle

The *pectoral girdle* forms the shoulder joint, which connects the arm to the thoracic cage (**Figure 10.6**). The body has two pectoral girdles: one on the left side and one on the right. Each pectoral girdle contains two bones: the *scapula* (shoulder blade) and the *clavicle* (collarbone).

pectoral girdle the shoulder joint, which connects an arm to the thoracic cage; consists of the scapula and clavicle

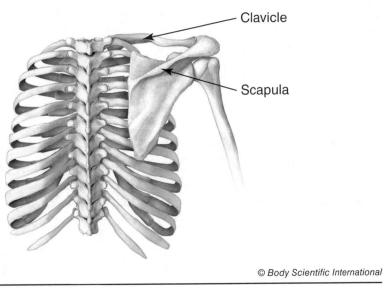

Clavicle

Scapula

© Body Scientific International

Figure 10.6 The pectoral girdle contains the scapula and clavicle.

Recall Activity

1. Which two bones make up the pectoral girdle? _____

2. The _____ girdle forms the shoulder joint.

Concept 7: Pelvic Girdle

The *pelvic girdle* forms the hip joints, which connect the legs to the spine. The pelvic girdle is composed of several fused bones known collectively as the *pelvis*. These are the *left ilium*, *left ischium*, *left pubis*, *right ilium*, *right ischium*, and *right pubis*.

pelvic girdle the hip joints, which connect a leg to the spine; consists of the pelvis (left ilium, left ischium, left pubis, right ilium, right ischium, and right pubis)

Recall Activity

1. The pelvic girdle forms the _____ joints.

2. *True or False.* The pelvic girdle bones are fused. _____

Concept 8: Upper Limbs

The bones of the upper limbs make up the arms and hands. From proximal to distal, the bones of the arms and hands are the *humerus* (upper arm), *radius* and *ulna* (forearm), *carpals* (wrist), *metacarpals* (hand), and *phalanges* (fingers).

Recall Activity

1. List the two bones of the forearm. _____

2. The bones of the upper limbs make up the _____ and

_____.

Concept 9: Lower Limbs

The bones of the lower limbs make up the legs and feet. The bones of the legs and feet, from proximal to distal, are the *femur* (upper leg), *tibia* and *fibula* (lower leg), *tarsals* (ankle), *metatarsals* (foot), and *phalanges* (toes).

Recall Activity

1. List the two bones of the lower leg. _____

2. The bones of the lower limbs make up the _____ and

_____.

Concept 10: Joints

joint a connection between bones; can be immovable, slightly movable, or freely movable; also called an *articulation*

Connections between bones are called *joints*, or *articulations*. Joints allow movement to varying degrees. Some joints are immovable (for example, joints in the skull), some are slightly movable (for example, rib joints), and some are freely movable (for example, arm and leg joints). There are six types of freely movable joints, as illustrated in **Figure 10.7**.

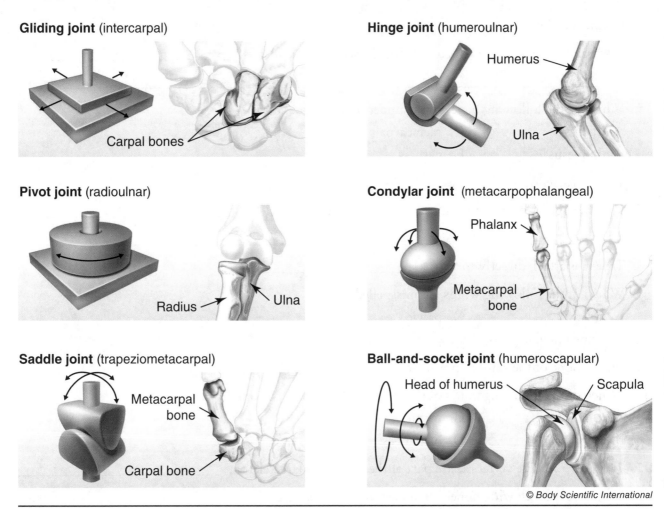

Gliding joint (intercarpal)

Carpal bones

Hinge joint (humeroulnar)

Humerus

Ulna

Pivot joint (radioulnar)

Radius

Ulna

Condylar joint (metacarpophalangeal)

Phalanx

Metacarpal bone

Saddle joint (trapeziometacarpal)

Metacarpal bone

Carpal bone

Ball-and-socket joint (humeroscapular)

Head of humerus

Scapula

© Body Scientific International

Figure 10.7 The six types of freely movable joints are the gliding joint, hinge joint, pivot joint, condylar joint, saddle joint, and ball-and-socket joint.

Recall Activity

1. Joints are _____ between bones.

2. Joints allow _____ to varying degrees.

3. List the types of freely movable joints. _____

_____

Section 10.2 Reinforcement

Answer the following questions using what you learned in this section.

1. The _____ girdle forms the hip joints.

2. Which of the following is *not* a type of freely movable joint?

    A. condylar joint   C. saddle joint

    B. ball-and-socket joint   D. cranial joint

3. Connections between bones are called _____.

4. Unscramble the letters: carlpeto. Define the word that is formed. _____
_____

5. Which of the following bones of the upper limbs is most distal?
   A. radius   C. metacarpals
   B. humerus   D. carpals

6. *True or False.* All of the bones in the skull are fused. _____

7. List the regions of the spine in order from superior to inferior. _____
_____

8. True ribs attach directly to the _____.

9. Which of the following words are misspelled?
   A. axial   C. palvic
   B. appendicular   D. pectral

10. Which bone of the skull is movable?_____

11. Which of the following bones of the lower limbs is most proximal?
   A. tibia   C. femur
   B. metatarsals   D. phalanges

12. *True or False.* The vertebrae are part of the appendicular skeleton. _____

13. Which of the following bones is *not* part of the pelvic girdle?
   A. clavicle   C. ischium
   B. ilium   D. pubis

14. Unscramble the letters: cupladeprain. Define the word that is formed. _____
_____

15. The _____ skeleton contains the spine and skull.

16. *True or False.* A pivot joint is freely movable. _____

17. Which two tissues make up most of the skeletal system?_____

18. The _____ girdle forms a shoulder joint.

19. Identify the functions of the skeletal system. _____
_____
_____

20. *True or False.* All of the bones in the pelvic girdle are fused. _____

21. List the bones of the pelvic girdle. _____
_____

Comprehensive Review (Chapters 1–10)

Answer the following questions using what you have learned so far in this book.

22. List two factors that can denature a protein. _____

23. How many nuclei does an anucleate cell have? _____

24. Science builds upon _____.

25. *True or False.* Contradicting evidence will cause the rejection of a scientific law. _____

26. Convert 0.2 m into mm. _____

27. *True or False.* Diffusion is a type of endocytosis. _____

28. Identify and define the prefix in the word *adduction*. _____

29. Name the four regions of the trunk. _____

_____

30. When muscle cells are stimulated, they _____, or shorten.

31. The deepest layer of skin is the _____.

Section 10.3   The Muscular System

All of the voluntary muscles in the body make up the muscular system. You have already learned about types of muscle tissue and muscle cells. In this section, you will learn about the muscular system as a whole, including its functions, structures, and directional movements.

The terms below are some of those that will be introduced in Section 10.3. To become familiar with these terms, reproduce each word on the line beside it. Pronounce each term as you write it. You will learn the definitions of these words as you complete this section.

1. muscular system _____

2. origin _____

3. insertion _____

4. flexion _____

5. extension _____

6. abduction _____

7. adduction _____

8. rotation _____

Concept 1: Functions of the Muscular System

muscular system a body system consisting of all of the skeletal muscles in the body; holds body parts in position, enables movement, helps maintain body temperature, and protects internal organs

The *muscular system* is composed of all the voluntary or skeletal muscles in the body. The muscular system performs several important functions in the human body:

- holds the parts of the body in position
- enables the movement of body parts
- helps maintain body temperature by producing heat
- protects the internal organs

The muscles work together to fulfill this group of functions.

Recall Activity

1. The muscular system is composed of all of the _____ muscles in the body.

2. List three functions of the muscular system._____

_____

Concept 2: Muscles of the Human Body

There are three types of muscle in the human body: skeletal muscle, smooth muscle, and cardiac muscle. *Smooth muscle* and *cardiac muscle* are involuntary. *Skeletal muscle* is voluntary and is attached to bone (**Figure 10.8**). Skeletal muscle makes up the muscular system. Some of the major skeletal muscles in the human body are illustrated in **Figure 10.9**. Knowing the locations of these muscles will help you understand how muscles produce movement.

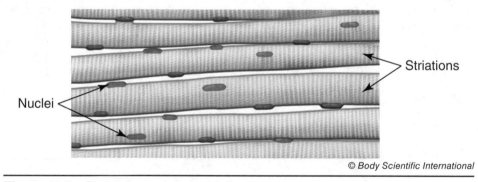

Nuclei

Striations

© Body Scientific International

Figure 10.8   Skeletal muscle has striations.

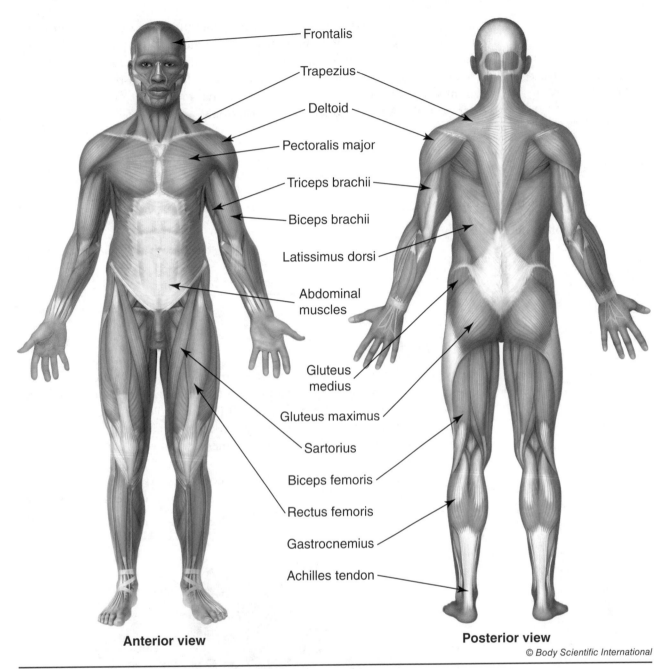

Frontalis

Trapezius

Deltoid

Pectoralis major

Triceps brachii

Biceps brachii

Latissimus dorsi

Abdominal
muscles

Gluteus
medius

Gluteus maximus

Sartorius

Biceps femoris

Rectus femoris

Gastrocnemius

Achilles tendon

Anterior view

Posterior view

© *Body Scientific International*

Figure 10.9 The major skeletal muscles of the human body are illustrated here.

Recall Activity

1. Identify the three types of muscle. _____

2. List two major skeletal muscles that make up the arm. _____

Concept 3: Muscle Contraction

Muscles *contract*, or shorten. When they are not contracting, they *relax*, or return to their resting length. For this reason, as you have learned, skeletal muscles operate in pairs. Skeletal muscles generally attach to two bones: one bone that moves and one bone that does not move. When a skeletal muscle contracts, it pulls the movable bone toward the immovable bone. The immovable bone is called the *origin*, and the movable bone is called the *insertion*. Skeletal muscles achieve several types of directional movement, including flexion, extension, abduction, adduction, and rotation.

origin the immovable bone to which a skeletal muscle is attached

insertion the movable bone to which a skeletal muscle is attached

Recall Activity

1. The immovable bone is called the _____.

2. The movable bone is called the _____.

3. List three types of directional movement that muscles achieve. _____

_____

Concept 4: Flexion

flexion a type of directional movement along the sagittal plane that reduces the angle between bones or between a limb and the body

One type of directional movement that muscles achieve is flexion. *Flexion* moves a body part along the sagittal plane and reduces the angle between bones or between a limb and the body (**Figure 10.10**). Examples of flexion are tilting your head toward your chest, bending your knee to raise your lower leg, and raising your arm forward. To feel this movement, wrap your hand around your upper arm and bring your forearm toward your upper arm. Feel the ventral side of your upper arm as the biceps brachii contracts. As the muscle shortens, it pulls the radius and ulna bones of the forearm toward the humerus in the upper arm. The elbow joint allows the ulna to pivot.

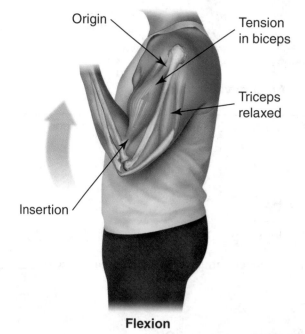

Origin

Tension in biceps

Triceps relaxed

Insertion

Flexion

© Body Scientific International

Figure 10.10 Flexion reduces the angle between bones or between the body and a limb.

Recall Activity

1. Flexion _____ the angle between bones or between a limb and the body.

2. During flexion, the elbow joint allows the _____ to pivot.

3. List two examples of flexion. _____

Concept 5: Extension

Extension also moves a body part along the sagittal plane; it increases the angle between bones or between a limb and the body. Examples of extension include raising your head from your chest, lowering your arm, and straightening your leg. To feel this movement, flex your forearm, wrap your hand around the dorsal surface of your upper arm, and extend your forearm. The triceps brachii contracts and causes the ulna to pivot at the elbow joint (**Figure 10.11**). Extension is the opposite of flexion. Because muscles only contract, one set of muscles moves a limb or bone one direction, and another set of muscles moves the limb or bone back.

extension a type of directional movement along the sagittal plane that increases the angle between bones or between a limb and the body

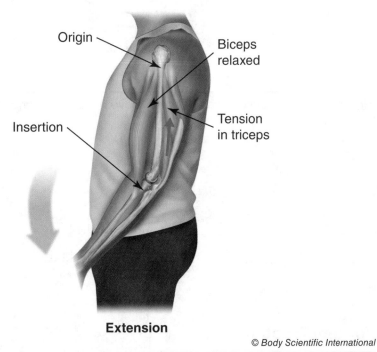

Extension

© Body Scientific International

Figure 10.11 Extension increases the angle between bones or between the body and a limb.

Recall Activity

1. Extension is the opposite of _____.

2. *True or False*. One muscle can both flex and extend a limb. _____

3. Extension _____ the angle between bones or between a limb and the body.

Concept 6: Abduction and Adduction

abduction a type of directional movement along the frontal plane that moves a body part away from the middle of the body

adduction a type of directional movement along the frontal plane that moves a body part toward the middle of the body

Abduction and adduction are directional movements away from or toward the middle (midsagittal plane) of the body. *Abduction* moves a limb along the frontal plane away from the middle of the body. *Adduction* is the opposite of abduction and moves a limb along the frontal plane toward the middle of the body (**Figure 10.12**). To feel these movements, stand in anatomical position and then practice abducting and then adducting your arm. The deltoid muscle abducts your arm. Several muscles, including the pectoralis and latissimus dorsi, adduct the arm.

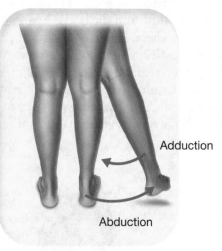

Adduction

Abduction

© Body Scientific International

Figure 10.12 Abduction and adduction move limbs in reference to the midsagittal plane.

Recall Activity

1. Abduction moves a limb _____ the middle of the body.

2. Adduction moves a limb _____ the middle of the body.

Concept 7: Rotation

rotation a type of directional movement along the transverse plane that moves a body part from side to side

In *rotation*, a body part moves from side to side along the transverse plane (**Figure 10.13**). Turning your head from side to side is an example of rotation. The left and right sternocleidomastoid muscles help turn the head from side to side. When the left sternocleidomastoid muscle contracts, the head rotates to the right. When the right sternocleidomastoid muscle contracts, the head rotates to the left.

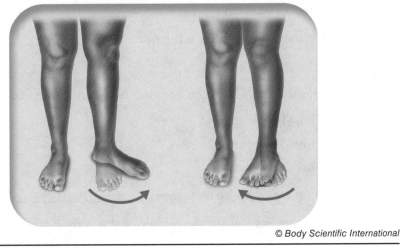

© Body Scientific International

Figure 10.13   Rotation moves a body part along the transverse plane.

Recall Activity

1. Turning your head from side to side is an example of _____.

2. When the left _____ muscle contracts, the head rotates to the right.

Section 10.3 Reinforcement

Answer the following questions using what you learned in this section.

1. When a skeletal muscle contracts, it _____ a movable bone toward an immovable bone.

2. Identify the three types of muscle found in the human body. _____

3. When you abduct your arm, you are moving your arm along the _____ plane away from the _____ plane.

4. The pectoralis and latissimus dorsi help _____ the arm.

5. *True or False.* Rotation moves a body part along the transverse plane. _____

6. In muscle contraction, the _____ bone is called the *insertion*.

7. Flexion is to extension as _____ is to adduction.

8. Which of the following directional movements reduces the angle between bones?
   A. flexion   C. extension
   B. rotation   D. adduction

9. Identify the four functions of the muscular system._____

   _____

   _____

10. *True or False.* The deltoid muscle adducts your arm. _____

11. Unscramble the letters: seentixon. Define the word that is formed. _____

_____

12. _____ increases the angle between bones or between a limb and the body.

13. Which of the following words are misspelled?
    A. flesion   C. adduction
    B. extension   D. rotatiun

14. *True or False.* Abduction and adduction are opposite movements. _____

15. In _____, a limb moves toward the middle of the body.

16. In flexion and extension, body parts move along the _____ plane.

17. Unscramble the letters: bonadutic. Define the word that is formed. _____

_____

18. In muscle contraction, the _____ bone is called the *origin*.

19. *True or False.* The triceps brachii muscle causes the extension of the forearm. _____

20. In _____, a limb moves away from the middle of the body.

21. When the right sternocleidomastoid muscle contracts, what direction does the head rotate? _____

Comprehensive Review (Chapters 1–10)

Answer the following questions using what you have learned so far in this book.

22. *True or False.* The pectoral girdle is part of the axial skeleton. _____

23. The prefix *af-* means "_____."

24. Breaking the high-energy bond in ATP is a(n) _____ reaction, meaning it _____ energy.

25. *True or False.* Scientific laws tell you that the natural world is unpredictable. _____

26. A volume measurement of 100 cc is the same as _____ L.

27. Science seeks _____ explanations to phenomena.

28. The complementary base of cytosine is _____.

29. The _____ is the control center of a cell.

30. Which of the following body parts is most lateral?
    A. hip   C. eye
    B. nose   D. thumb

31. Nerve cells that conduct electrical charges are known as _____.

Section 10.4   The Nervous System

The nervous system is responsible for sensory perception and electrical signaling in the body. Because of the nervous system, you can hear sounds, see images, and perceive changes in temperature. Because of the nervous system, your body breathes and moves. In this section, you will learn about the basic functions and structures of the nervous system.

The terms below are some of those that will be introduced in Section 10.4. To become familiar with these terms, reproduce each word on the line beside it. Pronounce each term as you write it. You will learn the definitions of these words as you complete this section.

1. nervous system _____

2. central nervous system (CNS)_____

3. peripheral nervous system (PNS)_____

4. brain _____

5. spinal cord_____

6. afferent nerve _____

7. efferent nerve _____

Concept 1: Functions of the Nervous System

The *nervous system* encompasses the brain, the spinal cord, and the nerves of the body. The functions of the nervous system include the following:

- receives external sensory information (for example, sound, smell, sight, and touch)
- processes and interprets sensory information
- responds to sensory information by transmitting impulses to control body parts

    The parts of the nervous system work together to perform these functions.

nervous system a body system consisting of the brain, spinal cord, and nerves of the body; receives sensory information, processes information, and transmits impulses to body parts

Recall Activity

1. Name the three components of the nervous system. _____

2. List two functions of the nervous system. _____

    _____

Concept 2: CNS and PNS

The nervous system is divided into two parts: the *central nervous system (CNS)* and the *peripheral nervous system (PNS)*. The CNS consists of the brain and spinal cord and is responsible for processing most information. The PNS includes all other nerves throughout the body and communicates impulses to and from the CNS.

Recall Activity

1. The two divisions of the nervous system are the _____ and the

   _____.

2. *True or False.* The PNS does not communicate with the CNS. _____

Concept 3: Brain

The *brain* is the center of nervous system function. This organ receives and integrates sensory information and then transmits commands to the rest of the body. It is responsible for reasoning, recalling, translating emotions, and coordinating movement. The brain consists of the brainstem, diencephalon, cerebellum, and cerebrum. The *brainstem* and *diencephalon* regulate vital unconscious processes (such as breathing and sleeping). The *cerebellum* coordinates balance and body movement. The *cerebrum* is responsible for most mental functions and is divided into four lobes (**Figure 10.14**).

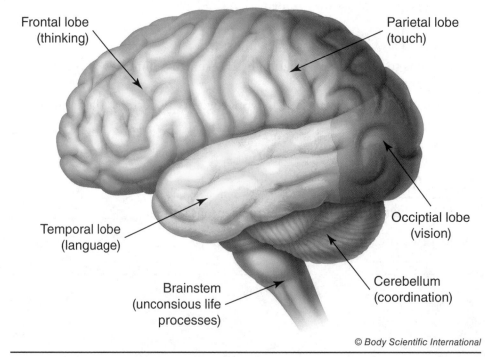

Frontal lobe
(thinking)

Parietal lobe
(touch)

Temporal lobe
(language)

Occiptial lobe
(vision)

Brainstem
(unconsious life
processes)

Cerebellum
(coordination)

© Body Scientific International

Figure 10.14 The four lobes of the brain participate in different functions within the body.

Recall Activity

1. Which organ is the center of nervous system function? _____

2. The _____ coordinates balance and body movement.

3. Identify the four lobes of the cerebrum. _____

Concept 4: Spinal Cord

The *spinal cord* is made of nervous tissue and is housed inside the vertebrae of the spine. Descending from the brain, the spinal cord attaches to and communicates with the nerves of the peripheral nervous system. The spinal cord also processes some sensory information and signals reflexes in the body.

spinal cord a cord of nervous tissue housed inside the vertebrae of the spine; descends from the brain and attaches to and communicates with the body's nerves

Recall Activity

1. The spinal cord is housed inside the _____ of the spine.

2. The spinal cord communicates with the _____ of the peripheral nervous system.

Concept 5: Afferent and Efferent Nerves

As you have learned, the PNS consists of all the nerves in the body. Nerves are made of *neurons*, which you learned about in Section 8.5. *Afferent nerves* transmit impulses *toward* the CNS. Afferent nerves are also called *sensory nerves* since they communicate information from the sensory organs (for example, the eyes) to the CNS. *Efferent nerves* transmit impulses *away from* the CNS. Efferent nerves are also called *motor nerves* since they communicate information from the CNS to the rest of the body, causing a response (for example, movement).

afferent nerve a nerve that transmits impulses from the sensory organs toward the central nervous system; also called a *sensory nerve*

efferent nerve a nerve that transmits impulses away from the central nervous system toward the rest of the body; also called a *motor nerve*

Recall Activity

1. Nerves that transmit impulses away from the CNS are called _____ nerves or _____ nerves.

2. Nerves that transmit impulses toward the CNS are called _____ nerves or _____ nerves.

Concept 6: Somatic and Autonomic Nerves

Efferent nerves (motor nerves) can be somatic and autonomic. *Somatic nerves* are consciously controlled and coordinate voluntary muscles (skeletal muscles). *Autonomic nerves* are not consciously controlled; they coordinate involuntary muscles and organs (for example, the adrenal gland).

Recall Activity

1. Somatic and autonomic nerves are types of _____ nerves.

2. Somatic nerves control _____ muscles.

3. Autonomic nerves control _____ muscles and _____.

Concept 7: Sympathetic and Parasympathetic Nerves

Autonomic nerves, which are not under conscious control, can be either sympathetic or parasympathetic. *Sympathetic nerves* help speed up the body and prepare it for action. *Parasympathetic nerves* slow down the body for rest. **Figure 10.15** summarizes the divisions of the PNS.

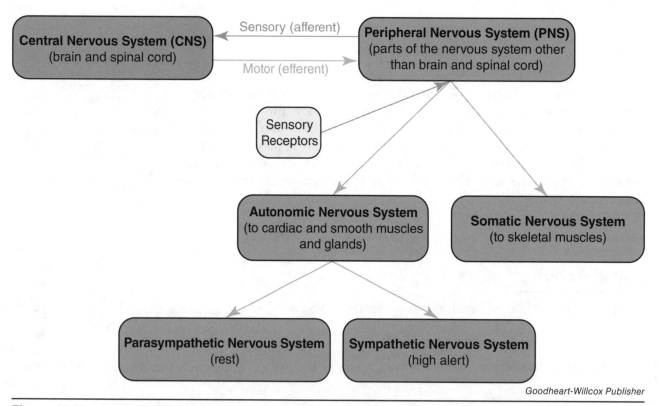

Goodheart-Willcox Publisher

Figure 10.15 The PNS can be divided into the autonomic and somatic nervous systems, and the autonomic nervous system is made up of the parasympathetic and sympathetic nervous systems.

Recall Activity

1. _____ nerves help prepare the body for action.

2. _____ nerves slow down the body for rest.

Section 10.4 Reinforcement

Answer the following questions using what you learned in this section.

1. What are the three functions of the nervous system?_____

   _____

2. Sensory nerves are to motor nerves as afferent nerves are to _____ nerves.

3. *True or False.* Autonomic nerves are consciously controlled. _____

4. The CNS consists of the _____ and _____.

5. Which of the following nerves is consciously controlled?
   - A. sympathetic nerve
   - B. autonomic nerve
   - C. parasympathetic nerve
   - D. somatic nerve

6. *True or False.* Afferent nerves transmit information from the sensory organs to the CNS._____

7. Which part of the brain is responsible for most mental functions? _____

8. *True or False.* The spinal cord lines the outside of the spine. _____

9. The nervous system encompasses the _____, the
   _____, and the _____ of the body.

10. Which of the following words are misspelled?
    - A. aferent
    - B. efferent
    - C. sympathic
    - D. parasympathetic

11. Which part of the brain coordinates balance and movement?_____

12. Nerves that transmit impulses toward the CNS are called _____ nerves or
    _____ nerves.

13. *True or False.* Sympathetic nerves prepare the body for action._____

14. Unscramble the letters: feerfant. Define the word that is formed. _____

    _____

15. Which part of the nervous system processes reflexes?_____

16. List the two types of efferent nerves. _____

17. Efferent nerves transmit impulses from the _____ to the
    _____.

18. *True or False.* Efferent and afferent nerves are part of the CNS. _____

19. Unscramble the letters: staprhymetapaci. Define the word that is formed. _____

_____

20. Which nerves control involuntary muscles? _____

21. _____ nerves communicate information from the CNS to the rest of the body, causing a response.

Comprehensive Review (Chapters 1–10)

Answer the following questions using what you have learned so far in this book.

22. What does the prefix *endo-* mean? _____

23. List the steps of the diagnostic scientific method. _____

_____

24. _____ is the science that studies life.

25. If 50 people (25% of a population) say "yes," how many people are in the population? _____

26. The process of cell respiration—transforming ADP into ATP—is a(n) _____ reaction.

27. Glands that release a product into the interstitial fluid surrounding a cell are called

_____ glands.

28. The heart and lungs are housed in the _____ cavity.

29. In _____, a limb moves toward the middle of the body.

30. How are functional proteins different from structural proteins? _____

_____

31. The bumps on RER are _____.

Section 10.5   The Endocrine System

Many of the body's processes are regulated by hormones. Hormones are secreted by glands throughout the body, and these glands make up the endocrine system. In this section, you will learn about the glands and hormones of the endocrine system and their functions in the body.

The following terms are some of those that will be introduced in Section 10.5. To become familiar with these terms, reproduce each word on the line beside it. Pronounce each term as you write it. You will learn the definitions of these words as you complete this section.

1. endocrine system _____

2. hormone _____

3. tropic hormone _____

4. nontropic hormone _____

5. pituitary gland _____

6. thyroid gland _____

7. parathyroid gland _____

Concept 1: Functions of the Endocrine System

The *endocrine system* consists of glands throughout the body. *Endocrine glands* secrete hormones, and these hormones signal diverse processes in the body. As you have learned, endocrine glands secrete hormones directly into interstitial fluid (not through a duct). The major functions of the endocrine system include the following:

endocrine system a body system consisting of glands throughout the body; releases hormones, maintains homeostasis, and helps regulate body function

- releases hormones to influence the functions of other organs
- maintains homeostasis
- helps regulate body functions

The body's endocrine glands are illustrated in **Figure 10.16**. These glands work together to regulate body processes.

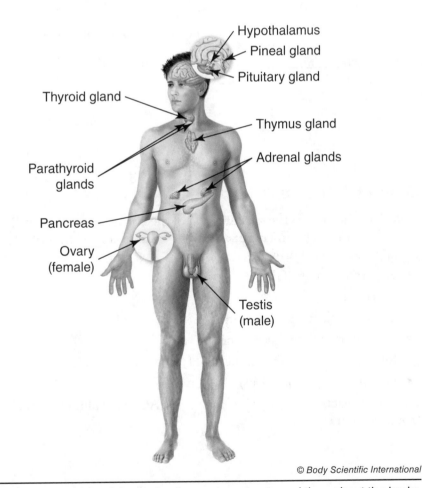

© Body Scientific International

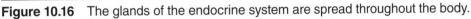

Figure 10.16   The glands of the endocrine system are spread throughout the body.

Recall Activity

1. Endocrine glands secrete _____.

2. List one function of the endocrine system. _____

3. Identify three endocrine glands. _____

Concept 2: Hormones

hormone a chemical message sent from an endocrine gland to a target

tropic hormone a chemical message sent from an endocrine gland that targets another endocrine gland

nontropic hormone a chemical message sent from an endocrine gland that targets a nonendocrine organ or tissue

Endocrine glands affect body functions by secreting hormones. A *hormone* is a chemical message sent from an endocrine gland to a target. The target can be another endocrine gland (such as the thyroid gland) or an organ (such as a kidney or tissue). The hormone received causes the target to respond. There are two types of hormones: tropic hormones and nontropic hormones. *Tropic hormones* target other endocrine glands. *Nontropic hormones* target nonendocrine organs or tissues. You have already learned about some hormones and their influence in the body. In the next few concepts, you will learn about a few more glands and their hormones.

Recall Activity

1. A(n) _____ is a chemical message sent from an endocrine gland to a target.

2. A hormone's target can be another _____ gland or a(n) _____.

3. List the two types of hormones. _____

Concept 3: Pituitary Gland

pituitary gland an endocrine gland at the base of the brain; also called the *master gland*

Commonly known as the *master gland* of the body, the *pituitary gland* is located at the base of the brain (**Figure 10.17**). The anterior portion of the pituitary gland produces six hormones:

- growth hormone (GH)
- prolactin
- adrenocorticotropic hormone (ACTH)
- thyroid-stimulating hormone (TSH)
- follicle-stimulating hormone (FSH)
- luteinizing hormone (LH)

GH and prolactin are nontropic hormones. ACTH, TSH, FSH, and LH are all tropic hormones.

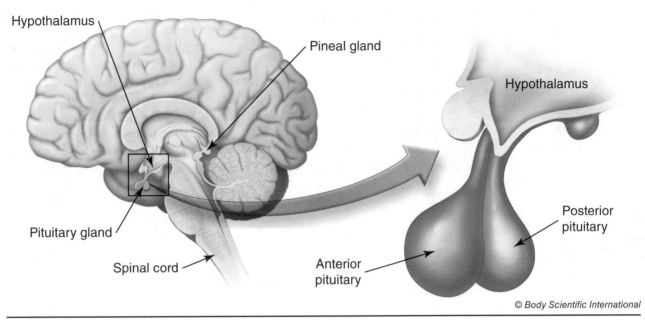

Figure 10.17 The pituitary gland is located at the base of the brain and contains anterior and posterior portions.

© Body Scientific International

Recall Activity

1. Where is the pituitary gland located? _____

2. List the six hormones produced by the anterior portion of the pituitary gland. _____

_____

Concept 4: Thyroid Gland

The anterior portion of the pituitary gland secretes *thyroid-stimulating hormone (TSH)*, which is also called *thyrotropin*. The target of TSH is another endocrine gland: the thyroid gland. The *thyroid gland* is located in the throat and is shaped like a butterfly (Figure 10.16). It releases the hormones triiodothyronine (T_3), thyroxine (T_4), and calcitonin. If there is not enough T_3 and T_4 in the blood, the anterior pituitary gland releases TSH to cause the thyroid gland to release more hormones. T_3 and T_4 control the *metabolic rate* (the rate at which cells transform energy) in the body.

thyroid gland an endocrine gland located in the throat that releases triiodothyronine (T_3), thyroxine (T_4), and calcitonin

Recall Activity

1. Thyroid-stimulating hormone (TSH) is also called _____.

2. What hormones does the thyroid gland release? _____

3. The rate at which cells transform energy is known as the _____.

Concept 5: Calcitonin

One of the hormones released by the thyroid gland is *calcitonin*. To understand the role of hormones in the body, this concept will discuss how calcitonin helps maintain the homeostasis of calcium in the body. Your thyroid gland releases calcitonin in response to a high level of calcium in the blood, and the targets of calcitonin are the bones, intestines, and kidneys. Calcitonin lowers the level of calcium in your blood by signaling your bone cells to remove calcium from the blood. Calcitonin also signals your intestines to stop absorbing calcium from food and signals your kidneys to take calcium out of the blood.

Recall Activity

1. The targets of calcitonin are the _____, _____, and
   _____.

2. Calcitonin signals bone cells to _____ calcium from the blood.

Concept 6: Parathyroid Glands

parathyroid gland an endocrine gland located on the dorsal surface of the thyroid gland that releases parathyroid hormone (PTH)

The level of calcium in the blood is also affected by a hormone released from the parathyroid glands. The *parathyroid glands* are small and are located on the dorsal surface of the thyroid gland. They release *parathyroid hormone* (*PTH*), which raises the level of calcium in the blood by targeting the bones, intestines, and kidneys. PTH signals bone cells to break down the bone matrix and release calcium into the blood. PTH also signals the intestines to absorb calcium from food and signals the kidneys to keep calcium in the blood. In this way, the thyroid gland and parathyroid glands work together to maintain homeostatic blood calcium levels.

Recall Activity

1. The _____ glands are small and are located on the dorsal surface of the thyroid gland.

2. Parathyroid hormone _____ the level of calcium in the blood.

Section 10.5 Reinforcement

Answer the following questions using what you learned in this section.

1. List the two hormones that target the bones, intestines, and kidneys to maintain homeostatic blood calcium levels. _____

2. Does calcitonin raise or lower the level of calcium in the blood? _____

3. List three functions of the endocrine system. _____

    _____

4. A(n) _____ is a chemical message sent from an endocrine gland to a target.

5. *True or False.* The targets of PTH are the bones, intestines, and kidneys. _____

6. Which hormone raises the level of calcium in the blood? _____

7. Which of the following hormones are produced by the thyroid gland?
    A. T_4 C. GH
    B. T_3 D. calcitonin

8. Identify five endocrine glands. _____

    _____

9. _____ is also called thyrotropin.

10. *True or False.* Tropic hormones target other endocrine glands. _____

11. Unscramble the letters: tlacocnini. Define the word that is formed. _____

    _____

12. *True or False.* Endocrine glands secrete hormones through ducts. _____

13. Which endocrine gland is located at the base of the brain? _____

14. Write the letters backward: dioryhtarap. Define the word that is formed. _____

    _____

15. *True or False.* Parathyroid hormone and calcitonin have the same targets. _____

16. Which of the following are nontropic hormones?
    A. prolactin   C. LH   E. PTH
    B. calcitonin   D. thyrotropin   F. FSH

17. The thyroid gland releases _____ in response to a high level of calcium in the blood.

18. What is the target of nontropic hormones? _____

19. Unscramble the letters: cdiereonn. Define the word that is formed. _____

    _____

20. *True or False.* Low levels of T_3 and T_4 in the blood cause the release of calcitonin. _____

21. Which endocrine gland is also known as the *master gland*? _____

Comprehensive Review (Chapters 1–10)

Answer the following questions using what you have learned so far in this book.

22. The prefix *intra-* means "_____."

23. *True or False.* There is only one scientific method. _____

24. Which subatomic particles do not leave the atom's core? _____

25. There are _____ layers of phospholipids in a cell's plasma membrane.

26. *True or False.* Oxygen and carbon dioxide can pass through a cell's lipid barrier. _____

27. Which part of the brain is responsible for most mental functions? _____

28. What is the strongest extracellular fiber? _____

29. Are the lungs superficial or deep to the thoracic cage? _____

30. Your _____ is your way of feeling, thinking about, and viewing a situation.

31. *True or False.* The metric unit of mass is the pound. _____

Section 10.6   The Respiratory System

Your respiratory system enables you to breathe—to inhale oxygen and exhale carbon dioxide. In the respiratory system, the exchange of gases maintains life. This section will discuss the major functions and structures of the respiratory system.

The terms below are some of those that will be introduced in Section 10.6. To become familiar with these terms, reproduce each word on the line beside it. Pronounce each term as you write it. You will learn the definitions of these words as you complete this section.

1. respiratory system _____

2. lung _____

3. diaphragm _____

4. inspiration _____

5. external respiration _____

6. internal respiration _____

7. expiration _____

respiratory system a body system consisting of the organs involved in breathing; inhales oxygen-rich air, exchanges respiratory gases, and exhales carbon dioxide

Concept 1: Functions of the Respiratory System

The *respiratory system* consists of the organs involved in breathing. Some of these organs include the lungs, trachea, and nasal cavities. The most important functions of the respiratory system include the following:

- inhales oxygen-rich air
- exchanges respiratory gases to bring oxygen into the body and discard carbon dioxide
- exhales carbon dioxide

The structures of the respiratory system work in concert to perform these functions. The respiratory gases involved in breathing are oxygen (O_2) and carbon dioxide (CO_2).

Recall Activity

1. The respiratory system consists of the organs involved in _____.

2. Identify the three functions of the respiratory system. _____
   _____

3. The respiratory gases involved in breathing are _____ and
   _____.

Concept 2: Volume and Air Pressure

The principles of volume and air pressure make the functions of the respiratory system possible. As you have learned, *air pressure* is the concentration of atoms that make up air. Air pressure in the atmosphere at sea level is always 760 mmHg. However, if you put air in a sealed container and then made the container larger (increasing volume), air pressure would decrease. If you put air in a sealed container and then made the container smaller (decreasing volume), air pressure would rise. You have learned that atoms tend to move from areas of high concentration to areas of low concentration. This also applies to air. The molecules in air tend to move from areas of high air pressure to areas of low air pressure.

Recall Activity

1. If you increase the volume of a container, will this make air pressure inside the container rise or fall?
   _____

2. If you decrease the volume of a container, will this make air pressure inside the container rise or fall?
   _____

3. Air pressure in the atmosphere at sea level is always _____ mmHg.

4. The molecules in air tend to move from areas of _____ air pressure to areas
   of _____ air pressure.

Concept 3: Lungs and Diaphragm

lung an organ located in the thoracic cavity that receives air and exchanges oxygen and carbon dioxide

diaphragm a dome-shaped muscle inferior to the thoracic cavity that contracts to lower the bottom of the thoracic cavity

The act of breathing depends on changes in lung volume. The *lungs* are organs that receive air and exchange oxygen and carbon dioxide (**Figure 10.18**). They are located in the thoracic cavity. For lung volume to increase, the thoracic cavity must expand. Lung volume then decreases when the thoracic cavity relaxes. Muscles are responsible for expanding the thoracic cavity. The muscles between your ribs contract, raising the ribs and causing the thoracic cavity to move up and out. The *diaphragm*, a dome-shaped muscle inferior to the thoracic cavity, also contracts to lower the bottom of the thoracic cavity and increase lung volume.

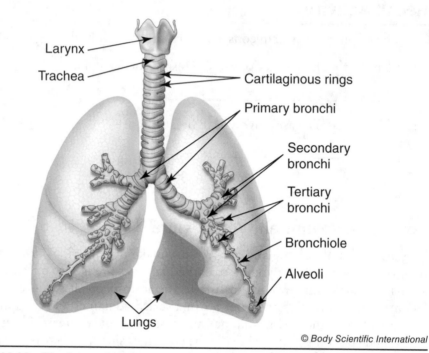

© Body Scientific International

Figure 10.18 The internal structures of the lungs are responsible for conducting and exchanging respiratory gases.

Recall Activity

1. Does muscle contraction in the diaphragm make the thoracic cavity larger or smaller? _____

2. The _____ is a dome-shaped muscle inferior to the thoracic cavity.

3. The act of breathing depends on changes in _____ volume.

Concept 4: Inspiration

inspiration the process of breathing in air as lung volume increases

The body breathes in air through a process known as *inspiration*. To inhale air, your thoracic cavity expands, increasing the volume of your lungs. As the volume of the lungs increases, *intrapulmonary pressure* (air pressure within the lungs) falls below atmospheric pressure (760 mmHg). As a result, air flows passively from high pressure to low pressure—from outside your lungs to inside your lungs (**Figure 10.19**).

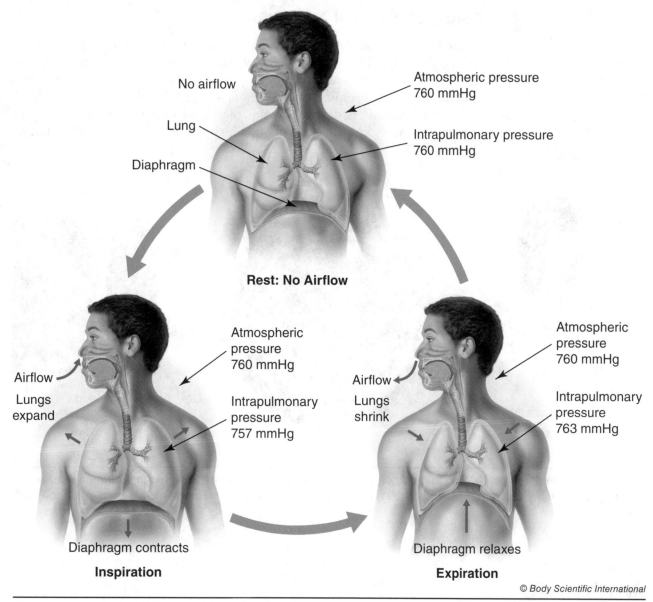

Rest: No Airflow

No airflow

Lung

Diaphragm

Atmospheric pressure
760 mmHg

Intrapulmonary pressure
760 mmHg

Airflow

Lungs
expand

Atmospheric
pressure
760 mmHg

Intrapulmonary
pressure
757 mmHg

Diaphragm contracts

Inspiration

Airflow

Lungs
shrink

Atmospheric
pressure
760 mmHg

Intrapulmonary
pressure
763 mmHg

Diaphragm relaxes

Expiration

© Body Scientific International

Figure 10.19 Notice how the size of the thoracic cavity changes air pressure in the lungs.

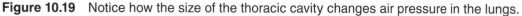

Recall Activity

1. Increasing the volume of the lungs _____ intrapulmonary pressure.

2. The body breathes in air through a process known as _____.

3. During inspiration, air flows _____ from outside your lungs to inside your lungs.

Concept 5: External Respiration

external respiration the exchange of oxygen and carbon dioxide between the air in the lungs and the blood; oxygen is loaded from the air into the blood, and carbon dioxide is unloaded from the blood into the air

In the lungs, *respiratory gases* (oxygen and carbon dioxide) move between the air and the blood. This is called *external respiration* because air is brought from the external environment into the lungs, where the air and blood have close contact. In external respiration, oxygen is loaded from the air into the blood, and carbon dioxide is unloaded from the blood into the air. This happens through a process known as *diffusion*, which you learned about in Section 7.3 (**Figure 10.20**).

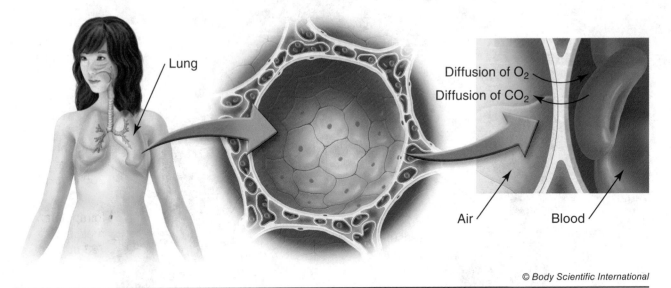

© *Body Scientific International*

Figure 10.20 In diffusion, oxygen and carbon dioxide both move from areas of high concentration to areas of low concentration. Oxygen moves from the air into the blood, and carbon dioxide moves from the blood into the air.

Recall Activity

1. In external respiration, respiratory gases move between the _____ and the _____.

2. Through diffusion, _____ is loaded from the air into the blood, and _____ is unloaded from the blood into the air.

Concept 6: Internal Respiration

internal respiration the exchange of oxygen and carbon dioxide between the blood and the cells of the body; oxygen in the blood is unloaded to body cells, and carbon dioxide is loaded from body cells into the blood

Once oxygen enters the blood, blood transports oxygen all throughout the body. The cells of the body use oxygen and produce carbon dioxide; they need a steady supply of oxygen for cell respiration. In *internal respiration*, the oxygen in the blood is unloaded to body cells, and carbon dioxide is loaded from body cells into the blood. Internal respiration occurs all throughout the body. After internal respiration, the carbon dioxide loaded into the blood travels back toward the lungs.

Recall Activity

1. Where does internal respiration occur? _____

2. In internal respiration, the _____ in the blood is unloaded to body cells, and _____ is loaded from body cells into the blood.

Concept 7: Expiration

Once internal and external respiration have taken place, the blood returned to the lungs contains a high concentration of carbon dioxide. External respiration takes place. Then you breathe out, in a process known as *expiration*. In expiration, the muscles that expanded the thoracic cavity relax, and the volume of your thoracic cavity decreases. Intrapulmonary pressure becomes higher than air pressure outside the lungs. As a result, air flows passively from inside your lungs to outside your lungs—from high pressure to low pressure (Figure 10.19).

expiration the process of breathing out air as lung volume decreases

Recall Activity

1. The body breathes out air through a process known as _____.

2. In expiration, the muscles that expanded the thoracic cavity _____.

3. During expiration, air flows passively from _____ your lungs to _____ your lungs.

Section 10.6 Reinforcement

Answer the following questions using what you learned in this section.

1. Will decreasing the volume of a container full of air make air pressure rise or fall? _____

2. The process of breathing _____ is known as expiration.

3. Where does external respiration take place? _____

4. In _____ respiration, oxygen and carbon dioxide move between the air and the blood.

5. *True or False.* Internal respiration takes place in the lungs. _____

6. Unscramble the letters: itroxpaine. Define the word that is formed. _____

_____

7. The process of breathing _____ is known as inspiration.

8. During inspiration, does the thoracic cavity shrink or expand? _____

9. *True or False.* The diaphragm contracts during expiration. _____

10. Air pressure in the atmosphere is always _____ mmHg.

11. Molecules in the air tend to move from areas of _____ pressure to areas of _____ pressure.

12. To lower intrapulmonary pressure, does lung volume need to increase or decrease? _____

13. *True or False*. External respiration takes place in the lungs. _____

14. Unscramble the letters: instairipon. Define the word that is formed. _____

_____

15. In _____ respiration, the oxygen in the blood is unloaded to body cells, and carbon dioxide is loaded from body cells into the blood.

16. *True or False*. Muscle contractions in the ribs and diaphragm make the thoracic cavity smaller. _____

17. Intrapulmonary pressure is pressure _____ the lungs.

18. Will increasing the volume of a container full of air make air pressure rise or fall? _____

19. During inspiration, where is air pressure higher: outside the lungs or inside the lungs? _____

20. Which of the following words are misspelled?
    A. inspirasion   C. expirasion
    B. respiration   D. thoracic

21. During expiration, where is air pressure higher: outside the lungs or inside the lungs? _____

22. List two functions of the respiratory system. _____

_____

Comprehensive Review (Chapters 1–10)

Answer the following questions using what you have learned so far in this book.

23. Which of the following terms indicates that a body part is closer to the head?
    A. superior   C. inferior
    B. medial   D. lateral

24. Which hormone lowers the level of calcium in the blood?_____

25. *True or False*. Students tend to like subjects at which they excel. _____

26. The _____ of a scientific article gives the background and observations that lead to the topic of the article.

27. Convert 2.44 m into cm. _____

28. A lipid with two or more double bonds between carbon atoms is a(n) _____ fat.

29. Identify and define the root word in the term *cardial*. _____

30. *True or False*. When water enters a cell, crenation occurs. _____

31. Which membrane junctions keep muscle cells in the heart from separating when the heart beats?

_____

32. List the three formed elements in blood. _____

Section 10.7   The Cardiovascular System

The cardiovascular system is responsible for circulating blood all throughout the body. It transports oxygen, carbon dioxide, nutrients, and other important substances among body parts. In this section, you will learn about the structures and major functions of the cardiovascular system.

The terms below are some of those that will be introduced in Section 10.7. To become familiar with these terms, reproduce each word on the line beside it. Pronounce each term as you write it. You will learn the definitions of these words as you complete this section.

1. cardiovascular system _____

   _____

2. heart _____

3. atrium _____

4. ventricle _____

5. atrioventricular (AV) valve _____

   _____

6. semilunar (SL) valve _____

   _____

7. artery_____

8. capillary _____

9. vein_____

10. pulmonary circulation _____

    _____

11. systemic circulation_____

    _____

Concept 1: Functions of the Cardiovascular System

The *cardiovascular system* consists of the heart and all of the blood vessels in the body. It is also known as the *circulatory system* since it circulates blood. The most important functions of the cardiovascular system include the following:

- transports oxygen-rich blood all throughout the body
- circulates nutrients, hormones, and other important substances in the blood
- collects and transports waste produced by cells
- helps regulate body temperature

The word *cardiovascular* is formed from the combining form *cardi/o* (meaning "heart") and the root word *vascul* (meaning "blood vessel"). The heart and blood vessels work together to perform cardiovascular functions.

cardiovascular system a body system consisting of the heart and blood vessels; transports blood, collects and transports waste, and helps regulate body temperature; also called the *circulatory system*

Recall Activity

1. The cardiovascular system consists of the _____ and all of the

   _____ in the body.

2. Name two functions of the cardiovascular system. _____

   _____

Concept 2: Heart

heart a muscular organ located in the thoracic cavity that receives oxygen-poor blood from the body, pumps it into the lungs for oxygenation, and then pumps oxygen-rich blood to the rest of the body

atrium an upper chamber of the heart

ventricle a lower chamber of the heart

The *heart* is a muscular organ found in the thoracic cavity; it is responsible for pumping blood to the rest of the body. The heart has four chambers: two *atria* (one right atrium and one left atrium) and two *ventricles* (one right ventricle and one left ventricle). The four chambers contract to move blood through the heart. Blood flows from the body into the right atrium and then into the right ventricle. From the right ventricle, blood is pumped to the lungs, where it gains oxygen. Then, from the lungs, blood flows into the left atrium. Blood then enters the left ventricle, where it is pumped to the rest of the body (**Figure 10.21**).

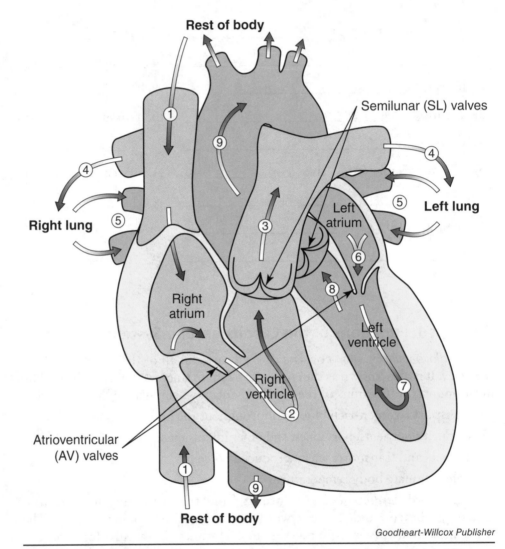

Figure 10.21 The arrows in this illustration indicate the direction of blood flow. Blue arrows represent oxygen-poor blood. Red arrows represent oxygen-rich blood. Follow the numbers (beginning with 1 and ending with 9) in the illustration to understand how blood flows through the heart.

Goodheart-Willcox Publisher

Recall Activity

1. Which organ is responsible for pumping blood to the rest of the body? _____

2. List the four chambers of the heart. _____

   _____

3. Describe blood flow through the heart. _____

   _____

   _____

   _____

Concept 3: Heart Valves

The four chambers of the heart contract to keep blood flowing. During contraction, *heart valves* open or close to keep blood moving in the right direction. *Atrioventricular (AV) valves* separate the atria and ventricles. When the ventricles contract, these valves close to prevent blood from flowing backward into the atria. *Semilunar (SL) valves* separate the ventricles from blood vessels that move blood out of the heart. These valves close when the atria contract and keep blood from flowing prematurely into the blood vessels (Figure 10.21). When the atria contract, SL valves are closed, and AV valves are open. When the ventricles contract, SL valves are open, and AV valves are closed.

atrioventricular (AV) valve a valve that separates an atrium and a ventricle; prevents blood from flowing backward into the atrium when the ventricle contracts

semilunar (SL) valve a valve that separates a ventricle from a blood vessel that moves blood out of the heart; keeps blood from flowing prematurely into a blood vessel when an atrium contracts

Recall Activity

1. During contraction, heart _____ open or close to keep blood moving in the right direction.

2. _____ valves separate the atria and ventricles, and _____ valves separate the ventricles from blood vessels that move blood out of the heart.

3. In the space below, draw and label the four chambers of the heart and the heart valves. Draw arrows to show circulation through the heart to the lungs and body.

Concept 4: Blood Vessels

Blood vessels carry blood between the heart and the rest of the body. There are three types of blood vessels in the body: arteries, capillaries, and veins. *Arteries* carry blood away from the heart toward the rest of the body. *Capillaries* are small blood vessels with thin walls that allow the exchange of nutrients and gases. *Veins* carry blood from the body back to the heart (**Figure 10.22**).

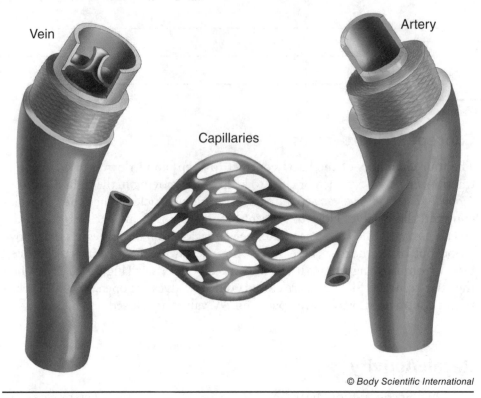

Vein   Artery   Capillaries

© Body Scientific International

Figure 10.22 Arteries, capillaries, and veins carry blood throughout the body.

Recall Activity

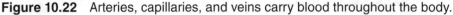

1. _____ carry blood away from the heart toward the rest of the body.

2. Veins carry blood from the _____ back to the _____.

3. _____ are small blood vessels with thin walls that allow the exchange of nutrients and gases.

Concept 5: Pulmonary Circulation

Two types of circulation occur in the cardiovascular system: pulmonary circulation and systemic circulation (**Figure 10.23**). *Pulmonary circulation* involves the heart and lungs. In pulmonary circulation, blood pumped from the right ventricle goes to the lungs. In the lungs, carbon dioxide is unloaded from the blood into the air in the lungs, and oxygen from the air is loaded into the blood. The blood, which now contains oxygen, leaves the lungs and travels to the left side of the heart. When oxygen-rich blood leaves the left side of the heart, systemic circulation begins.

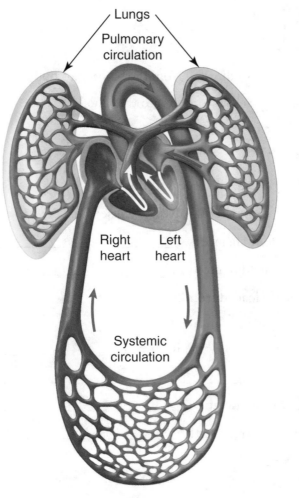

Lungs

Pulmonary circulation

Right heart

Left heart

Systemic circulation

Organs and tissues of the body

© Body Scientific International

Figure 10.23 Pulmonary circulation involves the heart and lungs. Systemic circulation involves the heart and the rest of the body.

Recall Activity

1. Pulmonary circulation involves the _____ and _____.

2. In the lungs, _____ is unloaded from the blood into the air in the lungs, and _____ from the air is loaded into the blood.

Concept 6: Systemic Circulation

Systemic circulation involves the heart and the rest of the body (Figure 10.23). In systemic circulation, the left side of the heart pumps blood to the organs and tissues of the body. In the body, oxygen is unloaded from the blood into body cells, and carbon dioxide produced by cells is loaded into the blood. The blood then carries carbon dioxide back to the right side of the heart.

systemic circulation the flow of blood from the heart to the rest of the body and back to the heart

Recall Activity

1. What does systemic circulation involve? _____

2. In the body, _____ is unloaded from the blood into body cells, and
   _____ produced by cells is loaded into the blood.

Section 10.7 Reinforcement

Answer the following questions using what you learned in this section.

1. When the _____ contract, SL valves are closed, and AV valves are open.

2. *True or False.* The heart is divided into four chambers. _____

3. In the heart, blood flows from the right atrium into the right _____.

4. During pulmonary circulation, oxygen is loaded from the _____ into the
   _____.

5. Unscramble the letters: nectliver. Define the word that is formed. _____
   _____

6. Why do heart valves open or close during contraction? _____

7. In the heart, blood flows from the right ventricle to the _____.

8. Which of the following words are misspelled?
   A. atrium   C. semilumar
   B. ventricals   D. atrioventricular

9. When the ventricles contract, are AV valves open or closed? _____

10. Identify two functions of the cardiovascular system. _____
    _____

11. When _____ contract, SL valves are open, and AV valves are closed.

12. *True or False.* Arteries carry blood from the body back to the heart. _____

13. Blood flows from the lungs to the _____ side of the heart.

14. Which side of the heart pumps blood from the heart to the rest of the body? _____

15. _____ are small blood vessels with thin walls that allow the exchange of
    nutrients and gases.

16. *True or False.* Systemic circulation involves the heart and the lungs. _____

17. Blood flows from the left atrium to the left _____.

18. *True or False.* Blood pumped from the left ventricle goes to the rest of the body. _____

19. Explain the difference between arteries and veins. _____
    _____

20. Blood flows from the left ventricle to the _____.

Comprehensive Review (Chapters 1–10)

Answer the following questions using what you have learned so far in this book.

21. A *trans* fat is made by adding _____ atoms to an unsaturated fat.

22. List the three arrangements of epithelial cells. _____

23. *True or False.* Interstitial fluid is the liquid inside a cell. _____

24. Which type of endocytosis is also known as *cell drinking*? _____

25. Identify the suffix that means "cell." _____

26. A scientific law is a general statement of _____.

27. If a circle is divided into 16 parts, and three parts are blue, what fraction of the circle is blue? _____

28. In which region of the trunk is the chest found? _____

29. Intrapulmonary pressure refers to pressure _____ the lungs.

30. *True or False.* You can only do one task well at a time. _____

Section 10.8   The Lymphatic System

The lymphatic system, like the cardiovascular system, circulates fluid throughout the body. This body system plays important roles in returning fluid to the cardiovascular system and defending the body against infection. In this section, you will learn about the structures and functions of the lymphatic system.

The terms below are some of those that will be introduced in Section 10.8. To become familiar with these terms, reproduce each word on the line beside it. Pronounce each term as you write it. You will learn the definitions of these words as you complete this section.

1. lymphatic system _____   4. spleen _____

   _____   5. thymus _____

2. lymph _____   6. lymphocyte _____

3. lymph node _____

Concept 1: Functions of the Lymphatic System

The *lymphatic system* includes lymphatic vessels, a fluid known as *lymph*, and lymphatic organs (spleen, thymus, and lymph nodes). The lymphatic system fulfills two important functions in the body:

- returns fluid leaked from capillaries back to the cardiovascular system
- defends the body against disease

The organs of the lymphatic system work together to perform these functions and coordinate with other body systems to protect the body.

lymphatic system a body system consisting of lymphatic vessels, lymph, and lymphatic organs; returns blood plasma to the cardiovascular system and defends the body against disease

Recall Activity

1. Name the components of the lymphatic system. _____

   _____

2. What two functions does the lymphatic system fulfill? _____

   _____

Concept 2: Lymph

lymph a fluid circulated through the lymphatic system that contains blood plasma and white blood cells

The lymphatic system circulates a fluid known as *lymph*. Lymph contains blood plasma leaked from the cardiovascular system's capillaries. It also contains white blood cells, which play a role in immunity. One function of the lymphatic system is returning the blood plasma leaked from capillaries back to the cardiovascular system (**Figure 10.24**). As lymph collects blood plasma, it travels through *lymphatic vessels*, which become larger and larger until they eventually connect to the cardiovascular system near the heart.

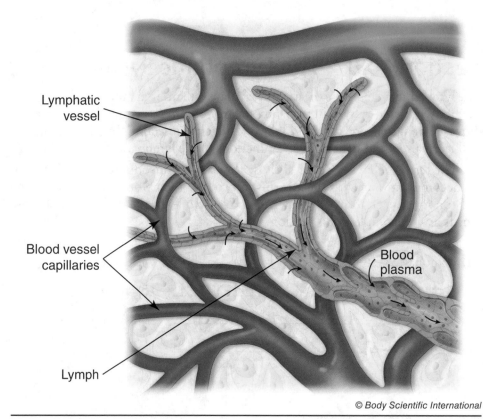

Lymphatic vessel

Blood vessel capillaries

Blood plasma

Lymph

© Body Scientific International

Figure 10.24 Lymph is composed of blood plasma leaked from capillaries.

Recall Activity

1. The lymphatic system circulates a fluid known as _____.

2. Lymph contains blood plasma leaked from the cardiovascular system's _____.

Concept 3: Lymph Nodes

As it travels through the lymphatic system and collects blood plasma, lymph may also collect harmful agents, such as bacteria or viruses. Lymph passes through several *lymph nodes* as it travels through the body (**Figure 10.25**). Each lymph node inspects lymph for harmful agents to destroy. This is why, if you have a sore throat, the lymph nodes in your neck may be swollen. Your lymph nodes are working hard to eliminate harmful agents.

lymph node a lymphatic organ that inspects lymph for harmful agents to destroy

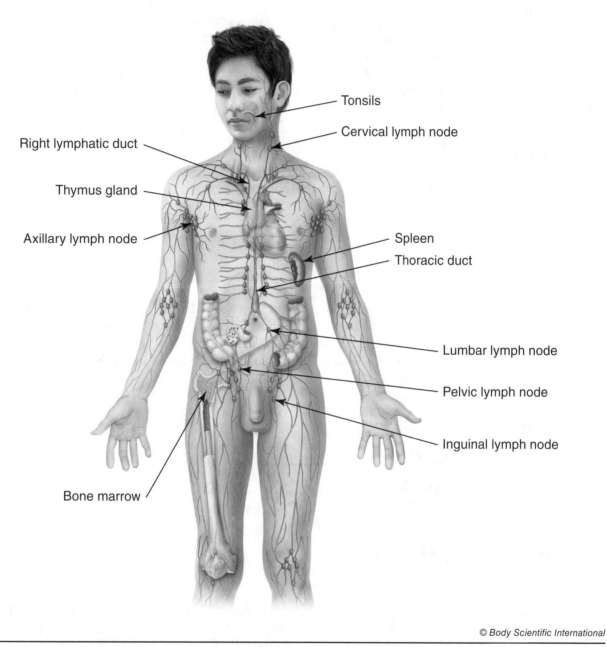

© Body Scientific International

Figure 10.25 Lymph nodes throughout the body destroy harmful agents.

Recall Activity

1. Lymph passes through several _____ as it travels through the body.

2. Each lymph node inspects lymph for harmful agents to _____.

spleen a lymphatic organ located in the abdominal cavity that helps control the amount of blood in the body, inspects lymph for harmful agents, and triggers the immune response

thymus a lymphatic organ located in the chest that houses white blood cells as they mature and signals bone marrow to produce white blood cells

Concept 4: Spleen and Thymus

The spleen and thymus are two important lymphatic organs. The *spleen* is located in the abdominal cavity and helps control the amount of blood in the body. This organ also inspects lymph for harmful agents and triggers the immune response. The *thymus* is located in the chest and houses white blood cells as they mature (Figure 10.25). It also signals the bone marrow to produce white blood cells.

Recall Activity

1. Which lymphatic organ triggers the immune response? _____

2. The _____ houses white blood cells as they mature.

Concept 5: Lymphocytes

lymphocyte a distinctive white blood cell of the lymphatic system; defends the body against infection

The lymphatic system's organs are made of distinctive cells known as *lymphocytes*. Lymphocytes are a type of white blood cell and play an active role in immunity. Like all white and red blood cells, they are produced in the bone marrow. Many lymphocytes circulate in the blood to help defend the body against infection.

Recall Activity

1. Lymphocytes are a type of _____ blood cell.

2. Where are lymphocytes produced? _____

Section 10.8 Reinforcement

Answer the following questions using what you learned in this section.

1. Lymph contains blood _____ leaked from the cardiovascular system's capillaries.

2. *True or False.* The lymphatic system returns lost blood plasma to the cardiovascular system. _____

3. As it travels through the lymphatic system and collects blood plasma, _____ also collects harmful agents, such as bacteria or viruses.

4. Unscramble the letters: plymh. Define the word that is formed. _____

_____

5. *True or False.* Lymphocytes are a type of red blood cell. _____

6. What are the two functions of the lymphatic system?_____

_____

7. Lymph travels through lymphatic vessels, which connect to the cardiovascular system near the

_____.

8. Which lymphatic organ helps control the amount of blood in the body? _____

9. Lymph nodes inspect _____ for harmful agents to destroy.

10. Write the letters backward: sumyht. Define the word that is formed. _____

_____

11. The lymphatic system's organs are made of distinctive cells known as _____.

12. *True or False.* Lymph contains white blood cells. _____

13. Where is the spleen located?_____

14. Why do lymph nodes become swollen when you have a sore throat? _____

_____

15. *True or False.* Many lymphocytes circulate in the blood. _____

16. Which of the following lymphatic organs triggers the immune response?
    A. thymus   C. lymphatic vessel
    B. spleen   D. lymph node

17. What fluid does the lymphatic system circulate?_____

18. *True or False.* The lymphatic system does not connect to the cardiovascular system. _____

Comprehensive Review (Chapters 1–10)

Answer the following questions using what you have learned so far in this book.

19. *True or False.* Mitosis is a type of cell division that produces haploid cells. _____

20. In the hierarchy of facts, scientific laws, and scientific theories, which ranks highest?

_____

21. Which types of muscle tissue are involuntary?_____

22. How you _____ a science class or subject will, to a great degree, determine
    your success or failure.

23. Convert 12/50 into a percentage. _____

24. If there are more H^+ than OH^- ions in a liquid, the liquid is a(n) _____.

25. Microvilli increase the surface area of a cell to allow for more _____.

26. *True or False.* Anatomy is the study of function. _____

27. _____ circulation involves the heart and lungs.

28. Does removing hydrogen ions (H^+) from the blood raise or lower blood pH? _____

Section 10.9   The Digestive System

The digestive system is responsible for the food you eat becoming energy for your body. The organs of the digestive system ingest food, break food down, and expel solid waste from the body. In this section, you will learn about the structures and functions of the digestive system.

The terms below are some of those that will be introduced in Section 10.9. To become familiar with these terms, reproduce each word on the line beside it. Pronounce each term as you write it. You will learn the definitions of these words as you complete this section.

1. digestive system _____

   _____

2. alimentary canal _____

   _____

3. peristalsis _____

4. ingestion _____

5. mechanical digestion _____

   _____

6. chemical digestion _____

   _____

7. absorption _____

8. defecation _____

Concept 1: Functions of the Digestive System

digestive system a body system consisting of the alimentary canal and several support organs; intakes and breaks down food, absorbs nutrients, and removes solid waste

The *digestive system* consists of organs that aid in ingestion, digestion, absorption, and defecation. It includes organs of the alimentary canal and several support organs. The major functions of the digestive system include the following:

- intakes food into the body
- breaks down food (mechanically and chemically) into nutrients
- absorbs nutrients into the bloodstream
- removes solid waste from the body through defecation

The organs of the digestive system coordinate to fulfill these functions.

Recall Activity

1. The digestive system consists of organs that aid in _____,

   _____, _____, and _____.

2. Name two functions of the digestive system. _____

   _____

Concept 2: Path of Food

The digestive system includes the alimentary canal and several support organs. The *alimentary canal* is the food path through the body; it includes the mouth, pharynx, esophagus, stomach, small intestine, colon, rectum, and anus. *Support organs* (for example, the liver and pancreas) aid in digestion, but food does not travel through them (**Figure 10.26**). Food does not move through the alimentary canal by gravity. Rather, a series of smooth muscle contractions known as *peristalsis* move food through the alimentary canal. Food moves when the muscles of the alimentary canal contract and push food along.

alimentary canal the food path through the body; includes the mouth, pharynx, esophagus, stomach, small intestine, colon, rectum, and anus

peristalsis smooth muscle contractions that move a substance through the body

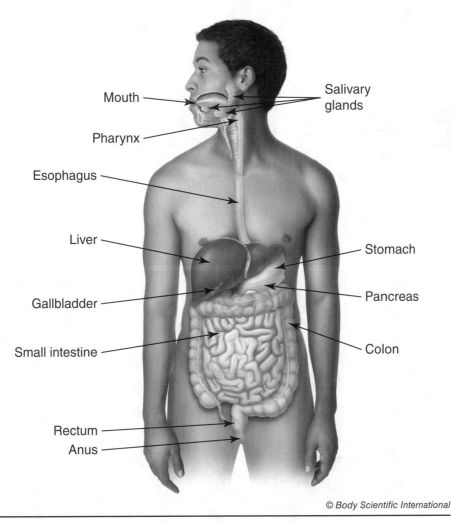

© Body Scientific International

Figure 10.26 Food travels through the alimentary canal.

Recall Activity

1. The digestive system includes the _____ canal and several support organs.

2. List the organs of the alimentary canal. _____

   _____

3. A series of smooth muscle contractions known as _____ move food through the alimentary canal.

Concept 3: Ingestion and Digestion

ingestion the process of taking food into the body

The first function of the digestive system is ingestion. In *ingestion*, food is brought into the body. Ingestion happens in the mouth. Once the teeth and tongue begin to break down food, digestion begins. *Digestion* means to break down food (solid or liquid) into macromolecules that can be absorbed by the blood. Think of the last meal you ate. Your body cannot benefit from that food until that food is broken into pieces that are too small to be seen with a microscope. There are two types of digestion: mechanical digestion and chemical digestion. You can follow the steps of ingestion, digestion, absorption, and defecation in **Figure 10.27**.

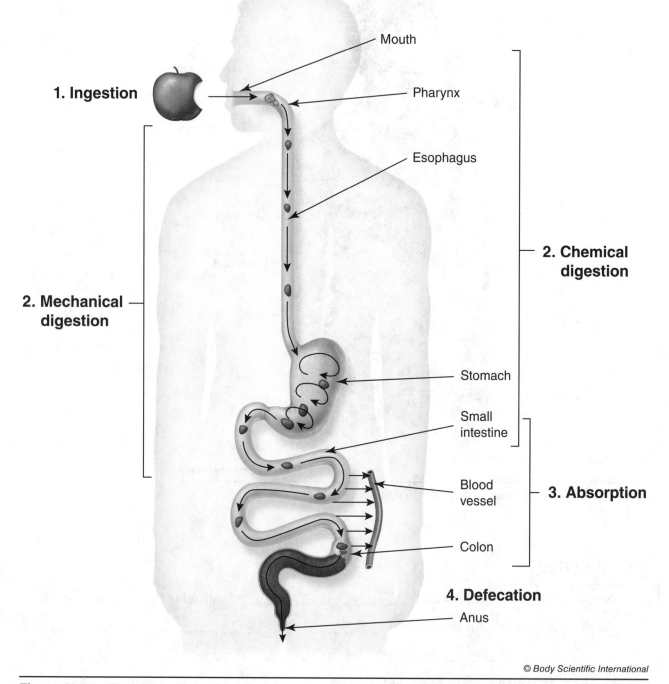

© *Body Scientific International*

Figure 10.27 The steps of ingestion, digestion, absorption, and defecation are illustrated here.

Recall Activity

1. Where does ingestion happen? _____

2. Digestion means to break down food into _____ that can be absorbed by the blood.

3. List the two types of digestion. _____

Concept 4: Mechanical Digestion

Mechanical digestion refers to physically tearing large pieces of food into smaller pieces (which are necessary for chemical digestion). You could say that mechanical digestion begins when you cut your food into bite-size pieces. Your teeth take chunks of food and grind them into smaller pieces for swallowing. The churning or mixing of food in the stomach and *segmentation* (the dividing and mixing of food) in the small intestine are other types of mechanical digestion.

mechanical digestion the process of physically tearing large pieces of food into smaller pieces

Recall Activity

1. _____ digestion tears large pieces of food into smaller pieces.

2. Your _____ take chunks of food and grind them into smaller pieces for swallowing.

3. Where does segmentation take place? _____

Concept 5: Chemical Digestion

In *chemical digestion*, enzymes and other chemicals break down food into macromolecules. Chemical digestion begins in the mouth with saliva and continues in the stomach with gastric juice. It is completed in the small intestine using chemicals from the small intestine brush border, pancreas, and gallbladder.

chemical digestion the process of breaking down food into macromolecules using enzymes and chemicals

Recall Activity

1. _____ digestion uses enzymes and other chemicals to break down food into macromolecules.

2. Chemical digestion begins in the mouth with _____.

3. Gastric juice continues chemical digestion in the _____.

Concept 6: Absorption

The goal of digestion is to deliver macromolecules to the blood. *Absorption* means to take macromolecules out of digested food and put them into the blood. Most absorption takes place in the small intestine, where microvilli

absorption the process of taking macromolecules out of digested food and putting them into the blood

increase cells' surface areas for absorption. Once absorbed by the blood, macromolecules travel to the liver. The liver then puts the macromolecules into general blood circulation for distribution throughout the body.

Recall Activity

1. The goal of _____ is to deliver macromolecules to the blood.

2. _____ means to take macromolecules out of digested food and put them into the blood.

3. Most absorption takes place in the _____.

Concept 7: Defecation

defecation the process of removing solid waste (feces) from the body

Not all of the substances that are ingested can be absorbed. Substances that cannot be absorbed exit the alimentary canal as *feces* through *defecation*. For example, humans do not have the enzymes needed to break down cellulose. When you eat vegetables, your body cannot break down the cellulose portion of the plant cell (called *fiber*). Even though it cannot be absorbed, fiber is beneficial; it helps move feces through the colon.

Recall Activity

1. Not all of the substances that are ingested can be _____.

2. Humans do not have the enzymes needed to break down _____.

Section 10.9 Reinforcement

Answer the following questions using what you learned in this section.

1. Most _____ takes place in the small intestine, where microvilli increase cells' surface areas.

2. Which body system includes the alimentary canal? _____

3. *True or False.* Food moves through the alimentary canal by gravity. _____

4. Which of the following parts of the alimentary canal is most superior?
   A. small intestine   C. esophagus
   B. stomach   D. colon

5. A series of smooth muscle contractions known as _____ move food through the alimentary canal.

6. List three functions of the digestive system. _____

_____

7. Substances that cannot be absorbed exit the alimentary canal as _____.

8. The digestive system includes the _____ canal and several support organs.

9. Which of the following organs is *not* part of the alimentary canal?
   A. small intestine
   B. pancreas
   C. esophagus
   D. anus

10. Unscramble the letters: dogistine. Define the word that is formed. _____
    _____

11. *True or False.* The digestive chemical in the stomach is gastric juice. _____

12. Which type of digestion involves physically tearing large pieces of food into smaller pieces?
    _____

13. *True or False.* All substances that are ingested can be absorbed. _____

14. Which of the following words are misspelled?
    A. peristalsis
    B. alimentry
    C. digestion
    D. absorbtion

15. *True or False.* Segmentation is a type of chemical digestion. _____

16. Unscramble the letters: boorpastin. Define the word that is formed. _____
    _____

17. Which type of digestion involves breaking down food into macromolecules using enzymes?
    _____

18. *True or False.* Chemical digestion begins in the mouth. _____

19. Once absorbed by the blood, macromolecules travel to the _____.

Comprehensive Review (Chapters 1–10)

Answer the following questions using what you have learned so far in this book.

20. The phospholipid bilayer is selectively _____, meaning that only certain materials can pass through it.

21. The kidney's tubules are composed of simple _____ epithelium.

22. *True or False.* The most basic skill in learning science is understanding the terminology. _____

23. The combining form *ren/o* means "_____."

24. Round 6.53 to the nearest whole number. _____

25. Lymph contains blood plasma leaked from the cardiovascular system's _____.

26. In proteins, amino acids are held together by _____ bonds.

27. Cells in the human body are _____, meaning that different types of cells have unique structures, components, or shapes.

28. *True or False.* The kidneys are medial to the spine. _____

29. A scientific _____ tells you why a result occurs.

Section 10.10   The Urinary System

The urinary system performs the important task of filtering blood and removing waste from the body. The kidneys, urinary bladder, and urethra are some of the organs that make up the urinary system. In this section, you will learn about the urinary system, its functions, and its structures in males and females.

The terms below are some of those that will be introduced in Section 10.10. To become familiar with these terms, reproduce each word on the line beside it. Pronounce each term as you write it. You will learn the definitions of these words as you complete this section.

1. urinary system _____

2. kidney _____

3. nephron _____

4. filtration _____

5. reabsorption _____

6. secretion _____

7. ureter _____

8. urinary bladder _____

9. urethra _____

Concept 1: Functions of the Urinary System

urinary system a body system consisting of the kidneys, ureters, urinary bladder, and urethra; filters blood, removes and stores waste, produces hormones, and maintains homeostasis

The *urinary system* includes the kidneys, ureters, urinary bladder, and urethra (**Figure 10.28**). All of these organs work together to perform the following functions:

- filters waste products out of blood
- removes and stores waste from the body
- produces hormones
- maintains homeostasis of pH and water levels

The organs of the urinary system coordinate to fulfill these functions in both males and females.

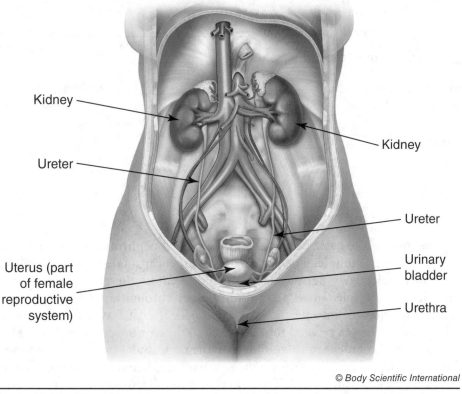

Kidney

Kidney

Ureter

Ureter

Uterus (part of female reproductive system)

Urinary bladder

Urethra

© Body Scientific International

Figure 10.28 The kidneys, ureters, urinary bladder, and urethra make up the urinary system.

Recall Activity

1. What organs are included in the urinary system? _____

2. List two functions of the urinary system. _____

_____

Concept 2: Kidneys

The first function of the urinary system involves filtering waste out of the blood. This process happens in the *kidneys*, which are located in the abdominal cavity. Blood flows into the kidneys, and blood and urine flow out of the kidneys. The kidneys regulate which molecules and ions remain in the blood and which molecules and ions become urine. The basic unit of the kidney is the *nephron*, which will be discussed in the next concept.

kidney an organ located in the abdominal cavity that filters waste out of the blood

Recall Activity

1. _____ flows into the kidneys, and _____ and

   _____ flow out of the kidneys.

2. The kidneys regulate which molecules and ions _____ in the blood and

   which molecules and ions become _____.

3. The basic unit of the kidney is the _____.

Concept 3: Nephrons

nephron the basic unit of the kidney; contains a glomerulus and renal tubule

The *nephron* is the basic unit of the kidney. Each nephron consists of a glomerulus and renal tubule. The *glomerulus* is an encapsulated ball of capillaries with thin, selectively permeable walls. Blood enters the glomerulus through an afferent arteriole (small artery) and leaves through an efferent arteriole, which branches off into *peritubular capillaries* after it leaves the glomerulus. The *renal tubule* is a twisted tube attached to the capsule containing the glomerulus. Renal tubules are surrounded by the peritubular capillaries and merge into *collecting ducts*. Nephrons remove waste, regulate the amount of water in the blood, and maintain pH. They do this through three processes: filtration, reabsorption, and secretion.

Recall Activity

1. The nephron's _____ is an encapsulated ball of capillaries with thin, selectively permeable walls.

2. The _____ is a twisted tube attached to the capsule containing the glomerulus.

3. What three processes do nephrons use to remove waste, regulate water levels in the blood, and

   maintain pH? _____

Concept 4: Filtration

filtration the process of removing molecules smaller than a protein from the blood; occurs in the glomerulus

The first process of nephron function is filtration. In *filtration*, products are removed from the blood. Blood enters the glomerulus through an afferent arteriole. In the glomerulus, any molecule smaller than a protein is pushed out of the blood into the glomerular capsule (**Figure 10.29**). The concentrations of molecules in the blood are not a factor in filtration; any molecule that is small enough to fit through the pores of the glomerulus is removed from the blood. Molecules pushed out of the blood are known as *filtrate*. After filtration, filtrate moves into the renal tubule.

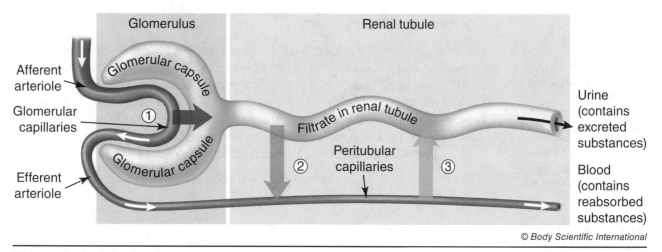

Figure 10.29 Filtration (1) happens in the glomerulus. Once filtrate moves into the renal tubule, reabsorption (2) and secretion (3) begin.

Recall Activity

1. In _____, products are removed from the blood.

2. In the glomerulus, any molecule smaller than a(n) _____ is pushed out of the blood into the glomerular capsule.

3. Molecules pushed out of the blood are known as _____.

Concept 5: Reabsorption and Secretion

After filtration, filtrate flows through the renal tubule, and blood flows through the nearby peritubular capillaries. Because the renal tubule and peritubular capillaries are close together, molecules can move between them by diffusion or active transport. When molecules move from the filtrate back into the blood, this is called *reabsorption*. Many molecules pushed out of the blood during filtration are needed in the blood (for example, glucose and amino acids); these molecules are put back into the blood during reabsorption.

When molecules move from the blood into filtrate, this is called *secretion*. Molecules that are secreted, such as urea and aspirin, are not needed in the blood. Once filtrate molecules have passed through the area of reabsorption, they become part of *urine*.

reabsorption the process of moving molecules from filtrate back into the blood; occurs in the renal tubule

secretion the process of moving molecules from the blood into filtrate after filtration has occurred; occurs in the renal tubule

Recall Activity

1. When molecules move from the filtrate back into the blood, this is called _____.

2. When molecules move from the blood into filtrate, this is called _____.

Concept 6: Urinary Tract

ureter a tubelike organ that transports urine toward the urinary bladder

urinary bladder a hollow, muscular organ that stores urine for a time before moving urine into the urethra

urethra a tubelike organ that transports urine out of the body

Once filtrate leaves the kidneys, it becomes urine and enters the *urinary tract* (ureters, urinary bladder, and urethra). From the kidneys, urine flows into two *ureters*, which transport urine through *peristalsis* (smooth muscle contractions) toward the urinary bladder. The *urinary bladder* stores urine for a time before moving urine into the urethra (Figure 10.28). The *urethra* then transports urine out of the body. The female urethra expels urine between the clitoris and the vagina. The male urethra expels urine through the penis.

Recall Activity

1. What organs make up the urinary tract? _____

2. Ureters transport urine toward the urinary bladder through _____.

Section 10.10 Reinforcement

Answer the following questions using what you learned in this section.

1. Nephrons remove waste, regulate the amount of water in the blood, and maintain

   _____.

2. *True or False.* The nephron is the basic unit of the kidney. _____

3. Blood enters the glomerulus through a(n) _____ arteriole and leaves through

   a(n) _____ arteriole.

4. Unscramble the letters: henpron. Define the word that is formed. _____

   _____

5. During _____, any molecule smaller than a protein is pushed out of the

   _____ into the glomerular capsule.

6. *True or False.* The concentrations of molecules in the blood are a factor in filtration. _____

7. Molecules pushed out of the blood during filtration are known as _____.

8. Which process moves molecules from the blood into the filtrate after filtration? _____

9. List one function of the urinary system. _____

   _____

10. After filtration, filtrate flows through the _____, and blood flows through

    the nearby peritubular _____.

11. Which organ transports urine out of the body? _____

12. Moving molecules from the _____ back into the _____ is called reabsorption.

13. Which organ stores urine before moving it into the urethra? _____

14. Does the renal tubule contain blood or filtrate? _____

15. The kidneys regulate which molecules and ions remain in the blood and which molecules and ions become _____.

16. Unscramble the letters: ecistrone. Define the word that is formed. _____
_____

17. Do peritubular capillaries contain blood or filtrate? _____

18. Which of the following words are misspelled?
    A. glomerulus   C. filtation
    B. kidney   D. reabsorbtion

19. *True or False.* Secretion takes place in the glomerulus. _____

20. Which organ transports urine from the kidneys to the urinary bladder? _____

21. During filtration, any molecule smaller than a(n) _____ is pushed out of the blood into the glomerular capsule.

Comprehensive Review (Chapters 1–10)

Answer the following questions using what you have learned so far in this book.

22. Which hormone causes the breakdown of glycogen in the liver? _____

23. A hypothesis is a prediction about the _____ of an experiment.

24. *True or False.* The metric unit of temperature is the degree Fahrenheit. _____

25. _____ are used as evidence to support scientific explanations.

26. What color is a leukocyte? _____

27. List the three basic parts of a cell. _____

28. Which cells are haploid in males and females? _____

29. At room temperature, which type of fat is solid? _____

30. Which type of digestion involves breaking down food into macromolecules using enzymes?
_____

31. *True or False.* Osteoblasts break down the bone matrix. _____

Section 10.11   The Reproductive Systems

The female and male reproductive systems are responsible for continuing the human species and reproducing life. The female and male reproductive systems perform different functions and contain different structures. In this section, you will learn about the reproductive systems of both females and males.

The terms below are some of those that will be introduced in Section 10.11. To become familiar with these terms, reproduce each word on the line beside it. Pronounce each term as you write it. You will learn the definitions of these words as you complete this section.

1. reproductive system _____

_____

2. ovary _____

3. fallopian tube _____

4. uterus _____

5. vagina _____

6. mammary gland _____

_____

7. testis _____

8. epididymis _____

9. ductus deferens _____

10. penis _____

Concept 1: Functions of the Reproductive Systems

reproductive system a body system involved in reproducing life; in females, consists of the ovaries, fallopian tubes, uterus, vagina, external genitalia, and mammary glands; in males, consists of the testes and scrotum, epididymis, ductus deferens, accessory organs, and penis

The *reproductive systems* are the body systems involved in reproducing life. The female and male reproductive systems are distinct from each other. The major functions of these body systems include the following:

- produces gametes (female and male)
- facilitates conception (female and male)
- protects and nourishes the developing fetus (female)
- expels a baby from the body (female)

The structures of the female and male reproductive systems work together to perform these functions.

Recall Activity

1. The reproductive systems are the body systems involved in reproducing _____.

2. List three functions of the reproductive systems. _____

_____

Concept 2: Ovaries

The *female reproductive system* consists of the ovaries, fallopian tubes, uterus, vagina, external genitalia, and mammary glands. *Egg cells* (female gametes) are released from the *ovaries*, which are located on either side of the uterus (**Figure 10.30**). A female is born with all of the egg cells she will ever have; these egg cells are in a resting stage between the two stages of meiosis. At the beginning of each menstrual cycle, an egg cell is selected to continue development with the release of FSH (follicle-stimulating hormone) from the anterior pituitary gland. When development is complete and the egg cell is ready to be released, the anterior pituitary gland releases LH (luteinizing hormone). Luteinizing hormone causes *ovulation*, the release of a mature egg cell from the ovary. FSH and LH also play a role in *menstruation*, which is the shedding of the innermost layer of the uterus each month.

ovary an organ in females that stores and releases egg cells; also secretes estrogen and progesterone

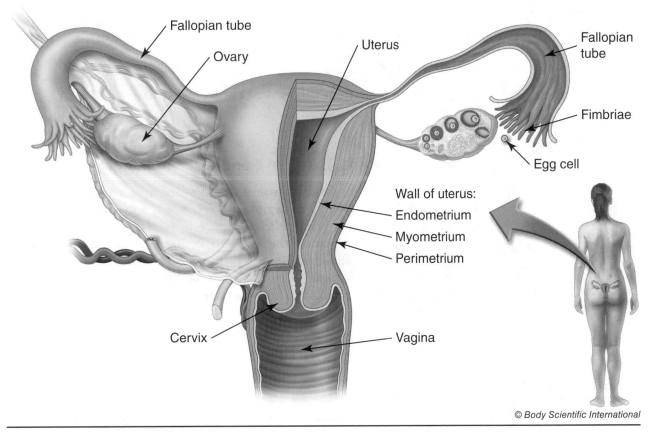

© Body Scientific International

Figure 10.30 The ovaries lie on either side of the uterus.

Recall Activity

1. Egg cells are released from the _____.

2. FSH and LH play a role in _____, which is the shedding of the innermost layer of the uterus each month.

Concept 3: Fallopian Tubes and Uterus

fallopian tube a hollow organ in females extending out from the uterus that receives the egg cell from an ovary

uterus a hollow, muscular organ in females that houses a developing fetus

Once an egg cell is released from an ovary, it travels through a *fallopian tube* toward the uterus. The *uterus* is a hollow, muscular organ that houses a developing fetus. If an egg cell is fertilized, it will implant in the *endometrium* (inner layer) of the uterus. The hormones *estrogen* and *progesterone*, which are secreted by the ovary after ovulation, cause the uterus to build up the endometrium. If the egg cell is not fertilized, the ovary will stop secreting estrogen and progesterone, and the endometrium will be shed during menstruation and lost outside the body.

Recall Activity

1. Once an egg cell is released from an ovary, it travels through a(n) _____ toward the uterus.

2. If an egg cell is fertilized, it will implant in the _____ of the uterus.

3. If an ovary stops secreting the hormones _____ and

   _____, the endometrium will be shed during menstruation.

Concept 4: Vagina, External Genitalia, and Mammary Glands

vagina a hollow organ in females that serves as the birth canal and receives sperm during intercourse

mammary gland a gland in females that produces milk after childbirth

During menstruation, material from the endometrium travels outside of the body through the *vagina*. The vagina also receives sperm during intercourse and serves as the birth canal when a female delivers a baby. The inside of the vagina is acidic to protect the female from bacteria. Outside the vagina, external genitalia include the *labia* (which protect the vaginal opening) and *clitoris* (female erectile tissue). The *mammary glands*, which produce milk after childbirth, are also part of the female reproductive system since they sustain a baby's new life.

Recall Activity

1. The inside of the vagina is _____ to protect the female from bacteria.

2. Which structure produces milk after childbirth? _____

Concept 5: Testes

testis an organ in males that produces sperm; hangs in the scrotum outside the body

epididymis an organ in males that stores sperm until ejaculation

The *male reproductive system* consists of the testes and scrotum, epididymis, ductus deferens, accessory organs, and penis. *Sperm* (male gametes) are produced in the *testes* through a process known as *spermatogenesis*. Because spermatogenesis cannot take place at body temperature, the testes are held outside the body in a skin sac called the *scrotum*. Once sperm complete their development, they are stored in the *epididymis*, which lies on the dorsal surface of a testis (**Figure 10.31**).

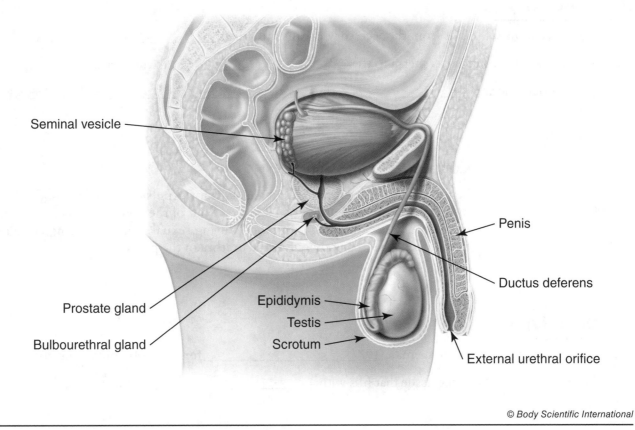

Seminal vesicle

Prostate gland

Bulbourethral gland

Epididymis

Testis

Scrotum

Penis

Ductus deferens

External urethral orifice

© Body Scientific International

Figure 10.31 Spermatogenesis begins in the testes.

Recall Activity

1. Spermatogenesis takes place in the _____.

2. Once sperm complete their development, they are stored in the _____.

Concept 6: Ductus Deferens and Accessory Organs

Sperm are stored in the epididymis until *ejaculation*, the process by which sperm exit the body. During ejaculation, sperm move out of the epididymis into the *ductus deferens*, which conveys sperm to the urethra in the penis. Along the ductus deferens are three accessory organs: the seminal vesicles, the prostate gland, and the bulbourethral gland. The *seminal vesicles* release *fructose*, a sugary substance. The *prostate gland* and the *bulbourethral gland* release alkaline fluids that protect sperm from the acidic male urethra and female vagina. Together, the sperm and fluids from the accessory organs are called *semen*.

ductus deferens an organ in males that conveys sperm from the epididymis to the urethra in the penis during ejaculation

Recall Activity

1. Together, sperm and fluids from the accessory organs are called _____.

2. The ductus deferens conveys sperm to the _____ in the penis.

3. What is ejaculation? _____

Concept 7: Penis

penis a structure in males that contains the urethra and is made of erectile tissue

Semen enters the urethra in the male *penis* for expulsion out of the body. The male urethra carries both semen and urine out of the body. The penis is made of erectile tissue that fills with blood during sexual arousal. During ejaculation, semen exits the body out of the urethra in the penis.

Recall Activity

1. Semen enters the urethra in the male _____ for expulsion out of the body.

2. The penis is made of erectile tissue that fills with _____ during sexual arousal.

Section 10.11 Reinforcement

Answer the following questions using what you learned in this section.

1. What is menstruation? _____

2. The prostate gland and the bulbourethral gland release _____ fluids that protect sperm from the _____ male urethra and female vagina.

3. List the two hormones that cause the uterus to build up the endometrium. _____

_____

4. *True or False.* FSH and LH play roles in ovulation. _____

5. The process by which sperm exit the body is called _____.

6. Once an egg cell is released from a(n) _____, it travels through a fallopian tube toward the _____.

7. What is the function of the mammary glands? _____

8. Once sperm complete their development, they are stored in the _____.

9. Unscramble the letters: simedipidy. Define the word that is formed. _____

_____

10. *True or False.* Spermatogenesis occurs at body temperature. _____

11. The testes are held outside the body in a skin sac called the _____.

12. Name the components of semen. _____

13. *True or False.* Sperm complete their development in the ductus deferens. _____

14. Unscramble the letters: ulovnatio. Define the word that is formed. _____

_____

15. If an egg cell is fertilized, it will implant in the _____ of the uterus.

16. List two functions of the reproductive systems. _____

_____

17. Which structure serves as the birth canal when a baby is delivered? _____

18. List the structures of the female reproductive system. _____

_____

19. *True or False.* A female is born with all of the egg cells she will ever have. _____

20. List the structures of the male reproductive system. _____

_____

21. Which of the following is *not* part of the male reproductive system?
    A. seminal vesicles   C. testes
    B. ovaries   D. epididymis

Comprehensive Review (Chapters 1–10)

Answer the following questions using what you have learned so far in this book.

22. What type of tissue has direct access to a blood supply? _____

23. In anatomy and physiology, body locations are described in reference to _____.

24. A(n) _____ is a physically observable fact or event.

25. Disassemble and define the word *physiology.* _____

26. Which organs are part of the urinary tract?_____

27. A scientific theory is the best _____ today for why a phenomenon occurs.

28. Which subatomic particle is involved in bonding? _____

29. *True or False.* Morphology is the study of structure or form. _____

30. Which of the following processes require energy?
    A. diffusion   C. exocytosis
    B. active transport   D. facilitated diffusion

31. To determine liquid volume, read a graduated cylinder at the _____ of the
    meniscus.

Chapter 10 Review

Answer the following questions using what you learned in this chapter.

1. In the nervous system, the CNS consists of the _____ and _____, and the PNS includes all other _____ throughout the body.

2. Which body system returns blood plasma leaked from capillaries to the cardiovascular system? _____

3. Which of the following is *not* a freely movable joint?
   A. hinge joint   C. saddle joint
   B. pivot joint   D. condyloid joint

4. What substance do sebaceous glands secrete? _____

5. List the two types of autonomic nerves. _____

6. The hormones calcitonin and PTH both target the _____, _____, and _____.

7. *True or False.* Female gametes are stored in the uterus. _____

8. Is segmentation a type of mechanical digestion or chemical digestion? _____

9. What organ regulates which molecules and ions remain in the blood and which molecules and ions become urine? _____

10. List one function of the endocrine system. _____

11. The making of sperm, known as _____, takes place in the testes.

12. *True or False.* When the ventricles contract, SL valves are open, and AV valves are closed. _____

13. When the thoracic cavity expands, the volume of the lungs _____.

14. When a skeletal muscle contracts, the _____ moves toward the origin.

15. Is the somatic nervous system made up of motor nerves or sensory nerves? _____

16. After filtration, molecules pushed out of the blood are known as _____.

17. In the lungs, which respiratory gas moves from the blood into the air? _____

18. The goal of digestion is to deliver macromolecules into the _____.

19. What organs are included in the lymphatic system? _____

20. *True or False.* Sensory and motor nerves are part of the CNS. _____

21. In internal respiration, the _____ in the blood is unloaded to body cells, and _____ is loaded from body cells into the blood.

22. _____ moves a limb along the frontal plane away from the middle of the body.

23. When the _____ contract, SL valves are closed, and AV valves are open.

24. During menstruation, material from the _____ travels outside of the body through the _____ .

25. Which of the following bones is *not* part of the axial skeleton?
   A. ribs   C. spine
   B. scapula   D. mandible

26. Which part of the brain coordinates balance and body movement?_____

27. Describe the flow of blood through the heart. _____

   _____

   _____

28. *True or False.* Lymph nodes inspect lymph for harmful agents to destroy. _____

29. List four endocrine glands. _____

30. Keratinocytes are pushed up to the apical surface of the _____ as superficial cells are shed.

Comprehensive Review (Chapters 1–10)

Using what you have learned so far in this book, match the following terms with their definitions.

_____ 31. A group of organs that work together to perform a group of functions

_____ 32. A structure that assembles amino acids into specific proteins

_____ 33. A group of different types of tissue that work together to do a job

_____ 34. The "then" part of a hypothesis

_____ 35. An area of biology that studies cells

_____ 36. A combination of many atoms held together by bonds

_____ 37. The flow of blood from the heart to the lungs and back to the heart

_____ 38. A state of relative stability

_____ 39. The values representing where a data point is placed on a graph

_____ 40. A combining form that means "function"

_____ 41. The flow of blood from the heart to the rest of the body and back to the heart

_____ 42. A combining form that means "life"

_____ 43. The average mass for an atom and all of its isotopes

A. homeostasis
B. ribosome
C. body system
D. relative atomic mass
E. macromolecule
F. coordinate pair
G. dependent variable
H. physi/o
I. cytology
J. organ
K. systemic circulation
L. pulmonary circulation
M. bi/o

Appendix A Word Parts

Many scientific words are composed of *word parts* (small segments of words). By disassembling terms into their word parts, you can better understand them. Word parts include *combining forms* (a root word plus its combining vowel), *prefixes*, and *suffixes*. For an overview of these word parts and how they combine, see Section 2.1. Following is a list of word parts introduced and used throughout this book.

Combining Forms

Combining Form	Meaning
alb/o	white
anter/o	front
appendic/o	appendix
arthr/o	joint
atri/o	atrium
axi/o	axis
bi/o	life
cardi/o	heart
cerebr/o	brain
cervic/o	neck
chlor/o	green
chondr/o	cartilage
coel/o	hollow
col/o	colon
cortic/o	outer region
cost/o	rib
crani/o	skull
cyan/o	blue
cyst/o	cyst
cyt/o	cell
delt/o	triangular
derm/o	skin
dist/o	far
dors/o	back (of body)
duct/o	to carry
enter/o	intestine

Combining Form	Meaning
erythr/o	red
faci/o	face
gastr/o	stomach
glob/o	round
hem/o	blood
hepat/o	liver
hydr/o	water
ili/o	ilium
is/o	same
ischi/o	ischium
lat/o	wide
later/o	side
leuk/o	white
lumb/o	lower back
lun/o	crescent shape
lute/o	yellow
lymph/o	lymph
medi/o	middle
melan/o	black
morph/o	form
my/o	muscle
neur/o	nerve
oste/o	bone
pector/o	chest
ped/o	foot
pelv/i	pelvis
physi/o	function
pod/o	foot
poster/o	back (of body)
proxim/o	near
pub/o	pubis
pulmon/o	lung
rect/o	straight

Combining Form	Meaning
ren/o	kidney
rubr/o	red
sacchar/o	sugar
sacr/o	sacrum
scapul/o	shoulder blade
sebace/o	sebum
serrat/o	jagged
spin/o	spine
spir/o	breathing
sten/o	narrow
strat/o	layer
system/o	system
tens/o	to stretch
thorac/o	chest
tub/o	tube
umbilic/o	navel
vascul/o	blood vessel
ventr/o	belly side (of body)
ventricul/o	ventricle

Prefixes

Prefix	Meaning
a-	not
ab-	away from
ad-	toward
af-	toward
an-	without
ana-	apart
anti-	against
bi-	two
centi-	1/100 of one unit
con-	together

Prefix	Meaning
de-	down from
di-	two
dis-	apart
ecto-	outside
ef-	away from
endo-	inside
epi-	upon
ex-	out of
hemi-	half
hetero-	different
hexa-	six
homo-	same
hyper-	above; beyond
hypo-	below
in-	into
infra-	under
inter-	between
intra-	within
kilo-	1000 units
macro-	large
mega-	large
meso-	middle
micro-	small
milli-	1/1000 of one unit
mono-	one
neo-	new
omni-	all
peri-	around
platy-	flat
poly-	many
post-	after
pre-	before
pseudo-	false

Prefix	Meaning
quadri-	four
semi-	half
sub-	below
super-	above
supra-	above
tetra-	four
tri-	three
ultra-	beyond
uni-	one

Suffixes

Suffix	Meaning
-ac	pertaining to
-al	character of
-algia	pain
-ar	pertaining to
-ary	pertaining to
-ation	process
-blast	developing cell
-ceps	heads
-clast	to break
-cyte	cell
-gen	producer
-genesis	production

Suffix	Meaning
-ia	condition
-iac	pertaining to
-ic	pertaining to
-ical	character of
-ion	process
-ior	pertaining to
-ist	specialist
-itis	inflammation
-logist	one who studies
-logy	study of
-lysis	breakdown
-oid	resembling
-oma	tumor
-osis	condition
-ous	nature of
-phage	eat
-philic	loving
-phobic	fearing
-plasm	formation
-plegia	paralysis
-stasis	stay or stop
-tic	pertaining to
-tomy	to cut
-ule	small
-um	structure

Appendix B Metric Conversions

In science, the *metric system* is used to take measurements. The metric system differs from the *English system of measurement*, which is used in the United States. Following is a guide for converting between the metric system and the English system of measurement. These operations are discussed in more detail in Section 4.9.

Length Conversions			
English to Metric		**Metric to English**	
Conversion	**Multiply by**	**Conversion**	**Multiply by**
inches to centimeters	2.54 cm/inch	centimeters to inches	0.39 inches/cm
feet to meters	0.30 m/foot	meters to feet	3.28 feet/m
yards to meters	0.91 m/yard	meters to yards	1.09 yards/m
miles to kilometers	1.61 km/miles	kilometers to miles	0.62 miles/km

Volume Conversions			
English to Metric		**Metric to English**	
Conversion	**Multiply by**	**Conversion**	**Multiply by**
gallons to liters	3.79 L/gallon	liters to gallons	0.26 gallons/L
quarts to liters	0.95 L/quart	liters to quarts	1.06 quarts/L
fluid ounces to milliliters	29.57 mL/fluid ounce	milliliters to fluid ounces	0.03 fluid ounces/mL

Mass Conversions			
English to Metric		**Metric to English**	
Conversion	**Multiply by**	**Conversion**	**Multiply by**
ounces to grams	28.35 g/ounce	grams to ounces	0.035 ounces/g
pounds to kilograms	0.45 kg/pound	kilograms to pounds	2.21 pounds/kg

Temperature Conversions			
English to Metric		**Metric to English**	
°Fahrenheit to °Celsius	$5/9 \times (F-32)$	°Celsius to °Fahrenheit	$(9/5 \times C) + 32$

The *periodic table of elements* lists atoms by atomic number. It also indicates atoms' names, symbols, and relative atomic masses. The periodic table is explained in more detail in Section 5.2.

Goodheart-Willcox Publisher

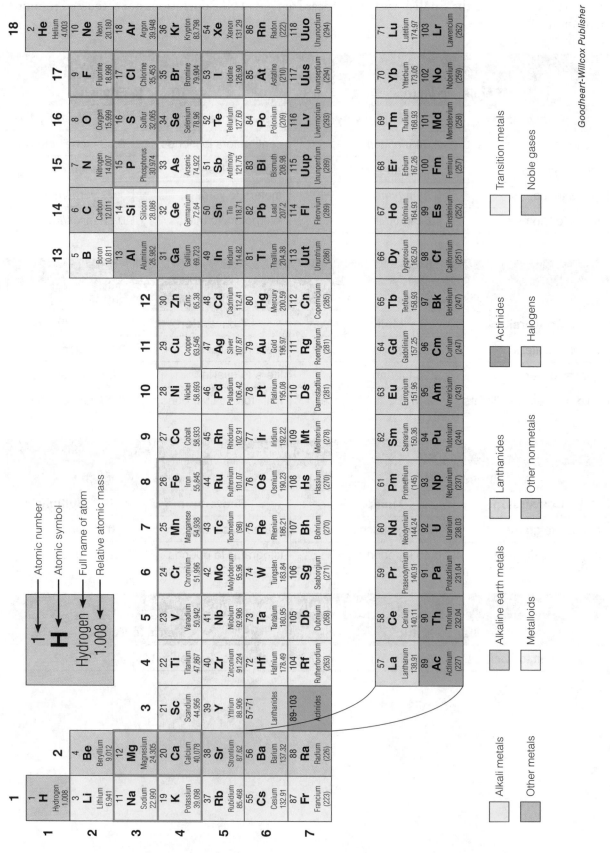

Glossary

A

a-: a prefix meaning "not."

ab-: a prefix meaning "away from."

abdominal cavity: the ventral body cavity that contains the stomach, liver, spleen, and intestines.

abdominal region: the belly area of the body.

abdominopelvic cavity: the abdominal and pelvic cavities; contains the stomach, liver, spleen, intestines, urinary bladder, and some reproductive organs.

abdominopelvic region: an area of the abdominopelvic cavity; the abdominopelvic cavity contains nine regions.

abduction: a type of directional movement along the frontal plane that moves a body part away from the middle (midsagittal plane) of the body.

absorption: the digestive process of taking macromolecules out of digested food and putting them into the blood; most absorption happens in the small intestine.

acid: a liquid that contains more H^+ ions than OH^- ions; has a pH value between 0 and 6.9.

action potential: an electrical charge that moves along the membranes of cells; causes muscle cells to shorten and nerve cells (neurons) to release neurotransmitters.

active learning: the practice of using one's hands or feet while studying material; for example, walking while studying.

active transport: the movement of atoms from areas of low concentration to areas of high concentration using a cell's solute pumps; requires energy.

ad-: a prefix meaning "toward."

adduction: a type of directional movement along the frontal plane that moves a body part toward the middle (midsagittal plane) of the body.

af-: a prefix meaning "toward."

afferent nerve: a nerve that transmits impulses from the sensory organs toward the central nervous system (CNS); also called a *sensory nerve*.

-al: a suffix meaning "character of."

alb/o: a combining form meaning "white."

-algia: a suffix meaning "pain."

alimentary canal: the food path through the body; includes the mouth, pharynx, esophagus, stomach, small intestine, colon, rectum, and anus.

an-: a prefix meaning "without."

ana-: a prefix meaning "apart."

anabolic reaction: a reaction in which molecules are joined together, requiring energy.

analysis: the fourth step in the experimental scientific method, in which data from an experiment is examined.

anatomical position: a body position in which a person stands upright with feet apart, arms at the sides, feet and palms facing forward, and thumbs pointing away from the body; all anatomical terms describe the body in reference to anatomical position.

anatomy: an area of biology that studies the parts of the body.

anemia: a condition in which the blood cannot carry enough oxygen to supply the body.

anti-: a prefix meaning "against."

anucleate: the quality of having no nucleus.

apical surface: the top layer of epithelial tissue that has contact with open space.

appendicular region: the limbs (arms and legs) of the body.

appendicular skeleton: the portion of the skeleton containing the pectoral girdle, pelvic girdle, upper limbs, and lower limbs.

aquaporin: a protein embedded in a cell's phospholipid bilayer that forms tunnels to help water move into or out of the cell.

-ar: a suffix meaning "pertaining to."

artery: a blood vessel that carries blood away from the heart toward the rest of the body.

arthr/o: a combining form meaning "joint."

atom: a core of protons and neutrons surrounded by orbiting electrons; an extremely small particle that, together with other atoms, makes up the universe; also called an *element*.

atomic diagram: an illustration of an atom that shows its core and electron shells; also called a *Bohr model*.

atomic mass: the number of protons plus the number of neutrons in an atom's core.

atomic number: the number of protons or electrons in an atom.

atomic symbol: an abbreviation used to refer to an atom.

ATP: adenosine triphosphate; a type of nucleic acid that is the energy storage molecule inside a cell; the main product of cell respiration.

atrioventricular (AV) valve: a valve that separates an atrium and a ventricle; prevents blood from flowing backward into the atrium when the ventricle contracts.

atrium: an upper chamber of the heart.

attitude: a way of feeling, thinking about, and viewing a situation.

attraction: the tendency of an atom to keep, donate, or accept an electron; also, a force that draws particles together.

avascular tissue: a type of tissue that does not have direct access to a blood supply.

axial region: the head, neck, and trunk of the body.

axial skeleton: the portion of the skeleton containing the skull, thoracic cage, and spine.

B

bar graph: a graph that visually compares information; uses narrow columns of different heights to show different amounts.

basal surface: the bottom layer of epithelial tissue that is attached to an acellular basement membrane.

base: a liquid that contains more OH⁻ ions than H⁺ ions; has a pH value between 7.1 and 14.

basement membrane: the acellular membrane beneath epithelial tissue through which nutrients and waste diffuse.

bi-: a prefix meaning "two."

bi/o: a combining form meaning "life."

biology: the science that studies life.

blood glucose concentration: the number of glucose molecules per a volume of blood; in homeostasis, is 90 mg/100 mL.

body cavity: a space within the body that contains organs; includes dorsal and ventral cavities.

body plane: an imaginary, flat surface that divides the body into sections; also called an *anatomical plane.*

body system: a group of organs that work together to perform several functions; also called an *organ system.*

body temperature: the temperature inside the body; in homeostasis, is 37°C (98.6°F).

Bohr model: an illustration of an atom that shows its core and electron shells; named for Niels Bohr; also called an *atomic diagram.*

bonding: an interaction in which electrons are exchanged or shared between atoms, joining the atoms together.

bone: a type of connective tissue that is hard like rock; has an extracellular matrix made of calcium salts reinforced with collagen fibers and is well supplied with blood.

brain: an organ that is the center of nervous system function; receives and integrates sensory information and transmits commands to the body; is located in the skull.

buffer: a molecule that can accept or donate H⁺ ions to resist changes in pH.

C

calorie: a measurement of the energy provided by macromolecules.

capillary: a small blood vessel with thin walls that allow the exchange of nutrients and gases.

carbohydrate: a type of macromolecule rich in energy that is a sugar; includes monosaccharides, disaccharides, and polysaccharides.

cardi/o: a combining form meaning "heart."

cardiovascular system: a body system consisting of the heart and blood vessels; transports blood, collects and transports waste, and helps regulate body temperature; also called the *circulatory system.*

carrier: a protein that spans a cell's phospholipid bilayer and moves large molecules, such as amino acids and glucose, through the plasma membrane.

cartilage: an avascular connective tissue with an extracellular matrix made of extracellular fibers, carbohydrates, and water.

catabolic reaction: a reaction in which molecules are broken apart, releasing energy.

cell: the basic structural unit of all living things.

cell respiration: the process inside a cell of adding one phosphate (P) molecule to one adenosine diphosphate (ADP) molecule to create adenosine triphosphate (ATP); occurs around or inside the mitochondria.

centi-: a prefix meaning "1/100 of one unit."

centimeter: a measurement of length equal to 1/100 of a meter.

central nervous system (CNS): the division of the nervous system that includes the brain and spinal cord; processes information.

cephalic region: the head area of the body.

-ceps: a suffix meaning "heads."

cerebr/o: a combining form meaning "brain."

cervical region: the neck area of the body.

chemical digestion: the process of breaking down food into macromolecules using enzymes and chemicals.

chlor/o: a combining form meaning "green."

cholesterol: a substance that separates individual phospholipids in a cell's phospholipid bilayer and helps the phospholipids shift location.

chondrocyte: a cartilage cell.

chromatin: a structure inside a cell's nucleus that contains packaged DNA when a cell is not dividing.

chromosome: a structure inside a cell's nucleus that contains packaged DNA during cell division.

cilia: hairs on the outside of a cell that move objects or liquid around the cell.

coel/o: a combining form meaning "hollow."

collagen fiber: a type of extracellular fiber that is white and contains the protein collagen; is especially strong; makes up irregular and regular dense connective tissue.

columnar cell: a tall epithelial cell.

combining form: a root word plus its combining vowel; often refers to a specific body part.

combining vowel: a vowel that is attached to a root word when a term is assembled; usually *o*.

compact bone: a type of bone tissue that looks solid.

complementary base: a nucleotide base that pairs with another base; purine and pyrimidine bases are complementary bases.

con-: a prefix meaning "together."

concentration: the number of atoms or molecules per one unit of volume; usually expressed in mg/L.

concentration gradient: the difference between concentrations inside the plasma membrane and outside the plasma membrane of a cell.

connective tissue: a type of tissue that fulfills the important functions of connection, support, and protection; contains an extracellular matrix; includes connective tissue proper and bone, cartilage, and blood.

connective tissue proper: a category of connective tissue that includes loose and dense connective tissue.

constant: an untested factor that could affect the dependent variable in an experiment; is kept the same across all groups in an experiment.

control group: the part of an experiment that does *not* receive the independent variable; the standard for comparison.

conversion: the process of changing a measurement from one unit to another unit.

conversion factor: a value that is multiplied to convert a unit from one measurement to another measurement.

coordinate pair: the values representing where a data point is placed on a graph; X, Y.

core: the center of an atom, which contains the atom's protons and neutrons.

cortic/o: a combining form meaning "outer region."

covalent bond: an atomic bond in which electrons are shared; includes single bonds (the sharing of two electrons) and double bonds (the sharing of four electrons).

cranial cavity: the dorsal body cavity formed by the skull; contains the brain.

crenation: the shrinking of a cell due to water leaving it.

cubic unit: a unit of measurement that results when three measurements of the same unit are multiplied together.

cuboidal cell: a square epithelial cell.

cyan/o: a combining form meaning "blue."

cyst: a root word meaning "cyst"; the combining form is *cyst/o.*

cyt/o: a combining form meaning "cell."

cytology: an area of biology that studies cells.

cytoplasm: all the material found inside a cell except for the nucleus; includes cytosol and organelles.

cytoskeleton: the structure that supports the cell; includes microfilaments, intermediate filaments, and microtubules.

D

de-: a prefix meaning "down from."

decide: the fifth step in the experimental scientific method, in which a hypothesis is accepted or rejected based on evidence.

decimal: a number that represents a value containing a fraction; is based on powers of 10.

deep: a term indicating that a body part is farther from the surface of the body.

defecation: the digestive process of removing solid waste (feces) from the body.

degree Celsius: the metric unit of temperature; is based on temperature variations of water.

dehydration: a condition characterized by lack of water in body tissues.

delt/o: a combining form meaning "triangular."

dense connective tissue: a type of connective tissue proper composed mostly of extracellular fibers with few cells; includes irregular dense connective tissue, regular dense connective tissue, and elastic connective tissue.

dependent variable: the "then" part of a hypothesis; hypothesized to depend on change in the independent variable.

dermis: the middle layer of skin; contains connective tissue, blood vessels, sweat and sebaceous glands, hair follicles, and nerve endings.

derm/o: a combining form meaning "skin."

desmosome: a locking joint between adjacent cells that prevents cells from being separated by force; consists of interlinked, anchoring proteins.

di-: a prefix meaning "two."

diabetes: a serious disease in which a person's body is unable to properly control levels of sugar in the blood because the body does not have enough insulin or cannot use it correctly.

diagnose: to identify and confirm the cause of an ailment.

diagnostic scientific method: a scientific method that collects facts from patient history and a physical exam of the patient; has four steps (facts, sift, test, and diagnose).

diameter: the longest measurement across a circle.

diaphragm: a dome-shaped muscle inferior to the thoracic cavity that contracts to lower the bottom of the thoracic cavity.

diffusion: the spreading out of atoms from areas of high concentration into areas of low concentration through the phospholipid bilayer of a cell; does not require energy.

digestive system: a body system consisting of the alimentary canal and several support organs; intakes and breaks down food, absorbs nutrients, and removes solid waste.

diploid: a human cell containing 23 pairs of chromosomes (46 total chromosomes); most human cells are diploid.

dis-: a prefix meaning "apart."

disaccharide: a type of carbohydrate containing two sugars bonded together.

distal: a term indicating that a body part is farther from the place where a limb is attached to the body's trunk.

DNA: deoxyribonucleic acid; a type of nucleic acid that makes up chromosomes.

dorsal: a term indicating that a body part is closer to the back of the body; also called *posterior*.

dors/o: a combining form meaning "back (of the body)."

double bond: a covalent bond in which four electrons are shared between two atoms.

downhill reaction: the movement of atoms down the concentration gradient, from high concentration to low concentration; does not require energy.

dry volume: the amount of space in a three-dimensional object.

duct: a root word meaning "to carry"; the combining form is *duct/o*.

ductus deferens: an organ in males that conveys sperm from the epididymis to the urethra in the penis during ejaculation.

E

ecto-: a prefix meaning "outside."

ef-: a prefix meaning "away from."

efferent nerve: a nerve that transmits impulses away from the central nervous system (CNS) toward the rest of the body; also called a *motor nerve*.

elastic fiber: a type of extracellular fiber that is made of the protein elastin and is yellow and thin; can stretch up to one and one-half times its resting length; makes up elastic connective tissue.

electrolyte: an acid, base, or salt that releases ions when added to water.

electron: a subatomic particle found in an atom's electron shells; has a negative charge, has no mass, and is involved in bonding.

electron capacity: the number of electrons an electron shell can hold; two electrons for the first shell, eight electrons for the second shell, and eight electrons for the third shell.

electronic balance: an instrument that measures the mass of an object in grams digitally.

electron shell: the outside part of an atom that contains the atom's orbiting electrons.

element: a core of protons and neutrons surrounded by orbiting electrons; an extremely small particle that, together with other elements, makes up the universe; also called an *atom*.

endo-: a prefix meaning "inside."

endocrine gland: a gland that releases a product into the interstitial fluid surrounding a cell; makes up the endocrine system; also called a *ductless gland*.

endocrine system: a body system consisting of glands throughout the body; releases hormones, maintains homeostasis, and helps regulate body function.

endocytosis: the movement of atoms into a cell; requires energy; includes phagocytosis, pinocytosis, and receptor-mediated endocytosis.

endoplasmic reticulum (ER): a network of membranes attached to a cell's nuclear envelope; can process, store, or digest some materials.

English system of measurement: the standard measurement system used in the United States.

enter/o: a combining form meaning "intestine."

enzyme: a protein catalyst; a substance produced by body cells that helps trigger or speed up reactions.

epi-: a prefix meaning "upon."

epidermis: the outermost, most superficial layer of skin; is made of stratified squamous epithelium and contains keratinocytes and melanocytes.

epididymis: an organ in males that stores sperm until ejaculation.

epithelial tissue: a type of tissue that covers the surfaces of the body and lines the body's internal hollow tubes and cavities; also called *epithelium*.

equilibrium: a state in which the concentrations of atoms on both sides of a cell's plasma membrane are equal.

erythr/o: a combining form meaning "red."

essential amino acid: an amino acid that the body cannot make and that must be included in a person's diet.

evidence: facts that relate to a possible cause; is used to test a hypothesis.

ex-: a prefix meaning "out of."

excitable tissue: a type of tissue that produces an electrical charge when stimulated; includes muscle and nerve tissue.

exocrine gland: a gland that releases a product through a duct.

exocytosis: the movement of atoms out of a cell; requires energy.

experiment: the third step in the experimental scientific method, in which actions are performed and their effects are carefully observed in order to learn about something.

experimental group: the part of an experiment that *does* receive the independent variable.

experimental scientific method: a scientific method that formulates a prediction and then tests the prediction to obtain data; has five steps (observation, hypothesis, experiment, analysis, decide).

expiration: the process of breathing out air as lung volume decreases.

extension: a type of directional movement along the sagittal plane that increases the angle between bones or between a limb and the body.

external respiration: the exchange of oxygen and carbon dioxide between the air in the lungs and the blood; oxygen is loaded from the air into the blood, and carbon dioxide is unloaded from the blood into the air.

extracellular matrix: a collection of material and fibers existing outside connective tissue cells; also called *ground substance*.

F

facilitated diffusion: the spreading out of atoms from areas of high concentration into areas of low concentration through protein channels and carrier proteins in a cell's plasma membrane; does not require energy.

fact: a confirmed observation; is used to test a hypothesis.

fallopian tube: a hollow organ in females extending out from the uterus that receives an egg cell from an ovary.

fiber: plant material that is eaten, but is indigestible; is made of cellulose.

fibroblast: a cell that secretes collagen and elastin.

filtration: the urinary process of removing molecules smaller than a protein from the blood; occurs in the glomerulus.

flagella: whip-like structures that propel a cell forward.

flexion: a type of directional movement along the sagittal plane that reduces the angle between bones or between a limb and the body.

fluid mosaic: a model used to describe how a cell's plasma membrane has many distinct parts that are not fixed in place.

fraction: a part of a whole number.

frontal plane: a body plane that divides the body into front (ventral) and back (dorsal) sections; also called the *coronal plane*.

full outer shell: an outermost electron shell that has the maximum number of electrons.

G

gamete: a human reproductive cell containing 23 total chromosomes; an egg cell in females and a sperm in males.

gap junction: a type of membrane junction that contains communication tunnels between adjacent cells.

gastr/o: a combining form meaning "stomach."

-gen: a suffix meaning "producer."

gene: a segment of DNA within a chromosome that codes for a particular trait.

-genesis: a suffix meaning "production."

genetics: an area of biology that studies inheritance.

gland: an epithelial tissue that produces and secretes products.

glob/o: a combining form meaning "round."

globular protein: a type of structure that forms channels that allow select molecules to pass through a cell's plasma membrane.

glucagon: a hormone produced by the alpha cells of the pancreas that signals the liver to break down stored glycogen into glucose and release glucose into the blood.

glycolipid: a carbohydrate chain attached to a lipid; found in a cell's plasma membrane.

glycoprotein: a carbohydrate chain attached to a globular protein; found in a cell's plasma membrane.

Golgi: an organelle within a cell that receives proteins from transport vesicles and packages them into secretory vesicles so they can travel out of the cell; looks like a stack of flattened sacks.

graduated cylinder: a narrow cylinder with milliliter increments; used for measuring liquid volume.

gram: the metric unit of mass.

graph: a visual representation of information.

H

hair: a strand of dead, protein-filled cells that grows from a hair follicle in the dermis.

haploid: a human cell containing 23 total chromosomes.

heart: a muscular organ located in the thoracic cavity that receives oxygen-poor blood from the body, pumps it into the lungs for oxygenation, and then pumps oxygen-rich blood to the rest of the body.

hemi-: a prefix meaning "half."

hem/o: a combining form meaning "blood."

hepat/o: a combining form meaning "liver."

hetero-: a prefix meaning "different."

hexa-: a prefix meaning "six."

high-energy bond: the bond with the third phosphate molecule in ATP; is broken when a cell requires energy.

histology: an area of biology that studies tissues.

homeostasis: a state of relative stability.

homo-: a prefix meaning "same."

hormone: a chemical message sent from an endocrine gland to a target.

humane: the quality of being kind and ethical.

hydr/o: a combining form meaning "water."

hydrogenation: the process of adding hydrogen atoms to an unsaturated or polyunsaturated fat; creates *trans* fat.

hydrogen bond: an atomic bond in which the partial charges of water molecules attract; the weakest type of atomic bond.

hydrophilic: the quality of being attracted to water.

hydrophobic: the quality of not being attracted to water.

hyper-: a prefix meaning "above; beyond."

hypertonic: a type of solution outside a cell that has a higher solute concentration than the solution inside a cell.

hypo-: a prefix meaning "below."

hypodermis: the deepest layer of skin that connects the dermis to muscles beneath the skin; helps insulate the body and protects deeper tissues.

hypothesis: a prediction about the outcome of an experiment; is proposed during the second step of the experimental scientific method and is tested with an experiment.

hypotonic: a type of solution outside a cell that has a lower solute concentration than the solution inside a cell.

I

-ia: a suffix meaning "condition."

-ic: a suffix meaning "pertaining to."

-ical: a suffix meaning "character of."

in-: a prefix meaning "into."

independent variable: the "if" part of a hypothesis; is manipulated to see if the dependent variable changes.

inferior: a term indicating that a body part is closer to the feet of the body.

infra-: a prefix meaning "under."

ingestion: the digestive process of taking food into the body.

insertion: the movable bone to which a skeletal muscle is attached.

inspiration: the process of breathing in air as lung volume increases.

insulin: a hormone produced by the beta cells of the pancreas that signals cells to take glucose out of the blood and signals the liver to draw glucose out of the blood and store it as glycogen.

integumentary system: a body system consisting of the skin, hair, and nails; protects the body, helps maintain homeostasis, makes vitamin D, removes waste, and perceives sensations.

inter-: a prefix meaning "between."

intermediate: a term indicating that a body part is between one medial and one lateral body part.

intermediate filament: a cytoskeleton component that holds some organelles in position within a cell; composed of several fibrous, long, and slender protein strands twisted around each other.

internal respiration: the exchange of oxygen and carbon dioxide between the blood and the cells of the body; oxygen in the blood is unloaded to body cells, and carbon dioxide is loaded from body cells into the blood.

interphase: a major phase in the life cycle of a cell in which the cell continues to perform its specific functions and does not divide, though it is preparing for cell division.

intra-: a prefix meaning "within."

involuntary muscle: a type of muscle that is not consciously controlled; includes smooth muscle and cardiac muscle.

-ion: a suffix meaning "process."

ion: an atom that has donated or accepted an electron or electrons so the number of protons and electrons is unequal; has a charge.

ionic bond: an atomic bond formed by the attraction between ions that have opposite charges.

isotonic: a type of solution outside a cell that has the same solute concentration as the solution inside a cell.

isotope: a form of an atom that has the same atomic number as, but a different atomic mass from, another form of that atom; atoms may have up to 10 different isotopes.

-ist: a suffix meaning "specialist."

-itis: a suffix meaning "inflammation."

J

joint: a connection between bones; can be immovable, slightly movable, or freely movable; also called an *articulation*.

K

key term: a word essential to understanding a concept.

kidney: an organ located in the abdominal cavity that filters waste out of the blood.

kidney stone: a rock-like structure that forms in the urinary system.

kilo-: a prefix meaning "1000 units."

L

lactic acid: a product of cell respiration in muscles that begins without oxygen; can cause tiredness and soreness in muscles.

lacuna: a cavity in the bone matrix; houses osteocytes.

lateral: a term indicating that a body part is farther from the middle (midsagittal plane) of the body.

later/o: a combining form meaning "side."

lat/o: a combining form meaning "wide."

leuk/o: a combining form meaning "white."

ligament: a band of regular dense connective tissue that connects bone to bone.

linear: the quality of being made up of, relating to, or resembling a straight line.

line graph: a graph that shows changes in information or values over time.

lipid: a macromolecule that is a fat, wax, or oil; one glycerol molecule bonded to three fatty acids.

lipid barrier: the lipid portion of a cell's phospholipid bilayer that prevents molecules that are not lipid soluble from passing through.

liquid volume: the amount of liquid in a three-dimensional object.

liter: the metric unit for measuring the volume of a liquid or gas.

literature: the body of scientific articles that are published in scientific journals.

-logist: a suffix meaning "one who studies."

-logy: a suffix meaning "study of."

loose connective tissue: a type of connective tissue proper composed of many cells with extracellular fibers winding through them; includes adipose connective tissue, areolar connective tissue, and reticular connective tissue.

lower limb: the leg and hip area of the body.

lun: a root word meaning "crescent shape"; the combining form is *lun/o*.

lung: an organ located in the thoracic cavity that receives air and exchanges oxygen and carbon dioxide.

lute/o: a combining form meaning "yellow."

lymph: a fluid circulated through the lymphatic system that contains blood plasma and white blood cells.

lymphatic system: a body system consisting of lymphatic vessels, lymph, and lymphatic organs; returns blood plasma to the cardiovascular system and defends the body against disease.

lymph node: a lymphatic organ that inspects lymph for harmful agents to destroy.

lymphocyte: a distinctive white blood cell of the lymphatic system; defends the body against infection.

lyse: to burst after swelling past maximum size; can occur in cells as water enters them.

-lysis: a suffix meaning "breakdown."

lysosome: a large bag of enzymes within a cell that prevents the enzymes from harming the cell and releases them to destroy bacteria.

M

macro-: a prefix meaning "large."

macromolecule: a combination of many atoms held together by bonds.

mammary gland: a gland in females that produces milk after childbirth.

manus: the hand area of the body.

mass: the amount of matter in an object.

mechanical digestion: the process of physically tearing large pieces of food into smaller pieces.

medial: a term indicating that a body part is closer to the middle (midsagittal plane) of the body.

medi/o: a combining form meaning "middle."

mega-: a prefix meaning "large."

meiosis: the process of cell division by which one diploid cell undergoes two sets of cell division to produce haploid cells; happens only in the testes and ovaries.

melan/o: a combining form meaning "black."

membrane junction: an attachment between nearby cells.

meniscus: the semicircular surface of liquid in a cylinder.

meso-: a prefix meaning "middle."

meter: the metric unit of length.

meter stick: a tool for taking linear measurements; is 1 meter in length.

metric system: the international system of measurement for the science and healthcare fields; based on powers of 10.

micro-: a prefix meaning "small."

microfilament: a cytoskeleton component that forms a net on the inside of a cell's plasma membrane; made of two globular protein chains wrapped around each other.

microtubule: a cytoskeleton component that organelles attach to and that forms the roadway on which organelles are moved throughout the cell; made of tubulins.

microvilli: finger-like projections of a cell's plasma membrane that increase the surface area of the cell to allow for more absorption.

midsagittal plane: a body plane that divides the body into equal left and right halves; also called the *median plane.*

milli-: a prefix meaning "$1/1000$ of one unit."

milliliter: a measurement of volume equal to $1/1000$ of a liter.

millimeter: a measurement of length equal to $1/1000$ of a meter.

mitochondrion: the powerhouse of the cell and the site of cell respiration.

mitosis: the process by which one diploid cell divides into two genetically identical diploid daughter cells; has four stages and happens in most cells in the human body.

mnemonic: a word, acronym, or phrase that can help one recall information.

molecule: a combination of atoms held together by bonds.

mono-: a prefix meaning "one."

monosaccharide: a type of carbohydrate containing one sugar; the simplest type of sugar.

morph/o: a combining form meaning "form."

morphology: the study of structure or form.

mucus: a substance that coats and moistens linings in the body.

multinucleate: the quality of having more than one nucleus.

muscle tissue: an excitable tissue composed of muscle cells; contracts when stimulated; includes smooth muscle, skeletal muscle, and cardiac muscle.

muscular system: a body system consisting of all of the skeletal muscles in the body; holds body parts in position, enables movement, helps maintain body temperature, and protects internal organs.

my/o: a combining form meaning "muscle."

myocyte: a muscle cell; also called a *muscle fiber.*

N

nail: a plate of keratin that protects the end of a phalanx (finger or toe).

natural: the quality of being observable and testable.

negative feedback: the cycle of taking action to correct a concentration or factor back to its set value within the body.

neo-: a prefix meaning "new."

nephron: the basic unit of the kidney; contains a glomerulus and renal tubule.

nerve tissue: an excitable tissue composed of neurons; communicates signals throughout the body.

nervous system: a body system consisting of the brain, spinal cord, and nerves of the body; receives sensory information, processes information, and transmits impulses to body parts.

neur/o: a combining form meaning "nerve."

neuroglia: a nonexcitable nerve cell that supports, insulates, and protects neurons.

neuron: a nerve cell that conducts an electrical charge; has a cell body, dendrites, and an axon.

neurotransmitter: a chemical released from the end of a nerve cell that causes a new action potential to start in an adjacent cell.

neutral: a liquid that contains equal amounts of OH^- ions and H^+ ions; is neither an acid nor a base; has a pH value of 7.0.

neutron: a subatomic particle found in the core of an atom; has no charge and a mass of 1 amu.

nonpolar: the quality of having no charge.

nontropic hormone: a chemical message sent from an endocrine gland that targets a nonendocrine organ or tissue.

nuclear envelope: the border of a cell's nucleus.

nucleic acid: a polymer that is a chain of nucleotides; the code for the genetic information in cells.

nucleolus: an area of a cell's nucleus that assembles the components needed to make organelles and ribosomes.

nucleotide: the basic unit of a nucleic acid; contains a phosphate, a sugar, and a base.

nucleus: the control center of a cell; contains genetic information.

O

OHEAD: an acronym for the five steps of the experimental scientific method: observation, hypothesis, experiment, analysis, and decide.

-oid: a suffix meaning "resembling."

-oma: a suffix meaning "tumor."

omni-: a prefix meaning "all."

organ: a group of different types of tissue that work together to do a job.

organism: a complex life form made of many interdependent parts.

origin: the immovable bone to which a skeletal muscle is attached.

-osis: a suffix meaning "condition."

osmosis: a type of diffusion in which water molecules move through a cell's phospholipid bilayer and aquaporins from areas with a high concentration of water to areas with a low concentration of water; does not require energy.

oste: a root word meaning "bone"; the combining form is *oste/o*.

osteoblast: a type of osteocyte that constructs the bone matrix.

osteoclast: a type of osteocyte that breaks down the bone matrix.

osteocyte: a bone cell that lives in a lacuna in the bone matrix; includes osteoblasts and osteoclasts.

-ous: a suffix meaning "nature of."

ovary: an organ in females that stores and releases egg cells; also secretes estrogen and progesterone.

P

parathyroid gland: an endocrine gland located on the dorsal surface of the thyroid gland that releases parathyroid hormone (PTH).

partial charge: a slight negative or positive charge in a part of a molecule.

pectoral girdle: the shoulder joint, which connects an arm to the thoracic cage; consists of the scapula and clavicle.

pedal: the foot area of the body.

pelvic cavity: the ventral body cavity formed by the pelvis that contains the urinary bladder and some reproductive organs.

pelvic girdle: the hip joints, which connect a leg to the spine; consists of the pelvis (left ilium, left ischium, left pubis, right ilium, right ischium, and right pubis).

pelvic region: the hip area of the body.

penis: a structure in males that contains the urethra and is made of erectile tissue.

percentage: a part of a whole number; a number of parts out of 100 parts.

peri-: a prefix meaning "around."

periodic table of elements: a grid that arranges elements by their atomic numbers and properties.

peripheral nervous system (PNS): the division of the nervous system that includes the body's nerves; receives information and communicates impulses; includes the somatic and autonomic nervous systems.

peristalsis: smooth muscle contractions that move a substance through the body.

permeable: the quality of a cell's plasma membrane that enables atoms and molecules to move through it.

peroxisome: a small bag containing enzymes within a cell that breaks down chemicals and free radicals.

pH: the measurement of acid or base in a liquid; pH values range from 0 to 14.

-phage: a suffix meaning "eat."

phagocytosis: a type of endocytosis in which the plasma membrane of a cell surrounds and engulfs an object; also called *cell eating*.

phenomenon: a physically observable fact or event; plural *phenomena*.

-philic: a suffix meaning "loving."

-phobic: a suffix meaning "fearing."

phospholipid: a molecule composed of one phosphate head and two lipid tails.

phospholipid bilayer: two layers of phospholipids that compose a cell's plasma membrane; forms the three-dimensional border around a cell.

physi/o: a combining form meaning "function."

physiology: an area of biology that studies the functions of body parts.

pi: a constant value rounded to 3.14; used for calculating the surface area of a circle.

pinocytosis: a type of endocytosis in which the plasma membrane of a cell surrounds and engulfs a liquid containing atoms; also called *cell drinking*.

pituitary gland: an endocrine gland at the base of the brain; also called the *master gland*.

-plasm: a suffix meaning "formation."

plasma: the extracellular matrix of blood; is primarily water, but also contains proteins.

plasma membrane: the selectively permeable barrier of a cell that acts as a gatekeeper and keeps molecules inside or outside of the cell.

platform balance: an instrument that measures the mass of an object in grams; has three beams with markings that indicate the number of grams.

platy-: a prefix meaning "flat."

-plegia: a suffix meaning "paralysis."

polar: the quality of having a charge.

poly-: a prefix meaning "many."

polypeptide: a combination of 10–49 amino acids.

polysaccharide: a type of carbohydrate containing many (more than two) sugars bonded together.

polyunsaturated fat: a lipid in which there is more than one double bond between carbon atoms, and far fewer than the maximum number of hydrogen atoms are bonded to each carbon atom; is liquid at room temperature.

post-: a prefix meaning "after."

pre-: a prefix meaning "before."

prefix: a letter or group of letters preceding a combining form; often describes time, location, or number.

pressure: the collisions of atoms with other atoms and with the sides of a container.

primary structure: a type of protein structure determined by the sequence of amino acids.

protein: a type of macromolecule that is a chain of amino acids; can be structural or functional.

protein buffer: a protein molecule that accepts all H^+ ions produced by chemical reactions inside a cell.

protein synthesis: the process of placing amino acids in the proper sequence to form a specific protein.

proton: a subatomic particle found in the core of an atom; has a positive charge and a mass of 1 amu.

proximal: a term indicating that a body part is closer to the place where a limb is attached to the body's trunk.

pseudo-: a prefix meaning "false."

pseudostratified arrangement: an epithelial cell arrangement consisting of one layer with cells with different heights.

pubic region: the groin and genital area of the body.

pulmonary circulation: the flow of blood from the heart to the lungs and back to the heart.

Q

quadri-: a prefix meaning "four."

R

radius: the measurement from one edge of a circle to the center; half the distance across a circle.

rate: the number of events that occur during a specific unit of time.

ratio: a comparison of numbers.

reabsorption: the urinary process of moving molecules from filtrate back into the blood; occurs in the renal tubule.

receptor-mediated endocytosis: a type of endocytosis in which a substance binds to a specific protein in a pit of a cell's phospholipid bilayer and is brought into the cell inside a vesicle.

rect/o: a combining form meaning "straight."

reinforce: to strengthen one's knowledge of material.

relative atomic mass: the average mass for an atom and all of its isotopes.

ren/o: a combining form meaning "kidney."

replication: the process of copying a cell's chromosomes to create twice as many chromatids; takes place during interphase before cell division.

reproductive system: a body system involved in reproducing life; in females, consists of the ovaries, fallopian tubes, uterus, vagina, external genitalia, and mammary glands; in males, consists of the testes and scrotum, epididymis, ductus deferens, accessory organs, and penis.

respiratory system: a body system consisting of the organs involved in breathing; inhales oxygen-rich air, exchanges respiratory gases, and exhales carbon dioxide.

reticular fiber: a type of extracellular fiber that is thin and white and is made of the protein collagen; forms a network in the extracellular matrix; makes up reticular connective tissue.

ribosome: a structure inside a cell that assembles amino acids into specific proteins.

RNA: ribonucleic acid; a type of nucleic acid involved in protein synthesis.

root word: the central component of a scientific term; often refers to a specific body part.

rotation: a type of directional movement along the transverse plane that moves a body part from side to side.

rough endoplasmic reticulum (RER): a type of endoplasmic reticulum covered with ribosomes inside a cell.

rubr/o: a combining form meaning "red."

ruler: a tool for taking linear measurements; is 30 centimeters in length.

S

sagittal plane: a body plane that divides the body into unequal left and right sections.

saturated fat: a lipid in which all bonds between carbon atoms are single bonds and each carbon atom has the maximum number of hydrogen atoms bonded to it; is solid at room temperature.

science: the body of knowledge and techniques that enables mankind to explain the natural world; is concerned with natural explanations.

scientific law: a general statement of fact that encourages the expectation of a result.

scientific method: a logical process for solving problems and answering questions about the natural world.

scientific theory: the best explanation today of why a phenomenon occurs; the basis for mankind's understanding of the natural world.

secondary structure: a type of protein structure resulting from the attraction between amino acids that are close together; determines the shape of the molecule (pleated sheet or helix).

secretion: the urinary process of moving molecules from the blood into filtrate after filtration has occurred; occurs in the renal tubule.

secretory vesicle: a sack that moves proteins out of a cell.

selective: the quality of a cell's plasma membrane that ensures not *all* atoms and molecules can move through it.

semi-: a prefix meaning "half."

semilunar (SL) valve: a valve that separates a ventricle from a blood vessel that moves blood out of the heart; keeps blood from flowing prematurely into a blood vessel when an atrium contracts.

sense strand: the strand of DNA containing assembly instructions for a specific protein; is copied to make mRNA during transcription.

serrat/o: a combining form meaning "jagged."

sift: to sort through collected facts very carefully in order to find something useful or valuable; is performed during the second step of the diagnostic scientific method.

simple arrangement: an epithelial cell arrangement consisting of one layer of cells.

single bond: a covalent bond in which two electrons are shared between two atoms.

skeletal system: a body system consisting of the bones and joints of the body; protects the body, provides support, produces red blood cells, facilitates movement, and stores calcium.

skin: an organ that forms the covering of the body; protects the body and contains organs that perceive sensory stimuli and cause perspiration.

skull: the cranial and facial bones that make up the head.

smooth endoplasmic reticulum (SER): a type of endoplasmic reticulum with smooth membranes that are not studded with ribosomes inside a cell.

sodium-potassium pump: a solute pump in a cell's plasma membrane that uses energy to push sodium ions out of a cell and potassium ions into the cell.

soluble: the quality of being capable of dissolving.

solute: the substance dissolved in a solution.

solute pump: a protein in a cell's phospholipid bilayer that uses energy to move specific ions into or out of a cell.

solvent: the liquid substance used to dissolve another substance in a solution.

specialized: a quality of cells that causes them to have unique structures, components, or shapes that enable them to perform a specific function.

spin: a root word meaning "spine"; the combining form is *spin/o*.

spinal cavity: the dorsal body cavity formed by the spine that contains the spinal cord.

spinal cord: a cord of nervous tissue housed inside the vertebrae of the spine; descends from the brain and attaches to and communicates with the body's nerves.

spine: a stack of block-like vertebrae that surround the spinal cord; also called the *vertebral column*.

spleen: a lymphatic organ located in the abdominal cavity that helps control the amount of blood in the body, inspects lymph for harmful agents, and triggers the immune response.

spongy bone: a type of bone tissue that looks like a honeycomb.

squamous cell: a flat epithelial cell; is so thin that macromolecules can move through it.

square unit: a unit of measurement that results when two measurements of the same unit are multiplied together.

-stasis: a suffix meaning "stay or stop."

sten/o: a combining form meaning "narrow."

stratified arrangement: an epithelial cell arrangement consisting of multiple layers of cells.

strat/o: a combining form meaning "layer."

studying: the process of concentrated learning; the deliberate effort to make long-term memories about subject matter.

sub-: a prefix meaning "below."

subject: an organism one is studying or on which one is experimenting.

substrate: the atoms involved in an enzymatic reaction.

suffix: a letter or group of letters following a combining form; usually describes certain types of diseases or procedures.

superficial: a term indicating that a body part is closer to the surface of the body.

superior: a term indicating that a body part is closer to the head of the body.

supernatural: the quality of not being testable or explainable by science or the laws of nature.

supra-: a prefix meaning "above."

surface area: the total area of the outer surface of an object.

systemic circulation: the flow of blood from the heart to the rest of the body and back to the heart.

T

tendon: a band of regular dense connective tissue that connects bone to muscle.

tens: a root word meaning "to stretch"; the combining form is *tens/o*.

terminology: the particular words or phrases used in a scientific field.

tertiary structure: a type of protein structure resulting from the attraction between distant amino acids; forms the three-dimensional shape of the molecule.

testis: an organ in males that produces sperm; hangs in the scrotum outside the body.

tetra-: a prefix meaning "four."

thoracic cage: the sternum and ribs that surround the thoracic cavity.

thoracic cavity: the ventral body cavity formed by the thoracic cage that contains the heart and lungs.

thoracic region: the chest or breast area of the body.

thymus: a lymphatic organ located in the chest that houses white blood cells as they mature and signals bone marrow to produce white blood cells.

thyroid gland: an endocrine gland located in the throat that releases triiodothyronine (T_3), thyroxine (T_4), and calcitonin.

-tic: a suffix meaning "pertaining to."

tight junction: a type of membrane junction that binds adjacent cells together to form an impermeable barrier; made by proteins.

tissue: a group of cells that work together to do a job.

-tomy: a suffix meaning "to cut."

transcription: the first stage of protein synthesis in which the sense strand of DNA is copied to make mRNA in a cell's nucleus.

trans fat: an unsaturated or polyunsaturated fat that has had hydrogen atoms added to it.

transitional cell: an epithelial cell that can stretch or relax, changing shape and thickness as needed.

translation: the second stage of protein synthesis in which amino acids are assembled in the order dictated by mRNA to create a protein.

transport vesicle: a sack that moves a product to another location inside a cell.

transverse plane: a body plane that divides the body into top and bottom sections; body sections divided by the transverse plane are called *cross-sections*.

tri-: a prefix meaning "three."

tropic hormone: a chemical message sent from an endocrine gland that targets another endocrine gland.

tub: a root word meaning "tube"; the combining form is *tub/o*.

turnover rate: the speed of enzymatic reactions.

U

-ule: a suffix meaning "small."

ultra-: a prefix meaning "beyond."

-um: a suffix meaning "structure."

uni-: a prefix meaning "one."

unsaturated fat: a lipid in which there is one double bond between carbon atoms and fewer than the maximum number of hydrogen atoms are bonded to each carbon atom; is liquid at room temperature.

uphill reaction: the movement of atoms up the concentration gradient, from low concentration to high concentration; requires energy.

upper limb: the arm and shoulder area of the body.

ureter: a tubelike organ that transports urine toward the urinary bladder.

urethra: a tubelike organ that transports urine out of the body.

urinary bladder: a hollow, muscular organ that stores urine for a time before moving urine into the urethra.

urinary system: a body system consisting of the kidneys, ureters, urinary bladder, and urethra; filters blood, removes and stores waste, produces hormones, and maintains homeostasis.

uterus: a hollow, muscular organ in females that houses a developing fetus.

V

vagina: a hollow organ in females that serves as the birth canal and receives sperm during intercourse.

vascular tissue: a type of tissue that has direct access to a blood supply; is permeated by blood vessels.

vein: a blood vessel that carries blood from the body back to the heart.

ventral: a term indicating that a body part is closer to the front of the body; also called *anterior*.

ventricle: a lower chamber of the heart.

ventr/o: a combining form meaning "belly side (of the body)."

voluntary muscle: a type of muscle that is consciously controlled; includes skeletal muscle.

W

weight: the force of gravity on the mass of an object.

X

x-axis: the horizontal side of a graph; tracks time when time is being measured.

Y

y-axis: the vertical side of a graph.

Z

zygote: the first cell of the human life cycle formed by the fusion of an egg cell and a sperm.

Index

nerve tissue, 419–420, 423
nervous system, 458–459, 495–498
    afferent nerves, 497–498
    autonomic nerves, 498
    brain, 496
    central nervous system, 496–497
    definition, 495
    efferent nerves, 497–498
    functions of, 495
    nerve tissue, 419–420, 423
    neuroglia, 423
    neurons, 423, 497
    parasympathetic nerves, 498
    peripheral nervous system,
        496–498
    somatic nerves, 498
    spinal cord, 497
    sympathetic nerves, 498
neuralgia, 70
neuroglia, 423
neurons, 423, 497
neurotransmitter, 419–420
neutral, pH value, 268–271
neutrons, 188–190, 199, 205
    atomic diagrams, 205
    atomic mass, 193
    definition, 188
    mass and charge, 190
    number of, 199
nonpolar, 323–324
nontropic hormone, 502. *See also*
    hormones
nuclear envelope, 294–296, 379
nuclear pores, 294
nucleic acids, 259–267
    adenosine triphosphate (ATP),
        267, 305, 351–354,
        357–358
    bases, 260–263
    complementary bases, 262–263
    definition, 259
    deoxyribonucleic acid (DNA),
        263–266, 292–293, 371,
        373, 376–381
    nucleotides, 259–261
    ribonucleic acid (RNA), 266,
        372–373

strands, 264
structure of, 259–263
nucleolus, 295
nucleoplasm, 294
nucleotide, 259–261
nucleus, 291–296
    anucleate cells, 294
    cell division, 296, 376–381
    chromosomes and chromatin,
        292–294, 371, 376–377
    definition, 280
    multinucleate cells, 294, 421
    nuclear envelope, 294
    nucleolus, 295
    protein synthesis, 371–373
number-related word parts, 44–48
numerator, 116
nutrition. *See* calories; digestive
    system; macromolecules

O

observation, step of experimental
    scientific method, 84, 89
OHEAD acronym, 84
opposing word parts, 34–37
opposite charges, 217, 227–228
    hydrogen bonding, 227–228
    ionic bonding, 217
organelles, 280, 295, 298–301,
    304–309, 352, 370–371, 373
    cytoplasm, 280, 304–309
    cytoskeleton, 307–309
    endoplasmic reticulum, 298–301
    Golgi, 302, 358, 373
    lysosomes, 302, 306
    mitochondria, 305, 352
    peroxisomes, 306
    ribosomes, 295, 300–301,
        370–371, 373
organism, level of body
    organization, 455, 461
organization of human body,
    455–461
organ, level of body organization,
    389, 457
organ systems. *See* body systems
origin, 490

osmosis, 344–348
    definition, 345
    effect on cell size, 348
    hypertonic, isotonic, and
        hypotonic solutions,
        346–347
    solute and solvent
        concentrations, 345,
        347
osteoblast, 413
osteoclast, 413
osteocyte, 413
ovary, 537
ovulation, 537
oxidase, 306
oxygen, 192, 226–228, 324, 337, 341,
    397, 506–511, 516–517
    blood circulation, 389–390, 510,
        516–517
    cell respiration, 352–354
    diffusion in the lungs, 341, 397,
        510
    lipid solubility, 324, 337
    respiratory system, 506–511
    water molecules, 226–228

P

parasympathetic nerves, 498
parathyroid gland, 501, 504
parathyroid hormone (PTH), 504
parietal cells, 456
partial charges, 227–228
particles, subatomic, 188–190, 199
passive transport. *See* diffusion;
    osmosis
patient history, 95, 100, 102
pectoral girdle, 483
pedal, body region, 444
pelvic cavity, 436, 441
pelvic girdle, 483
pelvic region, 441
pelvis, 483
penis, 534, 540
peptide bonds, 244, 373
percentages, 119–120
periodic table of elements, 195–200,
    209
periosteum, 66

pseudostratified columnar epithelium, 400

PTH. *See* parathyroid hormone (PTH)

pubic region, 441

published articles and journals, scientific, 110

pulmonary circulation, 516–517

purine bases, 260–262

pyrimidine bases, 260–262

R

R group. *See* remainder (R) group

radius, bone, 480, 484

radius, circle measurement, 138

range, 179

rate, 168

ratios, 145–150

reabsorption, 533

reading. *See* study skills

receptor-mediated endocytosis, 361

rectangle, 135–136
    measuring, 135
    surface area, 135–136

red blood cells, 51–52, 253, 255, 416–417, 522
    blood, 416–417
    hemoglobin, 253
    production, 51–52, 522

regions. *See* body regions

regular dense connective tissue, 409

reinforcement, of study material, 6–7

relative atomic mass, 196, 200

remainder (R) group, 245–247

renal tubule, 398–399, 532–533

repetition, 20

replication, 378

reproductive systems, 458, 460, 536–540
    definition, 536
    female reproductive system, 537–538
    functions of, 536
    gametes, 376, 380–381, 536–538
    male reproductive system, 538–540

RER. *See* rough endoplasmic reticulum (RER)

respiration, 510

respiratory gases, 507, 510

respiratory system, 458–459, 506–511
    definition, 506
    diaphragm, 508–509, 511
    expiration, 511
    functions of, 506–507
    inspiration, 508
    lungs, 341, 397, 508–511
    respiration, 510

results, section of scientific article, 110

reticular connective tissue, 408

reticular fiber, 406

rewards, 21

ribonucleic acid (RNA), 266
    definition, 266
    messenger (mRNA), 372–373
    ribosomal (rRNA), 300, 372–373
    role in protein synthesis, 372–373
    structure of, 259–263, 266
    transfer (tRNA), 372–373

ribose, 263

ribosomal RNA (rRNA), 300, 372–373

ribosomes, 295, 300–301, 370–371, 373

ribs, 481

right hyphochondriac region, 442

right iliac region, 443

right ilium, 483

right ischium, 483

right lumbar region, 443

right pubis, 483

RNA. *See* ribonucleic acid (RNA)

root word, 29. *See also* word parts

rotation, 492

rough endoplasmic reticulum (RER), 300, 373

rounding, 118

rRNA. *See* ribosomal RNA (rRNA)

rubrospinal tracts, 52

ruler, 129

S

saccharides, 233–237. *See also* carbohydrates

sacral region, 482

sagittal plane, 432

saturated fat, 240

scale, graph, 176

scale, measuring device. *See* balance

scapula, 483

science, 10–15, 28–71, 78–110
    changing nature of, 14, 109
    definition, 10
    explanations, 11–13, 78–79
    facts, 11, 81, 101–104, 107–108
    fields of, 14–15
    math, 117–127, 135–142, 145, 170–181
    measurement, 122–127, 135–141, 144–154, 158–162, 170–174
    methods, 78–110
    scientific laws, 106–109
    scientific theories, 107–109
    study skills, 4–7, 17–22
    vocabulary, 28–71

scientific laws, 107–109

scientific methods, 78–110
    definition, 81
    diagnostic scientific method, 94–105
    experimental scientific method, 83–93
    proving laws and theories false, 109

scientific terminology. *See* terminology

scientific theories, 107–109

scientific vocabulary. *See* terminology

scrotum, 538

sebaceous glands, 476

sebum, 476

secondary structure, protein, 249

secretion, 398, 533

secretory vesicles, 302, 358, 373

segmentation, 527

selective permeability, 284, 322

tarsals, 484
teaching others, 22
telophase, 379
temperature, 154–155, 173–174, 339
    converting between metric and English units, 173–174
    degrees Celsius, 154–155
    factor in diffusion speed, 339
tendon, 409
terminology
    assembling word parts, 31–32, 36, 41–42, 46, 51, 56, 61, 65, 70
    body-related word parts, 68–71
    color-related word parts, 49–52
    construction, 28–33
    definition, 18
    directional word parts, 39–42
    disassembling word parts, 28–30, 32, 37, 42, 47, 51, 56, 61, 66, 71
    location-related word parts, 64–67
    number-related word parts, 44–48
    opposing meanings, 34–37
    shape-related word parts, 59–62
    size-related word parts, 54–57
    terms of location, 447–452
    understanding from context, 33, 37, 42, 48, 52, 57, 62, 67, 71
    word parts, 29, 34–71
tertiary structure, protein, 249
testes, 538
test, step of diagnostic scientific method, 97, 101, 104
test taking, 7. See also study skills
theories, scientific, 107–108
thermometer, 154
thoracic cage, 481
thoracic cavity, 436
thoracic region, 441, 482
thymine (T), 261
thymus, 522
thyroid gland, 503
thyroid-stimulating hormone (TSH), 502–503

thyrotropin, 503
thyroxine (T$_4$), 503
tibia, 480, 484
tight junction, 314
tissue, level of body organization, 457
tissues, 388–423, 455, 457
    avascular, 390
    characteristics of, 388–390
    connective, 404–416
    definition, 388
    epithelial, 392–402
    excitable, 419–423
    muscle, 420–422
    nerve, 423
    types of, 388
    vascular, 390
title, graph, 176
trabecular bone. See spongy bone
trait, 266, 293–294
transcription, protein synthesis, 372–373
trans fat, 242
transfer RNA (tRNA), 372–373
transitional cell, 395, 401
transitional epithelium, 401
translation, protein synthesis, 372–373
transport vesicles, 300, 373
transverse plane, 433
triiodothyronine (T$_3$), 503
tRNA. See transfer RNA (tRNA)
tropic hormone, 502. See also hormones
true ribs, 481
trunk, 441, 481–482
TSH. See thyroid-stimulating hormone (TSH)
tube, surface area, 140–141
tubule, 56, 398–399, 532–533
tubulins, 308
turnover rate, 257

U

ulna, 480, 484
umbilical region, 443
uniform distribution, 338

units, 124–125, 136, 145, 170–174
    converting between metric and English units, 170–174
    cubic, 145
    metric, 122–127
    square, 136
unsaturated fat, 240
uphill reactions, 334–335, 356–361
upper limbs, 444, 484
uracil (U), 261
ureter, 534
urethra, 534
urinary bladder, 534
urinary system, 458, 460, 530–534
    definition, 530
    filtration, 532
    functions of, 530
    kidneys, 531
    nephrons, 531–533
    reabsorption, 533
    secretion, 533
    urinary tract, 534
urinary tract, 534
urine, 468, 533
uterus, 538

V

vagina, 538
valves, heart, 515
variables, experiment, 85, 90
vascular tissue, 390
vein, 516
ventral, anatomical term, 435, 448
ventricle, 514
vertebrae, 416, 435, 441, 482
vertebral column, 482
vocabulary. See terminology
volume, 146–153, 172, 507
    converting between metric and English units, 172
    dry, 144–150
    liquid, 151–153
    ratio of surface area to, 146–150
    relation to air pressure, 507
voluntary muscle, 421, 488–492

Answer Key

Chapter 1 Learning About Science

Section 1.1 Using This Book

Concept 5: Active Learning

1. active learning
2. short-term, long-term

Concept 6: Reinforcing Knowledge

1. strengthen
2. section reinforcement and comprehensive review sections

Concept 7: Checking Your Work

1. reread
2. because science builds upon itself

Concept 8: Testing Yourself

1. to help you retrieve information, to help you practice for an exam
2. memory, reinforces

Section 1.1 Reinforcement

1. 20–30
2. false
3. section reinforcement and comprehensive review
4. reinforce; to strengthen your knowledge of a topic
5. Basic, complicated
6. B
7. using your hands or feet—by writing, typing, or walking, for example—while studying material
8. false
9. red, italicized
10. where terms are introduced
11. Science builds on itself.
12. physical activity
13. chapter review, comprehensive review
14. false
15. reread, correct
16. writing, reading, hearing, speaking
17. five times a day
18. itself
19. C
20. Testing yourself at the end of each chapter will help you retrieve information you've learned and will hone your skills in test taking so you can excel in an anatomy and physiology course.

Comprehensive Review (Chapter 1)

21. 20–30 minutes

Section 1.2 What Is Science?

Concept 1: Defining Science

1. facts
2. Science
3. subatomic, atoms, molecules, cells, organisms

Concept 2: What Science Seeks

1. phenomenon
2. natural
3. phenomena

Concept 3: Facts

1. fact
2. opinion, people and opinions
3. connects

Concept 4: Natural Explanations

1. natural
2. measured, tested

Concept 5: Supernatural Explanations

1. supernatural
2. tested
3. Supernatural explanations are not science because they cannot be tested.

Concept 6: Science and the Supernatural

1. facts
2. science, supernatural
3. one

Concept 7: Explaining Observations

1. natural
2. supernatural

Concept 8: Acceptance Versus Belief

1. based
2. It is not correct to say you believe in science because science is not based on your opinions or feelings.

Concept 9: Science Changes

1. No. If, in the future, additional evidence leads to a better explanation, science will change.
2. change

Concept 10: Fields of Science

1. fields
2. life
3. Anatomy, physiology

Section 1.2 Reinforcement

1. confirmed
2. B, C, E
3. false
4. explanations
5. Accept. It is not correct to say you believe in science because science is not based on your opinions or feelings.
6. evidence
7. true
8. Scientific
9. false
10. natural; observable and testable
11. Science uses natural explanations because they can be observed and tested.
12. You can only see one side of a coin (science or the supernatural) at a time.
13. life
14. true
15. science
16. Supernatural
17. independent
18. certain

19. science; the body of knowledge and techniques that enables mankind to explain the natural world
20. true
21. feelings, opinions
22. true
23. Science is based on facts which are observable and testable.
24. observable, testable
25. evidence
26. genetics (study of inheritance), cytology (study of cells), histology (study of tissues), anatomy (study of the parts of the body), physiology (study of the functions of body parts)
27. C
28. A
29. D
30. B
31. E
32. G
33. H
34. I
35. J
36. F

Comprehensive Review (Chapter 1)

37. Active learning is using your hands or feet—by writing, typing, or walking, for example—while studying material.

Section 1.3 Study Skills

Concept 1: Studying

1. learning
2. studying
3. long-term

Concept 2: Understanding Terminology

1. success
2. vocabulary

Concept 3: Having a Good Attitude

1. attitude
2. success, failure

3. attitude

Concept 4: Thinking Positively

1. like, dislike
2. negative
3. like

Concept 5: Concentrating

1. one
2. varying

Concept 6: Using Mnemonics

1. mnemonic
2. blemn

Concept 7: Repetition, Repetition, Repetition

1. writing, reading, hearing, speaking
2. studying
3. five

Concept 8: Rewarding Yourself

1. value
2. intervals

Concept 9: Teaching Others

1. Teaching
2. mastered

Section 1.3 Reinforcement

1. success
2. attitude
3. true
4. successful; the character of achieving a goal
5. D
6. repetition; practicing repeatedly
7. scientific
8. a word, acronym, or phrase that can help you recall information
9. false
10. studying
11. attention
12. true
13. knowledge
14. attitude; your way of feeling, thinking about, and viewing a situation
15. true

16. terminology; the words used in science
17. true
18. one
19. view
20. writing, reading, hearing, speaking
21. Rewarding, celebrating

Comprehensive Review (Chapter 1)

22. Natural explanations are based on observable and testable facts. Supernatural explanations are based on feelings and opinions.

Chapter 1 Review

1. observation
2. because science builds upon itself
3. attitude
4. facts
5. 20–30
6. false
7. true
8. Facts
9. phenomenon
10. Studying
11. Yes. If, in the future, additional evidence leads to a better explanation, science will change.
12. true
13. active learning
14. No. Scientific evidence is based on facts. Opinions are based on people and feelings.
15. Science
16. location, time, duration, method
17. Supernatural explanations are not observable and testable.
18. natural
19. true
20. 10
21. natural
22. because science is not based on your opinions or feelings

23. You can only see one side of a coin (science or the supernatural) at a time.
24. true
25. knowledge
26. A, D
27. reward
28. Biology
29. Anatomy is the study of the parts of the body; physiology studies the functions of body parts.

Comprehensive Review (Chapter 1)

30. B
31. F
32. H
33. D
34. G
35. J
36. A
37. K
38. E
39. I
40. C
41. N
42. M
43. Q
44. L
45. P
46. O

Chapter 2 Scientific Vocabulary

Section 2.1 Word Construction

Concept 1: Scientific Words

1. descriptive
2. Disassembling
3. bones

Concept 2: Word Parts

1. prefix—a letter or group of letters preceding a combining form; combining form—a root word plus its combining vowel; suffix—a letter or group of letters following a combining form

2. -tic
3. life
4. not
5. pertaining to something that is not alive

Concept 3: Word Disassembly

1. bi/o + -logy
2. life; study of
3. A cut is made into the tonsils.

Concept 4: Word Assembly

1. biologist
2. physiologist
3. anatomist
4. physiological

Concept 5: Applying Word Disassembly and Assembly

1. cytology
2. derm/o + -lysis; breakdown of the skin
3. biomorphic
4. a- + morph + -ous; the nature of something without form
5. hydrogen
6. cardi + -um; heart structure
7. pseudomorph
8. an- + hydr + -ous; the nature of something without water
9. hydrostasis
10. hydr/o + morph + -ic; pertaining to the form of water
11. neoplasm
12. bi/o + -genesis; production of life

Concept 6: Word Context

1. new
2. condition
3. false

Section 2.1 Reinforcement

1. breakdown of cells
2. pseudopod
3. prefix
4. true
5. pseudo- + morph + -ic; pertaining to a false form
6. C
7. water
8. false
9. morphogenesis

10. A, B, D
11. cells
12. false
13. cyt
14. form
15. anti-
16. true
17. against
18. pertaining to formation
19. prefix, combining form, suffix

Comprehensive Review (Chapters 1–2)

20. because science builds upon itself
21. combining forms, prefixes, suffixes

Section 2.2 Word Parts with Opposite Meanings

Concept 1: Opposite Word Parts

1. before
   same
   after
   loving
   above; beyond
   inside
   fearing
   below
   outside
   different
   within
   between
2. endo-
   hypo-
   hetero-
   -philic
   pre-
   intra-
   ecto-
   hyper-
   homo-
   -phobic
   post-
   inter-
3. endo-—ecto-; intra-—inter-; hetero-—homo-; -philic—-phobic; pre-—post-; hyper-—hypo-

Concept 2: Assembling Terms

1. hydrophilic
2. hypoderm
3. intracytic
4. homomorph
5. endocardial

Concept 3: Disassembling Terms

1. endo- + cardi/o + -logist; one who studies the inside of the heart
2. cyt/o + -philic; loving cells
3. hetero- + morph; different form
4. hydr/o + -phobic; water fearing
5. ecto- + derm; outside the skin

Concept 4: Using Context

1. beyond
2. avoid or fear
3. between
4. outside

Section 2.2 Reinforcement

1. true
2. E
3. -phobic; fearing
4. hetero-; different
5. -phobic
6. C
7. after
8. true
9. ecto-; outside
10. true
11. outside
12. inter-
13. A
14. Hyper-; hypo-
15. -philic
16. false
17. intra-
18. intra-; within
19. false
20. hypo-

Comprehensive Review (Chapters 1–2)

21. one who studies
22. Science

Section 2.3 Word Parts Related to Directions

Concept 1: Direction Word Parts

1. epi-—upon; dis-—apart; ad-—toward; infra-—under; ex-—out of; con-—together; supra-—above; ef-—away from; in-—into
2. sub-
   con-
   ex-
   in-
   ad-, af-
   ab-, ef-
   supra-
   epi-
   dis-
   sub-
3. apart
   below
   into
   under
   away from
   away from
   toward
   upon
   above
   out of
   together
   toward

Concept 2: Assembling Terms

1. epicardium
2. distension
3. hyperextension
4. adduction
5. conduction

Concept 3: Disassembling Terms

1. hypo- + ex- + tens + -ion; the process of stretching out from the body below the normal range of movement
2. in- + duct + -ion; the process of carrying something in
3. supra- + duct + -ion; the process of carrying above
4. infra- + cyt/o + -logy; the study of things under (inferior to) the cell

5. sub- + derm + -al; the character of something below the skin

Concept 4: Using Context

1. away from; toward
2. toward
3. out; in
4. below
5. taken apart
6. above
7. below

Section 2.3 Reinforcement

1. false
2. B, F
3. infra-; under
4. above
5. E
6. B
7. supra-; above
8. false
9. dis-; apart
10. false
11. ab-, ad-, af-, con-, dis-, ef-, epi-, supra-
12. A
13. supra-
14. below
15. ad- and af-
16. true
17. away from
18. ab- and ef-
19. true
20. below

Comprehensive Review (Chapters 1–2)

21. true
22. B, C, E

Section 2.4 Word Parts Related to Numbers

Concept 1: Number Word Parts

1. hexa-
   omni-
   tri-
   quadri-, tetra-
   di-, bi-
   mono-, uni-
   poly-
   hemi-

2. one—uni-; two—di-; three—tri-; four—quadri-; six—hexa-; all—omni-; many—poly-

3. two
   one
   many
   one
   three
   four
   four
   all
   two
   half

Concept 2: Assembling Terms

1. triceps
2. monocyte
3. quadriplegia
4. quadriceps
5. omniology

Concept 3: Disassembling Terms

1. uni- + morph; one form
2. poly- + cyst + -ic; pertaining to many cysts
3. di- + -plegia; paralysis of two parts of the body
4. tetra- + -logy; the study of four things
5. bi- + cardi + -al; the character of having two hearts

Concept 4: Using Context

1. two
2. three
3. six
4. four

Section 2.4 Reinforcement

1. many
2. C, F
3. tetra-; four
4. four
5. A, C, D
6. B, E
7. poly-; many
8. two
9. mono-; one
10. true
11. two
12. D
13. hexa-; six

14. mono-, di-, tri-, quadri-, hexa-
15. one
16. false
17. hexa-, tetra-, tri-, bi-, uni-
18. quadri-; four
19. false
20. B
21. half

Comprehensive Review (Chapters 1–2)

22. attitude
23. loving

Section 2.5 Word Parts Related to Colors

Concept 1: Color Word Parts

1. blue
   red
   green
   yellow
   black
   white
   red
   white

2. erythr/o, rubr/o
   cyan/o
   alb/o, leuk/o
   lute/o
   chlor/o
   melan/o

3. chlor/o—green; leuk/o—white; lute/o—yellow; rubr/o—red; cyan/o—blue; melan/o—black

Concept 2: Assembling Terms

1. cyanosis
2. chlorophobic
3. melanoma
4. leukocytosis
5. luteolysis

Concept 3: Disassembling Terms

1. leuk + -osis; condition of whiteness (white blood cells)
2. lute + -um; yellow structure
3. melan/o + -genesis; production of black (melanin)
4. cyan/o + -gen; blue producer
5. erythr/o + -stasis; stoppage of red (blood cells)

Concept 4: Using Context

1. white
2. black
3. white
4. green

Section 2.5 Reinforcement

1. true
2. A, C
3. chlor/o; green
4. blue
5. B, D
6. E
7. chlor/o, cyan/o, erythr/o, leuk/o, melan/o, rubr/o
8. false
9. leuk/o; white
10. false
11. green
12. C
13. cyan/o
14. cyan/o; blue
15. alb/o and leuk/o
16. true
17. rubr/o and erythr/o
18. melan/o; black
19. true
20. B

Comprehensive Review (Chapters 1–2)

21. true
22. endo-; inside

Section 2.6 Word Parts Related to Sizes

Concept 1: Size Word Parts

1. large
   1/1000 of one unit
   small
   half
   large
   1000 units
   beyond
   small
   1/100 of one unit

2. kilo-
   micro-, -ule
   semi-
   macro-, mega-

milli-

ultra-

centi-

3. mega-—large; micro-—small; semi-—half; ultra-—beyond; kilo-—1000 units; centi-—$\frac{1}{100}$ of one unit; milli-—$\frac{1}{1000}$ of one unit

Concept 2: Assembling Terms

1. microphage
2. semihydrophilic
3. macrocytosis
4. megamorphology

Concept 3: Disassembling Terms

1. ultra- + hydr/o + -phobic; beyond fearing water
2. macro- + bi/o + -tic; pertaining to a large living thing
3. micro- + tens + -ion; the process of stretching a small amount
4. lun + -ule; small crescent shape

Concept 4: Using Context

1. large
2. small
3. 100
4. beyond
5. small
6. 2000
7. one-half
8. 1000

Section 2.6 Reinforcement

1. false
2. B
3. ultra-; beyond
4. small
5. macro-, mega-, micro-, semi-, ultra-
6. C, D
7. -ule; small
8. true
9. semi-; half
10. large
11. D
12. mega- and macro-
13. small
14. true
15. beyond

16. false
17. A, C
18. micro-; small
19. true
20. larger
21. small

Comprehensive Review (Chapters 1–2)

22. black
23. false

Section 2.7 Word Parts Related to Shapes

Concept 1: Shape Word Parts

1. wide

   flat

   jagged

   straight

   round

   layer

   narrow

   hollow

   triangular

2. platy-

   rect/o

   coel/o

   strat/o

   sten/o

   delt/o

   lat/o

   serrat/o

   glob/o

3. lat/o—wide; rect/o—straight; platy-—flat; glob/o—round; coel/o—hollow; strat/o—layer; delt/o—triangular; serrat/o—jagged; sten/o—narrow

Concept 2: Assembling Terms

1. serration
2. deltoid
3. stenosis
4. rectum

Concept 3: Disassembling Terms

1. sten + -osis; condition of narrowing
2. coel + -um; hollow structure
3. strat + -um; layer structure
4. platy- + morph + -ia; condition of a flat form

Concept 4: Using Context

1. round
2. hollow
3. triangular
4. jagged
5. straight
6. wide
7. flat
8. round

Section 2.7 Reinforcement

1. serrat/o; jagged
2. platy-; flat
3. lat/o
4. hollow
5. true
6. B
7. true
8. sten/o; narrow
9. false
10. lat/o
11. B, C
12. delt/o; triangular
13. D
14. round
15. true
16. glob/o; round
17. true
18. C

Comprehensive Review (Chapters 1–2)

19. life
20. hyper-; above or beyond

Section 2.8 Word Parts Related to Locations

Concept 1: Location Word Parts

1. belly side (of body)

   around

   middle

   down from

   back (of body)

   outer region

   side

   middle

2. dors/o

   later/o

   peri-

   meso-, medi/o

ventr/o

de-

cortic/o

3. meso-—middle; ventr/o—belly
   side (of body); dors/o—back (of
   body); cortic/o—outer region;
   later/o—side; peri-—around;
   de-—down from

Concept 2: Assembling Terms

1. pericardium
2. mesoderm
3. lateral
4. ventrolateral

Concept 3: Disassembling Terms

1. peri- + oste + -oma; tumor
   around a bone
2. meso- + morph; middle form
3. dors + -al; character of the
   back of the body
4. ventr/o + medi + -al; character
   of the middle belly of the body

Concept 4: Using Context

1. outer
2. around
3. back
4. sides
5. middle
6. belly
7. down

Section 2.8 Reinforcement

1. true
2. B
3. cortic/o; outer region
4. belly side (of the body)
5. peri-; around
6. D
7. medi/o, meso-
8. false
9. later/o; side
10. false
11. ventr/o; belly side (of the body)
12. D
13. medi/o; middle
14. around
15. cortic/o; outer region
16. true
17. later/o
18. B, E
19. false

20. side

Comprehensive Review (Chapters 1–2)

21. away from
22. One should accept an explana-
    tion because science is based
    on facts, not opinions.

Section 2.9 Word Parts Related to the Body

Concept 1: Body Word Parts

1. muscle
   kidney
   stomach
   joint
   intestine
   liver
   nerve
   blood
   brain
2. ren/o
   gastr/o
   hem/o
   arthr/o
   neur/o
   my/o
   cerebr/o
   hepat/o
   enter/o
3. neur/o—nerve; gastr/o—
   stomach; hem/o—blood;
   my/o—muscle; enter/o—
   intestine; hepat/o—liver;
   ren/o—kidney; cerebr/o—
   brain; arthr/o—joint

Concept 2: Assembling Terms

1. neurology
2. myogenesis
3. arthralgia
4. enterotomy
5. hemolysis

Concept 3: Disassembling Terms

1. arthr + -osis; condition of a
   joint
2. my/o + cyt/o + -lysis; breakdown of muscle cells
3. supra- + ren + -al; character of
   above the kidney
4. cerebr + -oma; tumor in the
   brain

5. gastr/o + enter + -itis; inflammation of the stomach and
   intestine
6. hepat/o + -logist; one who
   studies the liver

Concept 4: Using Context

1. brain
2. kidney
3. joint
4. stomach

Section 2.9 Reinforcement

1. enter/o; intestine
2. B
3. hepat/o; liver
4. kidney
5. gastr/o, hem/o, hepat/o, my/o,
   neur/o, ren/o
6. B
7. cerebr/o; brain
8. true
9. neur/o; nerve
10. true
11. gastr/o
12. E
13. B
14. false
15. cerebr/o
16. false
17. C
18. the stomach
19. false
20. B, D, E

Comprehensive Review (Chapters 1–2)

21. false
22. one

Chapter 2 Review

1. bi/o; life
2. morph
3. -stasis; stay or stop
4. bi- + later + -al; character of
   two sides
5. breakdown
6. a- + morph + -ous; the nature
   of something without form
7. liver
8. false
9. A, C

10. below
11. after
12. A
13. between
14. life
15. endocardiosis
16. physi/o; function
17. F
18. apart
19. hydr; water
20. hemi- + cerebr + -um; the structure of half the brain
21. B
22. brain
23. A
24. uni- and mono-
25. three
26. many
27. quadri- and tetra-
28. red
29. B
30. small
31. one-half
32. false
33. A
34. gastroenterology
35. glob/o
36. triangular
37. bone; joints

Comprehensive Review (Chapters 1–2)

38. C
39. E
40. D
41. J
42. F
43. B
44. I
45. G
46. A
47. H
48. K

Chapter 3 Scientific Methods

Section 3.1 Science Is Part of Everyday Life

Concept 1: An Everyday Problem

1. natural
2. natural—A, D; supernatural—B, C

Concept 2: Possible Cause

1. test
2. one

Concept 3: Test Results

1. is not
2. voltage

Concept 4: New Possible Cause

1. loose
2. Tightening

Concept 5: Steps in Everyday Science

1. logical
2. another
3. predicted, tested

Concept 6: Scientific Methods

1. logical
2. evidence
3. pathways

Concept 7: Testing with Facts

1. facts
2. rejected, modified
3. jigsaw puzzle

Section 3.1 Reinforcement

1. false
2. answer
3. true
4. facts
5. facts
6. logical
7. true
8. reject the solution and modify it to test again
9. rejected
10. method; a way of answering a question or solving a problem
11. true

12. evidence; facts that relate to a possible cause
13. true
14. logical
15. scientific method

Comprehensive Review (Chapters 1–3)

16. C
17. evidence
18. Science

Section 3.2 The Experimental Scientific Method Pathway

Concept 1: Steps in the Experimental Scientific Method

1. observation
2. observation, hypothesis, experiment, analysis, data

Concept 2: Hypothesis

1. prediction
2. this, that

Concept 3: Variables

1. independent, dependent
2. dependent, independent
3. independent
4. dependent
5. "if"

Concept 4: Experiment

1. experiment
2. control, experimental, constants
3. The experimental group receives the independent variable, but the control group does not.
4. control and experimental groups

Concept 5: Analysis

1. analysis
2. experimental, control
3. Did the independent variable cause the predicted change in the dependent variable?

Concept 6: Decide

1. decide
2. reject
3. accept

Concept 7: Beyond the Five Steps

1. accept
2. reject

Section 3.2 Reinforcement

1. predicts
2. independent
3. observation
4. accept, reject
5. true
6. untested
7. hypothesis
8. hypothesis
9. depends
10. analysis
11. true
12. constants
13. hypothesis
14. hypothesis
15. false
16. dependent
17. hypothesis; a prediction about the outcome of an experiment
18. hypothesis
19. experiment
20. false
21. D
22. F
23. C
24. A
25. B
26. E

Comprehensive Review (Chapters 1–3)

27. not
28. phenomena
29. evidence

Section 3.3 The Experimental Scientific Method in Action

Concept 1: Make an Observation

1. have more fat
2. humane

Concept 2: Develop a Hypothesis

1. high-fat diet
2. prediction
3. dependent

Concept 3: Perform an Experiment

1. control
2. tests
3. experimental
4. control

Concept 4: The Control Group

1. independent
2. calories

Concept 5: Understanding Constants

1. Constants
2. independent

Concept 6: Regulating Constants

1. uniform
2. random
3. dark
4. same

Concept 7: Analyze the Data

1. 64
2. 43
3. 12.8
4. 8.6

Concept 8: Accept or Reject the Hypothesis

1. If rats are fed a high-fat diet, then they will gain more fat.
2. yes
3. The hypothesis should be accepted. (Explanations will vary.)
4. high-fat diet and gain of fat

Section 3.3 Reinforcement

1. the same
2. subjects
3. have more fat
4. true
5. analysis; examining data
6. independent
7. reject
8. 100
9. false
10. fat
11. If, then
12. observation
13. independent
14. false

15. constants; untested factors that could affect the dependent variable
16. control group
17. constants
18. true
19. untested
20. dependent

Comprehensive Review (Chapters 1–3)

21. hypothesis
22. strat/o
23. natural

Section 3.4 Diagnostic Scientific Method Pathway

Concept 1: Steps in the Diagnostic Scientific Method

1. cause of, treatment for
2. patient history, physical exam
3. Facts, Sift, Test, Diagnose

Concept 2: Obtain Facts from Patient History

1. patient history
2. questionnaire

Concept 3: Obtain Facts from a Physical Exam

1. examining
2. blood pressure, temperature, pulse, respiratory rate

Concept 4: Sift Facts

1. sifts
2. likely
3. ranks
4. 3, 5, 2, 4, 1

Concept 5: Perform Tests

1. biopsy
2. ultrasound
3. CT scan

Concept 6: Diagnose

1. confirm
2. diagnose
3. 100%
4. uncertainty
5. certain

Section 3.4 Reinforcement

1. cause
2. facts
3. true
4. facts, sift, test, diagnose
5. facts
6. facts
7. true
8. most, least
9. likely
10. rejected
11. diagnosis
12. true
13. Sifting
14. vital
15. test
16. ultrasound
17. false
18. diagnostic
19. patient history, physical exam
20. some
21. sift
22. diagnose

Comprehensive Review (Chapters 1–3)

23. white
24. false
25. understanding

Section 3.5 The Diagnostic Scientific Method in Action

Concept 1: Case 1—Gathering Facts from Patient History

1. 21, female
2. tired, thirsty, always going to the bathroom
3. heart attacks, high blood pressure, high cholesterol, diabetes, obesity

Concept 2: Case 1—Gathering Facts from the Patient Exam

1. 140/95
2. dark patches

Concept 3: Case 1—Sifting Facts

1. fatigue, hunger, thirst, frequent urination
2. anemia, cardiovascular system disease

Concept 4: Case 1—Performing Tests

1. sugar
2. 7.0%

Concept 5: Case 1—Making a Diagnosis

1. 7.0%
2. diabetes

Concept 6: Case 2—Gathering Facts from Patient History

1. 18, male
2. vomiting and belly pain
3. high cholesterol, kidney stones

Concept 7: Case 2—Gathering Facts from the Patient Exam

1. 130/85
2. dehydration

Concept 8: Case 2—Sifting Facts

1. kidney stones, appendicitis
2. gastroenteritis, colitis

Concept 9: Case 2—Performing Tests

1. CT
2. a kidney stone in the left kidney

Concept 10: Case 2—Making a Diagnosis

1. kidney stones
2. appendicitis
3. gastroenteritis, colitis

Section 3.5 Reinforcement

1. hemoglobin A1C
2. fatigue, hunger, thirst, frequent urination
3. true
4. pain, fever, nausea, vomiting
5. C
6. type 1, type 2
7. patient history, physical exam
8. true
9. CT scan
10. true
11. blood pressure
12. true
13. diagnosis; confirmation of the cause of an ailment
14. Test

15. false
16. normal
17. 10
18. confirmed; tested and found to be true
19. no
20. Pinching

Comprehensive Review (Chapters 1–3)

21. joint
22. supernatural
23. observation

Section 3.6 Laws and Theories

Concept 1: Scientific Laws

1. law
2. expectation
3. predictable

Concept 2: Scientific Theories

1. theory
2. understanding
3. evidence

Concept 3: Facts, Laws, and Theories

1. fact
2. law
3. theory

Concept 4: The Hierarchy of Facts, Laws, and Theories

1. laws
2. fact
3. theories

Concept 5: Proving Laws and Theories False

1. can
2. Contradicting
3. modified

Concept 6: Scientific Journals

1. literature
2. build
3. published

Concept 7: Scientific Articles

1. abstract
2. materials and methods
3. supporting

Section 3.6 Reinforcement

1. theory
2. fact
3. literature cited
4. Scientists
5. They can if contradicting evidence is found.
6. explanation
7. false
8. hierarchy
9. results
10. summary
11. scientific theories
12. true
13. theories
14. introduction
15. true
16. support
17. One fact, by itself, may not tell you much.
18. articles
19. abstract
20. results
21. (Answers will vary.)
22. scientific law

Comprehensive Review (Chapters 1–3)

23. around
24. fields
25. patient history, physical exam

Chapter 3 Review

1. false
2. facts
3. analysis
4. control
5. "then"
6. Constants
7. facts
8. facts, diagnose
9. diagnosis
10. natural
11. scientific theory, scientific law, fact
12. scientific article
13. accept, reject
14. accept
15. rejected
16. independent variable, dependent variable

17. Observation, Hypothesis, Experiment, Analysis, Decide
18. scientific method
19. literature cited
20. dependent
21. independent variable—temperature; dependent variable—whether water freezes
22. false
23. C
24. "then"
25. The experimental group receives the independent variable, and the control group does not.
26. independent
27. true
28. independent
29. abstract, introduction, materials and methods section, results section, discussion section, literature cited section
30. scientific journals

Comprehensive Review (Chapters 1–3)

31. E
32. B
33. G
34. I
35. D
36. J
37. H
38. A
39. F
40. C
41. O
42. L
43. M
44. N
45. K

Chapter 4 Math and Measurement

Section 4.1 Fractions, Decimals, and Percentages

Concept 1: Fractions

1. four

2. three, ¾
3. one, ¼

Concept 2: Decimals

1. 0.001, 0.01, 0.1, 1, 10, 1000
2. two
   three
   one
   zero
   two
   one
3. largest number—1000, smallest number—0.001
4. 0.002
5. $^{67}/_{100}$

Concept 3: Converting Fractions into Decimals

1. 0.2
2. 0.5
3. 3.5

Concept 4: Rounding

1. 2.8
2. 93
3. 0.24
4. 0.676
5. 28

Concept 5: Percentages

1. 30%
2. 25%
3. 40%
4. 75%
5. 50%
6. 75%
   25%
   100%

Concept 6: Calculating Percentages from Data

1. 50 people
2. 64% of people
3. 32% of people
4. 4% of people

Concept 7: Converting Percentages into Other Numbers

1. 45 people
2. 150 questions
3. 2285.71 mg sodium
   27.27 g fiber
   1000 mg calcium

Section 4.1 Reinforcement

1. 33%
2. ¼, ⅜, ½
3. true
4. ⅞ of the circle
5. 125 people
6. 24 people
7. 75 people
8. 75% of the circle
9. false
10. percentage; the number of parts out of 100 parts
11. 60% of students
12. 20%
13. 7/16 of the circle
14. 50 students
15. false
16. 10% of the class
17. 25% of the circle
18. 25% of the people
19. ¾ of the circle
20. ⅝, ½, ⅜, ¼, ⅛
21. ⅙
22. ⅜ of the rectangle is shaded; ⅝ of the rectangle is not shaded
23. a part of a whole number
24. percentage

Comprehensive Review (Chapters 1–4)

25. Fractions represent a part of any whole number, while percentages specifically describe the number of parts out of 100 parts.
26. di-
27. hypothesis
28. Anatomy is the study of body parts, and physiology is the study of functions of body parts.

Section 4.2 The Metric System

Concept 1: Powers of 10

1. 100
2. one
3. 10
4. 10
5. 200
6. 1.5 dollars
7. 120
8. one
9. 692 pennies

Concept 2: Moving the Decimal Point

1. larger
2. Dividing
3. right, left
4. multiply
5. left
6. 2, right
   3, left
   3, right
   2, left
7. left, 3
   left, 2
   left, 1
   (neither left nor right), 0
   right, 3
   right, 1
   right, 2

Concept 3: Metric Units

1. meter
2. gram
3. liter
4. degree Celsius
5. milliliters
6. centigrams
7. smallest unit—millimeter, largest unit—kilometer
8. meter
   centimeter
   kilogram
   gram
   kilogram
   liter
9. milligram
   milliliter
   centimeter
   millimeter
   milligram

Concept 4: Conversion Direction

1. small to large
   small to large
   small to large
   large to small
   large to small
   small to large
   large to small
   large to small
   small to large
   small to large
2. multiply
   divide
   divide
   divide
   multiply
   multiply
3. right
   left
   right
   right
   left
   right

Concept 5: Converting Between Metric Units

1. small to large
   large to small
   large to small
   small to large
   small to large
   small to large
2. multiply, 1000, right
   divide, 1000, left
   multiply, 1000, right
   divide, 1000, left
   multiply, 1000, right
   divide, 1000, left
3. 0.1 kilograms
4. 10,000 milliliters
5. 10 millimeters
6. 0.1 meters
7. 100,000 grams

Section 4.2 Reinforcement

1. C
2. right
3. false
4. 1000
5. 0.5 mm, 1 mm, 6 mm, 1 cm, 7 cm
6. 0.5 m
7. 1000
8. E
9. smaller
10. 100
11. 1.7 cm
12. 1500 milliliters

13. true
14. liter; the metric unit of volume
15. false
16. 200 mL, 0.3 L, 1000 mL, 2.4 L, 4 L
17. 1000
18. A, C, E, F
19. gram
20. 20 cm, 186 mm, 0.15 m, 1.7 cm, 16 mm
21. 30 mm
22. 1000
23. false
24. A
25. false
26. C
27. D
28. F
29. G
30. B
31. E
32. A

Comprehensive Review (Chapters 1–4)

33. inside
34. $^{31}/_{100}$
35. true
36. independent

Section 4.3 Linear Measurements

Concept 1: Meters
1. meter
2. line
3. 1
4. 30

Concept 2: Centimeters and Millimeters
1. 8, 80
2. 1000, 100, 1

Concept 3: Reading Linear Measurements
1. 27.8 cm
2. 16.6 cm
3. (Draw a line 10 cm in length and label cm and mm.)

Concept 4: Measuring Lines
1. 31 mm

2. 7 cm
3. 10 mm
4. (Draw a line 5.4 cm in length.)
5. (Draw a line 32 mm in length.)

Section 4.3 Reinforcement
1. D
2. 7
3. 0.07 m
4. 1000
5. 20
6. 1000
7. true
8. 10
9. 100
10. divide
11. 100
12. 10
13. 1000
14. A
15. true
16. 65 cm
17. 1000
18. 10
19. false
20. 1.24 m

Comprehensive Review (Chapters 1–4)
21. red
22. degrees Celsius
23. independent
24. false

Section 4.4 Surface Area

Concept 1: Measuring the Width and Height of a Rectangle or Square
1. 40 mm, 4 cm
2. 20 mm, 2 cm

Concept 2: Calculating the Surface Area of a Rectangle or Square
1. surface area
2. cm^2
3. 6 cm × 2 cm = 12 cm^2

Concept 3: Calculating the Surface Area of a Cube
1. width: 4 cm, height: 4 cm, surface area: 96 cm^2

2. (Draw a 1 cm × 1 cm cube); surface area: 6 cm^2

Concept 4: Measuring the Radius and Diameter of a Circle
1.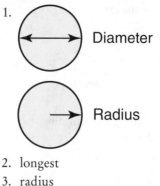

2. longest
3. radius
4. ½
5. 19 mm, 1.9 cm
   9.5 mm, 0.95 cm
6. 21 mm, 2.1 cm
   10.5 mm, 1.05 cm

Concept 5: Calculating the Surface Area of a Circle
1. 11
2. 3.14 × (2 cm)^2 = 3.14 × 4 cm^2 = 12.56 cm^2
3. 3.14 × (54 mm)^2 = 3.14 × 2916 mm^2 = 9156.24 mm^2

Concept 6: Calculating the Surface Area of a Tube
1. 30 mm
2. 60 mm
3. 60 mm
4. 11,304 mm^2

Concept 7: Calculating the Surface Area of a Cylinder
1. the surface area of the tube, the surface area of the top, the surface area of the bottom
2. surface area of the tube: 2 × 2 cm × 3.14 × 7 cm = 87.92 cm^2
   surface area of the top: 3.14 × (2 cm)^2 = 3.14 × 4 cm^2 = 12.56 cm^2
   surface area of the bottom: 3.14 × (2 cm)^2 = 3.14 × 4 cm^2 = 12.56 cm^2
   surface area of the cylinder: 87.92 cm^2 + 12.56 cm^2 + 12.56 cm^2 = 113.04 cm^2
3. 2.4 cm
   1.2 cm

0.8 cm

15 cm²

Section 4.4 Reinforcement

1. radius; the measurement from one edge of a circle to the center
2. false
3. A, B, D, F
4. 24 cm²
5. 3.14
6. width
7. 314 cm²
8. diameter
9. circle
10. area; the measurement of the outer surface of an object
11. 50
12. false
13. A, C
14. 8
15. true
16. 2110.08 cm²
17. 60
18. six sides
19. diameter; the longest measurement across a circle
20. 150 cm²
21. C
22. B
23. A

Comprehensive Review (Chapters 1–4)

24. 300
25. true
26. fact
27. true

Section 4.5 Dry Volume

Concept 1: Calculating the Dry Volume of a Cube

1. depth, width, height
2. Cubic
3. cubic centimeters
4. volume
5. 8 cm³

Concept 2: Ratios

1. 9:1
2. 6:1
3. 3:1

4. 1.5:1

Concept 3: Ratio of Surface Area to Volume

1. **Large cube**
   surface area: 216 cm²
   dry volume: 216 cm³
   ratio of surface area to dry volume: 216:216 (1:1)
   There is one unit of surface area for each unit of volume.

   Small cube
   surface area: 54 cm²
   dry volume: 27 cm³
   ratio of surface area to dry volume: 54:27 (2:1)
   There are two units of surface area for each unit of volume.
2. small
3. larger
4. 6:1
5. large cube: 1 unit
   small cube: 2 units
   smallest cube: 6 units

Concept 4: Cells and the Ratio of Surface Area to Volume

1. Raw materials, products, waste
2. plasma membrane
3. surface
4. small
5. large

Section 4.5 Reinforcement

1. B
2. 24 cm²
3. false
4. volume; the amount of space in a three-dimensional object
5. false
6. A, B
7. Raw materials
8. area
9. B
10. cubic; three measurements of the same units multiplied together
11. true
12. surface area
13. false

14. waste
15. large cube
16. volume; the amount of space in a three-dimensional object
17. A
18. microscopic
19. true
20. volume

Comprehensive Review (Chapters 1–4)

21. 30
22. sten/o
23. true
24. theories

Section 4.6 Liquid Volume and Temperature

Concept 1: Cubic Centimeters and Milliliters

1. 10 mL
2. equal to

Concept 2: Reading a Meniscus

1. meniscus
2. bottom
3. cylinder
4. 25
5. 14 mL
6. 36 mL

Concept 3: Celsius Scale

1. 0
2. degrees Celsius
3. 100

Concept 4: The Celsius Thermometer

1. degrees Celsius
2. nine marks
3. an individual
4. 42°C
5. −4°C
6. 24°C

Section 4.6 Reinforcement

1. meniscus; the semicircular surface of liquid in a cylinder
2. true
3. 100
4. 1000
5. degrees Celsius
6. A

7. Celsius
8. meniscus; the semicircular surface of liquid in a cylinder
9. 100
10. 0
11. false
12. A, D
13. 100
14. A, B, C, F
15. true
16. C, D, F
17. true
18. 10
19. water
20. milliliter; ⅟₁₀₀₀ of 1 liter
21. Liquid volume
22. meniscus

Comprehensive Review (Chapters 1–4)
23. C
24. 54 cm²
25. theory
26. view

Section 4.7 Mass

Concept 1: Mass Versus Weight
1. Mass
2. gravity
3. less

Concept 2: Grams
1. gram
2. nickel
3. 1
4. 1000, 1000, 1

Concept 3: The Platform Balance
1. three beams
2. individual, hundreds of, tens of

Concept 4: Using the Platform Balance
1. zero
2. platform
3. beams
4. weights
5. zero

Concept 5: Reading a Platform Balance
1. 352.8 g
2. 79 g

3. 135.9 g

Concept 6: Using an Electronic Balance
1. grams
2. to subtract the mass of the container from the mass of the object being measured

Section 4.7 Reinforcement
1. true
2. 0.5 kg
3. true
4. three
5. balance; an instrument that measures mass or weight
6. true
7. 168.5 g
8. gram
9. 100 g, 710 g, 0.75 kg, 1120 g, 1.2 kg
10. 96.4 g
11. false
12. platform balance; an instrument that measures the mass of an object in grams; has three beams with markings that indicate the number of grams
13. An object weighs more on the earth than on the moon. This is because the force of gravity on the moon is less than the force of gravity on the earth.
14. zero
15. weight; the force of gravity on the mass of an object
16. zero
17. 400 g, 30 g, 2.6 g
18. No, the three beams of a platform balance cannot read 0 g, 50 g, and 66 g. This is because one beam measures hundreds of grams, one measures tens of grams, and the last one measures individual grams.
19. mass
20. 412.3 g
21. mass
22. weight
23. An electronic balance measures mass digitally.
24. zero, tare

Comprehensive Review (Chapters 1–4)
25. pre-
26. 10
27. Studying
28. patient history, physical exam of patient

Section 4.8 Concentration, Pressure, and Rate

Concept 1: Concentration
1. A
2. A
3. three dots
4. equal

Concept 2: Concentration Units
1. salt
2. water
3. 5 mg/L
4. 2 mg/L
5. 3 mg/L

Concept 3: Pressure
1. increases
2. decreases
3. increases
4. increases

Concept 4: Blood Pressure
1. millimeters of mercury (mmHg)
2. ¹²⁰/₈₀ mmHg
3. ¹⁴⁰/₉₀ mmHg
4. increase
5. pressure when the heart is contracting, pressure when the heart is relaxing

Concept 5: Rate and Heart Rate
1. (Answers will vary.)
2. 40
3. time

Section 4.8 Reinforcement
1. solution; a liquid that has atoms dissolved in it
2. true
3. rate
4. solute
5. C
6. decreases
7. B, C

8. false
9. pressure; the collisions of atoms with other atoms and with the sides of a container
10. milligrams per liter (mg/L)
11. solute
12. A, B, C
13. moving
14. 10 mg
15. concentration; the number of atoms or molecules per one unit of volume
16. false
17. a volume
18. solvent
19. 95 mmHg
20. solvent
21. E
22. C
23. D
24. B
25. A

Comprehensive Review (Chapters 1–4)

26. bone, joint
27. 100 cm^2
28. questionnaire
29. natural

Section 4.9 Converting Between Metric and English Units of Measurement

Concept 1: Metric and English Measuring Systems

1. English
2. metric

Concept 2: Length Conversions

1. 12.7 cm
2. 15.24 cm
3. 0.45 m
4. 6.54 yards
5. 6.2 miles
6. 5.72 cm
7. 2.93 inches

Concept 3: Volume Conversions

1. 7.58 L
2. 14.79 mL
3. 9.5 L
4. 5.3 quarts
5. 0.14 fluid ounces
6. 1.56 gallons

Concept 4: Mass Conversions

1. 3.5 ounces
2. 22.1 pounds
3. 2.25 kg
4. 56.7 g

Concept 5: Temperature Conversions

1. 10°C
2. 68°F
3. 37.8°C
4. 95°F
5. 18.9°C
6. 32°F

Section 4.9 Reinforcement

1. 1.04 gallons
2. true
3. 30.48 cm
4. 45.48 liters
5. A
6. false
7. A, B, F, G, H
8. English
9. 3.28 feet/m
10. conversion; changing a measurement from one unit to another unit
11. 62 miles
12. 11.05 pounds
13. meter
14. 3 m
15. false
16. B, D, E, F
17. true
18. 161 km
19. 1.8 kg
20. false

Comprehensive Review (Chapters 1–4)

21. meniscus
22. one cell
23. diagnose
24. Biology

Section 4.10 Graphs

Concept 1: Parts of a Line Graph

1. title
2. y
3. scale

Concept 2: Reading a Line Graph

1. Daily Plant Height
2. centimeters
3. 7 cm
4. day 10
5. day 9
6. daily
7. No, plant height does not increase the same amount each day.
8. days 7–8
9. 14 cm
10. 0–14 days
11. 27 cm
12. days 5–6

Concept 3: Placing Points on a Line Graph

1. (Answers will vary.)

2–3.

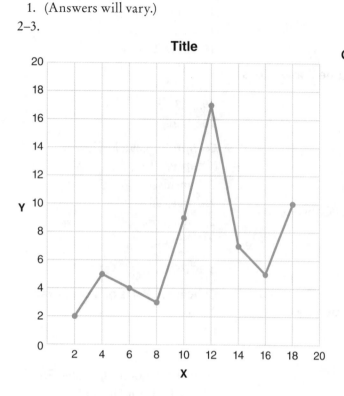

Title

Concept 4: Setting Up a Line Graph

1. smallest, largest

2. range

3.

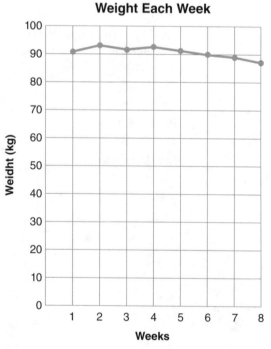

Weight Each Week

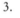

4. 87.2 kg, 93.1 kg

Concept 5: Reading a Bar Graph

1. October 20

2. 129 mmHg–141 mmHg

3. 82 mmHg–91 mmHg

Concept 6: Drawing a Bar Graph

1. 35

2. 68 bpm–121 bpm

3. x

4.

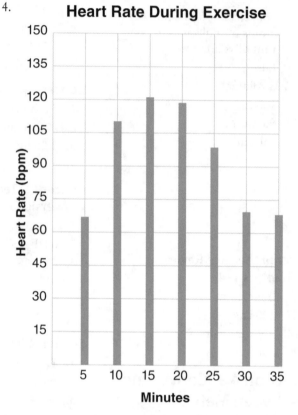

Section 4.10 Reinforcement

1. axes

2. graph; a visual representation of information

3. 2 mm–27 mm

4. false

5. x

6. graph; a visual representation of information

7. x

8. true

9. horizontal; running from left to right

10. y

11. y

12. 0.3 g–1.5 g

13. false

14. title

15. x

16. 2 g–11 g

17. B

18. numbers

**Comprehensive Review
(Chapters 1–4)**

19. 50 cm
20. true
21. true
22. Both sides of the coin exist, but you can see only one side at a time.

Chapter 4 Review

1. B, D
2. 3.4 cm
3. A
4. right
5. true
6. 1.5 cm
7. radius
8. diameter
9. false
10. C, E
11. 83 mm
12. cc
13. 96 cm²
14. Volume
15. the cubic centimeter
16. 150
17. boils
18. false
19. mass
20. An object weighs more on the earth than on the moon. This is because the force of gravity on the moon is less than the force of gravity on the earth.
21. 127.5 g
22. 1.5 kg
23. 200 g, 10 g, 3.1 g
24. 0.52 gallons
25. 1 inch
26. 30 m
27. false
28. 1–14
29. measured
30. x
31. line
32. ¾ of the circle
33. 20
34. 43%
35. Concentration

36. solute
37. true

**Comprehensive Review
(Chapters 1–4)**

38. E
39. J
40. H
41. B
42. A
43. D
44. F
45. I
46. C
47. G

Chapter 5
Chemistry

Section 5.1 Atoms

Concept 1: Subatomic Particles

1. (See Figure 5.1 in the text.)
2. proton, neutron, electron
3. protons, electrons
4. core
5. electron shell

Concept 2: Mass and Charge

1. 1 amu, positive
2. 1 amu, no
3. 0 amu, negative
4. atomic mass units
5. (See Figure 5.1 in the text.)
6. electron shell
7. core
8. core

Concept 3: Bonding

1. core, neutrons, electrons
2. proton, neutron
3. electron
4. Electrons can be donated to another atom, accepted from another atom, or shared between atoms.

Concept 4: Atomic Symbol

1. atomic symbol
2. elements
3. letter
4. nitrogen

oxygen

carbon

hydrogen

Concept 5: Atomic Number

1. atomic number
2. atomic number
3. neutron
4.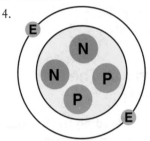

Concept 6: Atomic Mass

1. neutron, proton
2. electron
3. electron
4. plus
5. 4 amu
6. 7 amu

Section 5.1 Reinforcement

1. C
2. electron
3. true
4. A, B
5. A, B
6. atomic mass
7. true
8. electron shell
9. N
10. equal to
11. false
12. To determine atomic mass, add the number of protons to the number of neutrons.
13. electron; a subatomic particle found in an atom's electron shells; has a negative charge and no mass
14. false
15. C
16. H
17. A, C
18. proton
19. true
20. C
21. E

22. B
23. D
24. A
25. F

Comprehensive Review (Chapters 1–5)

26. atomic mass units
27. B
28. 1000 mL
29. scientific law
30. true

Section 5.2 The Periodic Table of Elements

Concept 1: Reading the Periodic Table of Elements

1.

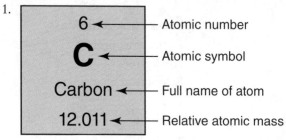

6 ←	Atomic number
C ←	Atomic symbol
Carbon ←	Full name of atom
12.011 ←	Relative atomic mass

2. atomic number
3. atomic symbol
4. relative atomic mass
5. whole number
6. 12 amu

Concept 2: Atoms of the Periodic Table

1. iron
   hydrogen
   silicon
   boron
   calcium
   magnesium
   sodium
   sulfur
2. (Answers will vary. See Figure 5.6 in the text.)
3. (Answers will vary. See Figure 5.6 in the text.)

4.

Name	Atomic Symbol	Atomic Number	Relative Atomic Mass
Hydrogen	H	1	1
Carbon	C	6	12
Nitrogen	N	7	14
Oxygen	O	8	16
Sodium	Na	11	23
Sulfur	S	16	32
Chlorine	Cl	17	35
Potassium	K	19	39
Calcium	Ca	20	40

Concept 3: Number of Neutrons

1. two (4 – 2)
2. 10 (19 – 9)
3. 16 (32 – 16)
4. 12 (23 – 11)
5. 20 (40 – 20)

Concept 4: Construct a Brief Periodic Table

1.

1 H 1.008							2 He 4.003
3 Li 6.941	4 Be 9.012	5 B 10.811	6 C 12.011	7 N 14.007	8 O 15.999	9 F 18.998	10 Ne 20.180
11 Na 22.990	12 Mg 24.305	13 Al 26.982	14 Si 28.086	15 P 32.065	16 S 32.065	17 Cl 35.453	18 Ar 39.948

2. atomic number
3. silicon
4. aluminum
5. oxygen
6. boron

Concept 5: Isotopes

1. mass
2. protons, neutrons
3. isotope
4. 12
5. different
6. whole

Section 5.2 Reinforcement

1. Si
2. 47 amu
3. Na
4. Li, N, Mg, Cl
5. three
6. true
7. neutron; a subatomic particle found in the core of an atom; has no charge and a mass of 1 amu
8. 3 amu
9. Li
10. Al
11. Boron
12. Cl
13. number
14. phosphorus
15. isotope; a form of an atom that has the same atomic number but a different atomic mass than another form of that atom
16. false

17. 13
18. 1
19. false
20. neon
21. isotopes
22. Si
23. 18
24. D
25. true

Comprehensive Review (Chapters 1–5)

26. nitrogen
27. A natural explanation is observable and testable. A supernatural explanation cannot be tested.
28. patient history, physical examination of the patient
29. C
30. away from

Section 5.3 Atomic Diagrams

Concept 1: Electron Shells

1. first electron shell
2. third electron shell
3. teal

Concept 2: Electron Shell Capacity

1. first electron shell
2. second electron shell, third electron shell
3. (See Figure 5.10 in the text.)

Concept 3: Core Diagram

1. diagramming the core

2. Neutrons

Concept 4: Place Electrons

1. two
2. eight
3. two in the first shell, three in the second shell
4. first electron shell
5. four
6. 10
7. two

Concept 5: Diagram Lithium and Fluorine

1.–5.

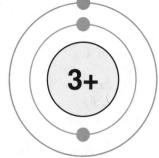

6.

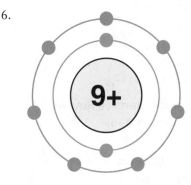

Concept 6: Diagram Phosphorus

1. 15
2. 15
3. three

Concept 7: Diagram Chlorine and Sodium

1.–7. (See Figure 5.14 in the text.)
  8. (See Figure 5.15 in the text.)

Concept 8: Electron Shells and the Periodic Table

1. hydrogen (H) 1; helium (He) 2
2. lithium (Li) 3; beryllium (Be) 4; boron (B) 5; carbon (C) 6; nitrogen (N) 7; oxygen (O) 8; fluorine (F) 9; neon (Ne) 10
3. sodium (Na) 11; magnesium (Mg) 12; aluminum (Al) 13; silicon (Si) 14; phosphorus (P) 15; sulfur (S) 16; chlorine (Cl) 17; argon (Ar) 18

Section 5.3 Reinforcement

1. lithium
2. false
3. one
4. four
5. electron; a subatomic particle found in an atom's electron shells; has a negative charge and no mass
6. six
7. false
8. B
9. Si
10. false
11. lithium (Li), beryllium (Be), boron (B), carbon (C), nitrogen (N), oxygen (O), fluorine (F), neon (Ne)
12. periodic table; a grid that arranged elements by their atomic numbers and properties
13. neon
14. S
15. false
16. Si
17. Be, N, Mg, Cl

Comprehensive Review (Chapters 1–5)

18. Cl
19. 12.4 centimeters
20. a-; not
21. dependent
22. Anatomy, physiology

Section 5.4 Ionic Bonding

Concept 1: How Atoms Bond

1. full
2. outermost electron shell
3. donate electrons, accept electrons, share electrons

Concept 2: Chlorine's Outer Shell

1. seven
2. one
3. outermost electron shell

Concept 3: Sodium's Outer Shell

1. one
2. one
3. outermost electron shell
4. second electron shell
5. second

Concept 4: Chlorine and Sodium Interact

1. donates
2. accepts
3. chlorine
4. one
5. one

Concept 5: Full Outer Shells

1. 11
2. 10
3. 17
4. 18

Concept 6: Ions and Charges

1. donated
2. accepted
3. ions
4. charge
5. 11, 10
6. 17, 18

Concept 7: Ionic Symbols

1. positive
2. negative
3. two
4. Ca^{++}

Concept 8: Opposite Charges Attract

1. attract
2. opposite
3. positive
4. negative

5. ionic
6. molecule

Section 5.4 Reinforcement

1. disappear, outermost
2. true
3. donate
4. full
5. If sodium donates the electron, the second shell will become its outer shell.
6. negative
7. ions
8. chlorine
9. ionic; related to the attraction between ions with opposite charges
10. positive
11. opposite
12. electron
13. false
14. molecule; a combination of many atoms held together by bonds
15. true
16. molecule
17. ionic
18. accept
19. 2
20. false
21. accept

Comprehensive Review (Chapters 1–5)

22. 235 cm, 0.09 m, 75 mm, 15 mm
23. 2
24. accept, reject
25. physi/o ("function") + -logy ("study of")
26. confirmed

Section 5.5 Covalent Bonding

Concept 1: Equal Attraction

1. one
2. four
3. share
4. share

Concept 2: Forming a Covalent Bond

1. four, one

2. covalent
3. eight
4. full
5. shared

Concept 3: Molecular Symbols
1. one, four
2. one
3. three, eight

Concept 4: Stick Diagrams
1. four
2. two
3. eight
4. one
5. eight
6. two

Concept 5: Single and Double Covalent Bonds
1. two
2. four
3. four
4. one
5. two
6. four
7. one stick (–)
8. two sticks (=)
9. two
10. four, 10

Concept 6: Construct a Stick Diagram
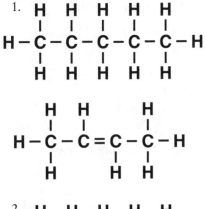
1.
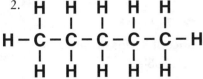
2.

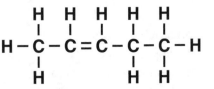

Section 5.5 Reinforcement
1. Carbon has five sticks instead of four.
2. share
3. covalent; relating to the bond formed by sharing electrons between atoms
4. four
5. four
6. false
7. six, 14
8. one
9. false
10. covalent
11. share; the process of atoms sharing electrons to achieve full outer shells
12. double bond
13. two
14. Electrons are shared between atoms in a covalent bond; protons are in the core of the atom and are not shared or transferred between atoms.
15. one stick
16. true
17. single covalent bond, double covalent bond
18. four
19. true
20. A

Comprehensive Review (Chapters 1–5)
21. two
22. 1560 mm
23. untested
24. anti-
25. false

Section 5.6 Hydrogen Bonding

Concept 1: Water Molecule
1. one, two
2. covalent
3. chin (oxygen atom), ears (hydrogen atoms)
4. negative
5. negative
6. positive

Concept 2: Forming a Hydrogen Bond
1. chin
2. attract
3. weaker
4. ~
5. negative (~–)
6. (See Figure 5.25 in the text.)

Concept 3: Hydrogen Bonds and Water Characteristics
1. ionic
2. charges
3. Ions
4. negative charge, chin, positive charge, ear
5. cohesive
6. less
7. resists

Concept 4: Types of Bonds
1. ionic bonds—the attraction between ions with opposite charges; covalent bonds—the sharing of electrons between atoms; hydrogen bonds—the attraction of partial charges between molecules made of hydrogen atoms and atoms with an especially intense attraction for electrons
2. hydrogen

Concept 5: Chemical Formulas
1. three
2. one
3. two, one, four
4. three, three
5. two, two, two, six
6. eight, four

Section 5.6 Reinforcement

1. five
2. eight, four, 16
3. ionic, covalent, and hydrogen bonds
4. hydrogen
5. A, B
6. ear
7. false
8. covalent bonds
9. hydrogen; relating to a bond in which the partial charges of water molecules attract
10. 16, eight
11. false
12. A
13. true
14. partial; a slight negative or positive charge in a part of a molecule
15. covalent
16. A, C
17. attract
18. oxygen
19. true
20. weaker
21. weak; lacking strength, liable to break or give way under pressure
22. 12
23. A hydrogen bond is an atomic bond in which the partial charges of water molecules attract. It is the weakest type of atomic bond.

Comprehensive Review (Chapters 1–5)

24. four
25. 1.567 km
26. life
27. false
28. In an experiment, the experimental group receives the independent variable, whereas the control group does not.

Section 5.7 Carbohydrates

Concept 1: Macromolecules

1. carbohydrates, lipids, proteins, nucleic acids
2. macromolecule

Concept 2: Sugars

1. sugars
2. monosaccharides, disaccharides, polysaccharides
3. sugars

Concept 3: Monosaccharides

1. mono-
2. sacchar/o
3. monosaccharides
4. glucose
5. carbohydrates, glucose
6. cells
7. hexagon
8. $C_6H_{12}O_6$

Concept 4: Disaccharides

1. disaccharide
2. maltose
3. table
4. monosaccharides

Concept 5: Polysaccharides

1. hexagon
2. monosaccharides
3. poly-
4. glycogen, cellulose, starch
5. glycogen
6. glucose

Concept 6: Fiber

1. cellulose
2. monosaccharides
3. fiber

Concept 7: Complex Carbohydrates

1. complex
2. simple
3. complex
4. simple
5. simple

Concept 8: Calories in Carbohydrates

1. calories, kilocalories
2. four

Section 5.7 Reinforcement

1. A
2. A, C
3. complex

4. sugar; a carbohydrate; also known as saccharide
5. glycogen
6. disaccharides, monosaccharides, polysaccharides
7. monosaccharides
8. C, D
9. Glycogen
10. carbohydrate; a sugar
11. true
12. polysaccharide
13. glucose
14. C, D
15. monosaccharides
16. hexagon; a shape with six equal sides
17. simple
18. fiber
19. saccharide; sugar
20. C
21. B
22. D
23. A

Comprehensive Review (Chapters 1–5)

24. two
25. D
26. independent, dependent
27. false
28. long-term

Section 5.8 Lipids

Concept 1: Types of Lipids

1. fats, waxes, oils
2. glycerol, fatty acids
3. fats
4. saturated fat, unsaturated fat, polyunsaturated fat, *trans* fat

Concept 2: Saturated Fat

1. single
2. maximum
3. solid
4. fat on meat

Concept 3: Unsaturated Fat

1. double
2. fewer
3. liquid
4. olive

Concept 4: Polyunsaturated Fat

1. polyunsaturated
2. liquid
3. corn
4. hydrogen

Concept 5: *Trans* Fat

1. *trans*
2. hydrogenation
3. easier
4. hydrogen

Concept 6: Calories in Lipids

1. Fats
2. nine

Section 5.8 Reinforcement

1. unsaturated
2. polyunsaturated
3. maximum
4. *trans*
5. poly-; a prefix which means "many"; in reference to fats, polyunsaturated
6. solid
7. easier
8. polyunsaturated; fat with multiple double bonds between carbon atoms
9. hydrogen
10. single
11. saturated; fat with single bonds between carbon atoms; solid at room temperature
12. hydrogenation
13. saturated, unsaturated, poly-unsaturated, *trans*
14. D
15. C
16. B
17. A

Comprehensive Review (Chapters 1–5)

18. false
19. false
20. observation
21. 100
22. mnemonic

Section 5.9 Proteins

Concept 1: What Is a Protein?

1. amino acids

2. 20
3. peptide bond

Concept 2: Amino Acids

1. central carbon atom, hydrogen atom, carboxyl group, amino group, remainder group
2. (See Figure 5.33 in the text.)

Concept 3: Types of Amino Acids

1. 20
2. glycine
3. (List three:) alanine, leucine, threonine, valine, methionine, isoleucine

Concept 4: Essential Amino Acids

1. essential
2. diet

Concept 5: Primary Protein Structure

1. primary, secondary, tertiary
2. sequence

Concept 6: Secondary Protein Structure

1. attraction
2. pleated sheet, helix (twisted)

Concept 7: Tertiary Protein Structure

1. tertiary structure
2. hydrogen, covalent
3. three
4. distant, fold

Concept 8: Denaturing

1. protein
2. high heat, low pH
3. protein
4. denatures

Concept 9: Calories in Proteins

1. 4
2. amino

Section 5.9 Reinforcement

1. B, C
2. 4
3. C
4. R
5. tertiary; in reference to protein structures, the result of attraction between distant amino acids, resulting in a hydrogen

or covalent bond; takes a three-dimensional shape
6. primary
7. peptide; the bonds that hold amino acids together
8. high heat, low pH
9. lipid
10. primary, secondary, tertiary
11. carboxyl; the group within an amino acid structure that has one carbon atom and two oxygen atoms
12. A, B
13. true
14. Peptide
15. amino
16. tertiary
17. false
18. primary, secondary, tertiary
19. B
20. false
21. protein; a chain of amino acids
22. D
23. protein

Comprehensive Review (Chapters 1–5)

24. two
25. C
26. false
27. rejected, modified
28. true

Section 5.10 Enzymes

Concept 1: Structural Proteins

1. structural, functional
2. keratin
3. collagen
4. tough

Concept 2: Functional Proteins

1. carry oxygen in the blood, regulate the movement of materials through the cell membrane, speed up reactions in the body
2. hemoglobin

Concept 3: What Are Enzymes?

1. functional
2. Enzymes
3. speeds

4. substrate
5. active

Concept 4: Active Site

1. shape
2. catalyze

Concept 5: Enzyme-Substrate Complex

1. enzyme-substrate
2. enzymatic reaction
3. active site
4. enzymatic reaction

Concept 6: Enzyme Names

1. Hydrolases
2. *ase*
3. oxygen

Concept 7: Types of Enzymatic Reactions

1. synthesis, degradative
2. synthesis
3. degradative

Concept 8: Turnover Rate

1. turnover rate
2. heat
3. cold (lack of heat)

Section 5.10 Reinforcement

1. sucrase
2. catalyst; a substance that speeds up a chemical reaction
3. turnover rate
4. B
5. active site
6. lactase
7. shape
8. degradative, synthesis
9. keratin
10. enzymatic reaction
11. Hyrdolases
12. synthesis; an enzymatic reaction that binds two substrates together
13. *ase*
14. A
15. true
16. A
17. C
18. false
19. enzyme; a protein catalyst

20. synthesis
21. enzyme

Comprehensive Review (Chapters 1–5)

22. isotope
23. false
24. 73°C
25. independent
26. theory

Section 5.11 Nucleic Acids

Concept 1: Nucleotides

1. nucleotide
2. phosphate, sugar, base

Concept 2: Bases

1. phosphate, sugar, base
2. pyrimidines, purines
3. pyrimidines
4. purines
5. (See Figure 5.44 in the text.)

Concept 3: Purines and Pyrimidines

1. adenine, guanine
2. cytosine, thymine, uracil
3. cytosine
4. adenine
5. thymine
6. guanine

Concept 4: Base Pairing

1. T
2. A
3. G
4. C
5. pyrimidine
6. purine
7. complementary

Concept 5: Base Bonding

1. hydrogen
2. three
3. two

Concept 6: DNA

1. deoxyribose
2. nucleic acid
3. deoxyribonucleic acid
4. down

Concept 7: Two Strands

1. complementary

2. hydrogen
3. phosphate, sugar, base

Concept 8: Double Helix

1. double helix
2. strands
3. coiled

Concept 9: Genes

1. proteins
2. Chromosomes
3. segment
4. gene, chromosome

Concept 10: RNA

1. DNA, RNA, ATP
2. ribonucleic acid
3. protein synthesis
4. DNA
5. uracil, thymine
6. RNA
7. ribose

Concept 11: ATP

1. nucleic acid
2. adenosine triphosphate
3. stores energy inside a cell
4. carbohydrates, lipids, amino acids

Section 5.11 Reinforcement

1. purine
2. guanine
3. adenine
4. phosphate, sugar, base
5. traits
6. B
7. complementary
8. purine; a base (either adenine or guanine) drawn as a hexagon combined with a pentagon
9. deoxyribose
10. ribonucleic acid; the strand of nucleotides that stores energy inside cells
11. pyrimidine
12. nucleic acid
13. false
14. deoxyribonucleic acid
15. nucleic acid
16. C
17. D

18. A
19. B

Comprehensive Review (Chapters 1–5)

20. positive
21. explanations
22. false
23. meter
24. summary

Section 5.12 pH

Concept 1: What Is pH?

1. OH^-
2. H^+
3. pH
4. hydrogen, hydroxide
5. acid
6. base
7. neutral
8. an acid, a base

Concept 2: pH Values

1. 0, 14
2. acid
3. base
4. neutral

Concept 3: Strong and Weak Acid Bases

1. strong base
2. strong acid
3. weak base
4. weak acid
5. weak acid

Concept 4: pH Scale

1. OH^- ions
2. H^+ ions

Concept 5: pH Values of Liquids

1. acids
2. bases
3. neutral
4. 1
5. sodium hydroxide

Concept 6: Buffers

1. buffer
2. changes
3. H^+
4. release
5. water

6. H_2O

Concept 7: Electrolytes

1. H^+
2. OH^-
3. Na^+, Cl^-
4. electrolyte
5. acids, bases, salts

Section 5.12 Reinforcement

1. hydrogen ion
2. acid
3. most acidic—2.5; most basic—10.1
4. strong base
5. weak acid
6. strong acid, weak acid, neutral, weak base, strong base
7. hydroxide ion
8. A
9. true
10. weak base
11. neutral
12. D
13. B
14. true
15. pH
16. buffer
17. A
18. C
19. B

Comprehensive Review (Chapters 1–5)

20. weaker
21. 1
22. true
23. measured, tested
24. false

Chapter 5 Review

1. 2.1, 3.4, 4.9, 5.6
2. false
3. synthesis
4. essential
5. base
6. C
7. false
8. four
9. lactose
10. Al
11. hydrogen

12. hydrogen
13. protons
14. B
15. shared
16. proton, neutron
17. covalent, hydrogen, ionic
18. strong acid
19. Mg
20. true
21. 12
22. He, O, Al, S
23. B
24. one
25. false
26. protons, electrons
27. B
28. glycerol, fatty acids
29. false
30. three
31. eight
32. helium
33. share
34. false
35. A
36. 20
37. oxygen
38. electron
39. neutron

Comprehensive Review (Chapters 1–5)

40. D
41. A
42. E
43. N
44. K
45. J
46. I
47. G
48. C
49. B
50. F
51. H
52. L
53. M

Chapter 6 Cell Morphology

Section 6.1 Overview of the Cell

Concept 1: What Are Cells?

1. community
2. cells

Concept 2: The Morphology of Cells

1. Morphology
2. bag, bags, fluid

Concept 3: Cell Size

1. surface area
2. surface area
3. magnification

Concept 4: Cell Diversity

1. specialized
2. function

Concept 5: Cell Activities

1. cells
2. activities

Concept 6: Basic Parts of a Cell

1. cytosol
2. plasma membrane
3. cytosol, interstitial
4. cytosol, organelles
5. DNA
6. cytosol
7. plasma membrane, nucleus, cytoplasm
8. organelles
9. nucleus

Concept 7: Cells and Life

1. cell
2. alive

Section 6.1 Reinforcement

1. cells
2. organelle; a specialized structure that performs a specific function inside the cell
3. C
4. nucleus, organelles
5. magnification
6. Different types of cells have unique structures, components, or shapes that enable them to do a specific function.
7. false
8. A, B, E
9. cytosol; the fluid inside a cell
10. false
11. cytosol, interstitial fluid
12. chemical reactions
13. plasma membrane
14. enter, exit
15. water
16. B, C
17. true
18. plasma membrane, nucleus, cytoplasm
19. surface-area-to-volume
20. false
21. structure, form
22. B
23. E
24. F
25. D
26. C
27. A

Comprehensive Review (Chapters 1–6)

28. masses
29. false
30. concentration
31. B, C
32. interstitial fluid
33. genetics (study of inheritance), cytology (study of cells), histology (study of tissues), anatomy (study of the parts of the body), physiology (study of the functions of body parts)

Section 6.2 Plasma Membrane

Concept 1: Gatekeeper

1. gatekeeper
2. in, out, leaving, entering
3. permeable
4. selective

Concept 2: Components of the Plasma Membrane

1. phospholipid bilayer, globular proteins, glycolipids, glycoproteins, cholesterol
2. cholesterol, globular proteins, glycolipids, glycoproteins, phospholipid bilayer

Concept 3: Phospholipids

1. head, tails
2. (See Figure 6.4 in the text.)
3. a negative, is
4. tails, are not
5. hydrophobic, hydrophilic

Concept 4: Phospholipid Bilayer

1. two
2. lipid tails, phosphate heads
3. three-dimensional

Concept 5: Globular Proteins and Cholesterol

1. channels
2. Cholesterol

Concept 6: Glycoproteins and Glycolipids

1. glycoprotein
2. glycolipid
3. fingerprint

Concept 7: Fluid Mosaic Model

1. phospholipid bilayer, globular proteins, cholesterol, gylcoproteins, glycolipids
2. They are not. The parts constantly move around the surface of the cell.
3. oil

Section 6.2 Reinforcement

1. glucose
2. Globular proteins
3. C
4. mosaic; a structure composed of many parts
5. phospholipids
6. glycolipid; a carbohydrate chain attached to a lipid
7. false
8. glycoproteins, glycolipids
9. fluid
10. true

11. phosphate heads, lipid tails
12. phospholipid; a molecule composed of one phosphate head and two lipid tails
13. phospholipids
14. phosphate head
15. B
16. lipid
17. true
18. phospholipid, glycolipid
19. globular proteins
20. true
21. B, D
22. C
23. A
24. E
25. B
26. D

Comprehensive Review (Chapters 1–6)

27. thymine
28. independent
29. C
30. 600 cm²
31. the study of structure or form
32. long-term

Section 6.3 Nucleus

Concept 1: Control Center

1. nucleus
2. histones
3. processes

Concept 2: Chromosomes and Chromatin

1. chromosomes
2. chromatin
3. true
4. true

Concept 3: Genes on Chromosomes

1. 23 pairs
2. chromosomes
3. proteins

Concept 4: Multinucleate and Anucleate Cells

1. false
2. Anucleate
3. many

Concept 5: Nuclear Envelope

1. nucleoplasm
2. pores
3. envelope, cytoplasm

Concept 6: Nucleoli

1. nucleolus, ribosomes
2. may not

Concept 7: The Nucleus During Cell Division

1. One, two
2. dissolves

Section 6.3 Reinforcement

1. envelope
2. chromosomes
3. C
4. nucleoplasm
5. true
6. nuclear envelope
7. false
8. nucleolus; a structure inside the nucleus that assembles the components needed to make organelles and ribosomes
9. red blood cell
10. true
11. skeletal muscle cell
12. chromatin; the form in which DNA is usually packaged
13. histones
14. chromatin
15. chromosome; the form in which DNA is packaged during cell division
16. A, B, D
17. true
18. channels
19. DNA
20. chromosomes
21. B
22. E
23. A
24. F
25. C
26. D
27. B

Comprehensive Review (Chapters 1–6)

28. false
29. monosaccharide
30. constants
31. B
32. to separate the individual phospholipids in the bilayer and help them shift location
33. -philic

Section 6.4 Endoplasmic Reticulum and Golgi

Concept 1: Endoplasmic Reticulum

1. endoplasmic reticulum
2. process, store, digest

Concept 2: Types of Endoplasmic Reticulum

1. smooth endoplasmic reticulum, rough endoplasmic reticulum
2. connected

Concept 3: Smooth Endoplasmic Reticulum

1. SER
2. drugs, alcohol, lipids
3. calcium
4. fats
5. SER

Concept 4: Rough Endoplasmic Reticulum

1. rough endoplasmic reticulum
2. ribosomes
3. transport vesicles

Concept 5: Ribosomes

1. ribosome
2. cytoplasm
3. nuclear envelope, RER

Concept 6: Ribosome Structure

1. nucleoli
2. enzymes

Concept 7: Ribosome Proteins

1. Free
2. Bound

Concept 8: Golgi

1. Golgi
2. transport, secretory
3. plasma membrane
4. lysosomes

Section 6.4 Reinforcement

1. Secretory
2. tubes
3. true
4. reticulum; a network of membranes
5. ribosomes
6. no
7. ribosome; a structure that assembles amino acids into specific proteins
8. drugs, alcohol, lipids
9. ribosome
10. true
11. rough endoplasmic reticulum
12. Golgi; a structure that receives proteins from transport vesicles and packages them into secretory vesicles
13. transport
14. within
15. RNA
16. Ribosomes
17. true
18. Free
19. Golgi
20. false
21. A, B
22. B
23. C
24. E
25. A
26. D

Comprehensive Review (Chapters 1–6)

27. two, two
28. volume
29. fact
30. around
31. none
32. D

Section 6.5 Cytoplasm

Concept 1: Mitochondria

1. mitochondria
2. muscle cell
3. ATP

Concept 2: Mitochondria Structure

1. kidney beans
2. cristae

Concept 3: Lysosomes

1. lysosome
2. enzymes

Concept 4: Peroxisomes

1. Peroxisomes
2. oxidase, catalase

Concept 5: Cytoskeleton

1. no
2. microfilaments, intermediate filaments, microtubules
3. microtubule

Concept 6: Microfilaments

1. Microfilaments
2. two globular (round) protein chains wrapped around each other

Concept 7: Intermediate Filaments

1. hold organelles in position and reinforce cell shape
2. disassembled and reassembled

Concept 8: Microtubules

1. microtubules
2. tubulins
3. roadways

Section 6.5 Reinforcement

1. A
2. peroxisomes
3. Golgi
4. mitochondria; organelles that serve as the powerhouse of the cell
5. Intermediate filaments
6. Intermediate filaments
7. false
8. microfilaments, intermediate filaments, microtubules
9. lysosome; an organelle that is a large bag of enzymes
10. false
11. plasma membrane
12. cytoskeleton; the structure that supports the cell
13. Peroxisomes
14. microfilaments, microtubules
15. mitochondrion
16. Microtubules
17. false
18. mitochondrion
19. microfilaments
20. true
21. A, B, D
22. D
23. B
24. C
25. A

Comprehensive Review (Chapters 1–6)

26. 9/16
27. unsaturated
28. confirmed
29. ventr/o
30. within
31. observation

Section 6.6 Outside the Cell

Concept 1: Membrane Extensions

1. Cilia, flagella
2. Microvilli

Concept 2: Cilia

1. hairs
2. microtubules
3. windpipe, fallopian tubes

Concept 3: Flagella

1. Flagella
2. flagellum

Concept 4: Microvilli

1. Microvilli, absorption
2. brush border

Concept 5: Membrane Junctions

1. false
2. tight junctions, desmosomes, gap junctions

Concept 6: Tight Junctions

1. Tight junctions, impermeable
2. liquid
3. stomach

Concept 7: Desmosomes

1. Desmosomes

2. true
3. Desmosomes

Concept 8: Gap Junctions
1. Connexons
2. gap junction
3. Ions

Section 6.6 Reinforcement
1. true
2. flagellum; a whip-like extension of the plasma membrane
3. C
4. cilia, flagella, microvilli
5. A
6. B, C
7. true
8. desmosome; a locking joint between adjacent cells
9. B
10. false
11. hairs
12. microvilli
13. C
14. gap junction
15. microvilli; finger-like projections of the plasma membrane that increase the surface area of the cell
16. gap junction
17. B, C
18. tight junction, desmosome, gap junction
19. B, C
20. A, B, C
21. false
22. C
23. B
24. A
25. D
26. F
27. E

Comprehensive Review (Chapters 1–6)
28. Science
29. below
30. two
31. 1000 milliliters
32. microfilaments, intermediate filaments, microtubules
33. "if"

Chapter 6 Review
1. shorten, contract
2. organelles
3. plasma membrane
4. false
5. structure, form
6. life
7. false
8. carbohydrate, lipid
9. true
10. The phosphate head is hydrophilic, which means it is attracted to water.
11. nucleoli
12. cell division
13. false
14. plasma membrane, nucleus, cytoplasm
15. true
16. tubulins
17. false
18. channels
19. true
20. C
21. true
22. A
23. false
24. Microfilaments
25. energy
26. lysosome
27. microtubules
28. true
29. roadways
30. false
31. B
32. Desmosomes

Comprehensive Review (Chapters 1–6)
33. A
34. D
35. B
36. E
37. C
38. F
39. G
40. I
41. H
42. J
43. K

Chapter 7 Cell Physiology

Section 7.1 Movement Through the Plasma Membrane

Concept 1: Selective Permeability
1. permeable
2. harm

Concept 2: Molecules Entering the Cell
1. oxygen, glucose, amino acids, ions
2. blood

Concept 3: Molecules Exiting the Cell
1. Carbon dioxide, nitrogen
2. factories, enzymes, hormones

Concept 4: Polarity of Molecules
1. polar, polar
2. nonpolar
3. polarity

Concept 5: Lipid Solubility
1. lipid barrier
2. nonpolar
3. soluble

Concept 6: Passing Through the Lipid Barrier
1. lipid-soluble, hydrophobic, and nonpolar molecules
2. hydrophilic and polar molecules
3. Water

Concept 7: Protein Channels
1. channels
2. small, polar molecules, such as sodium ions, calcium ions, chloride ions, and potassium ions

Concept 8: Aquaporin Channels
1. Aquaporins
2. lipid barrier

Concept 9: Carrier Proteins
1. Carriers, large
2. amino acids, glucose

Concept 10: Solute Pumps

1. energy
2. Solute pumps

Section 7.1 Reinforcement

1. aquaporin; a channel through which water enters or exits a cell
2. water
3. A, C
4. glucose, amino acids
5. true
6. phospholipid
7. true
8. lipid
9. A, B
10. true
11. C
12. Yes, they can. Hydrophobic molecules are lipid soluble.
13. B
14. cell respiration
15. C
16. A, D
17. false
18. out of
19. hydrophilic; attracted to water
20. permeable
21. lipid
22. Solute pumps
23. C
24. A
25. B
26. D

Comprehensive Review (Chapters 1–7)

27. nucleoplasm
28. homo-; same
29. false
30. 0.25 kg
31. protein channels, carrier proteins, aquaporins, solute pumps
32. confirmed
33. evidence

Section 7.2 Areas of High and Low Concentration

Concept 1: Reviewing Concentration

1. A
2. A

Concept 2: Comparing Concentrations

1. 14.7 lbs/in², 32 lbs/in²
2. plasma membrane

Concept 3: Concentration Gradient

1. the difference between concentrations inside the plasma membrane and outside the plasma membrane
2. higher

Concept 4: Moving Between Concentrations

1. out of
2. high, low

Concept 5: High to Low Concentration

1. (See Figure 7.7 in the text.)
2. downhill
3. energy input

Concept 6: Equilibrium

1. difference
2. equilibrium

Concept 7: Low to High Concentration

1. (See Figure 7.20 in the text.)
2. energy
3. low, high

Section 7.2 Reinforcement

1. true
2. low, high
3. higher
4. Concentration
5. top
6. A, B
7. moving, colliding
8. Equilibrium
9. downhill
10. false

11. equilibrium; a state in which concentrations inside the cell and outside the cell are equal
12. false
13. up
14. equal
15. volume
16. gradient; the difference between concentrations
17. false
18. concentration gradient
19. high, low
20. uphill
21. C
22. E
23. B
24. A
25. D

Comprehensive Review (Chapters 1–7)

26. 16
27. A
28. false
29. protein
30. cilia, flagella, microvilli
31. "if"
32. facts

Section 7.3 Diffusion

Concept 1: What Is Diffusion?

1. high, low
2. Diffusion
3. less
4. oxygen, carbon dioxide, water

Concept 2: Uniform Distribution

1. highly, low
2. uniformly

Concept 3: Effect of Temperature on Diffusion

1. temperature
2. high
3. low
4. quickly
5. slowly

Concept 4: Effect of Size on Diffusion

1. more quickly
2. size

3. lithium
4. brown dye
5. blue dye

Concept 5: Diffusion in the Lungs

1. highly, less
2. highly, less
3. blood, air, air, blood

Concept 6: Facilitated Diffusion

1. facilitated diffusion
2. charged ions, such as sodium, calcium, chloride, and potassium ions; large molecules

Section 7.3 Reinforcement

1. semisolid
2. false
3. large molecule
4. facilitated; aided by other structures
5. No energy input is required. Atoms naturally tend to do this.
6. temperature, size
7. true
8. protein, carrier
9. visible
10. true
11. Facilitated diffusion requires the actions of protein channels and carrier proteins.
12. hydrogen
13. from, into
14. true
15. drop of dye
16. diffusion
17. true
18. high, low
19. B
20. oxygen
21. diffusion; the spreading out of atoms from areas of high concentration into areas of low concentration
22. facilitated diffusion
23. In facilitated diffusion, atoms are still moving from areas of high concentration to areas of low concentration.

Comprehensive Review (Chapters 1–7)

24. Yes. Contradicting evidence will cause the rejection of a scientific law.
25. hydrogen bond
26. 84 people
27. water
28. B
29. high, low
30. fields

Section 7.4 Osmosis

Concept 1: What Is Osmosis?

1. phospholipid bilayer, aquaporins
2. high, low
3. Water molecules are moving from areas of high concentration to areas of low concentration.

Concept 2: Solute and Solvent Concentrations

1. 97%
2. 7%
3. inside, outside

Concept 3: Hypertonic, Isotonic, and Hypotonic Solutions

1. below
   same
   above
2. hypertonic
3. hypotonic
4. isotonic

Concept 4: Comparing Solute and Solvent Concentrations

1. 95
2. 8
3. solute, solvent

Concept 5: Movement of Water During Osmosis

1. hypertonic, out of
2. hypotonic, into
3. isotonic, net
4. D

Concept 6: Effect of Osmosis on Cell Size

1. enters
2. swelling

3. leaves
4. crenation

Section 7.4 Reinforcement

1. B
2. leaves
3. C
4. hypertonic; having a higher solute concentration
5. B
6. phospholipid bilayer, aquaporins
7. true
8. is/o
9. A, C
10. true
11. above
12. solute
13. C
14. solute
15. swell
16. hypo-
17. true
18. phospholipid bilayer, aquaporins
19. solvent
20. true
21. 4
22. true
23. F
24. H
25. E
26. G
27. C
28. B
29. A
30. D

Comprehensive Review (Chapters 1–7)

31. 12.56 cm^2
32. constants
33. In both diffusion and osmosis, atoms move from areas of high concentration to areas of low concentration. Osmosis refers specifically to the movement of water molecules.
34. C
35. true
36. half
37. life

Section 7.5 Cell Respiration

Concept 1: Anabolic and Catabolic Reactions

1. requires, releases
2. anabolic, catabolic

Concept 2: Energy Transformation

1. transformed
2. carbohydrates
3. mitochondria

Concept 3: Glucose and Oxygen

1. glucose
2. Glucose, oxygen

Concept 4: ADP to ATP

1. ATP
2. anabolic

Concept 5: Steps in Cell Respiration

1. ATP, ADP
2. glycolysis, prep reaction, citric acid cycle, electron transport chain
3. oxygen

Concept 6: No Oxygen

1. cannot
2. lactic acid

Concept 7: Other Energy Sources

1. fats, protein
2. only if carbohydrate and fat sources are lacking

Concept 8: ATP to ADP

1. high-energy
2. catabolic

Section 7.5 Reinforcement

1. glucose, oxygen
2. They are joined together.
3. C
4. oxygen
5. true
6. releases
7. false
8. carbohydrates
9. catabolic
10. false
11. releases

12. lactic acid
13. catabolic reaction
14. ADP, P
15. glycolysis, prep reaction, citric acid cycle, electron transport chain
16. true
17. tiredness, soreness
18. high-energy
19. true
20. false
21. ADP, P
22. up
23. B
24. C
25. A

Comprehensive Review (Chapters 1–7)

26. false
27. 12, 28
28. to push molecules into or out of a cell using energy
29. plasma membrane, nucleus, cytoplasm
30. D
31. bottom
32. varying

Section 7.6 Energy-Required Reactions

Concept 1: Uphill Reactions

1. Energy
2. breaking, phosphate
3. adenosine, phosphates
4. ADP

Concept 2: Active Transport

1. uphill, solute pumps
2. energy, ATP

Concept 3: Exocytosis

1. exocytosis
2. true
3. separate

Concept 4: Endocytosis

1. endocytosis
2. energy
3. phagocytosis, pinocytosis, receptor-mediated endocytosis

Concept 5: Phagocytosis

1. cell eating
2. pocket
3. phagocytes

Concept 6: Pinocytosis

1. liquid
2. In both processes, the plasma membrane forms a pocket and surrounds the liquid or object entering the cell, encasing it in a membrane within the cell.
3. cell drinking

Concept 7: Receptor-Mediated Endocytosis

1. receptor-mediated endocytosis
2. pit
3. phagocytosis, pinocytosis, receptor-mediated endocytosis

Section 7.6 Reinforcement

1. adenosine, phosphates
2. false
3. C
4. Solute, energy
5. endocytosis
6. Phagocytosis
7. true
8. endocytosis; moving atoms into a cell
9. phagocytosis, pinocytosis, receptor-mediated endocytosis
10. true
11. B, C, D
12. drinking
13. In receptor-mediated endocytosis, only certain substances can enter a cell. To enter, a substance must bind with a specific protein within a pit in the phospholipid bilayer.
14. Active transport uses solute pumps and requires energy.
15. receptor-mediated
16. endocytosis
17. secretory vesicles
18. phosphate
19. C
20. F
21. D
22. E
23. B

24. A

Comprehensive Review (Chapters 1–7)

25. dependent
26. 272.3 g
27. true
28. ions
29. true
30. Water molecules move from areas of high concentration to areas of low concentration.
31. mnemonic

Section 7.7 Maintaining Homeostasis

Concept 1: Homeostasis

1. Homeostasis
2. constant
3. adjusting

Concept 2: Sodium and Potassium in Homeostasis

1. enter, leave
2. high, low
3. outside, inside
4. homeostasis

Concept 3: Sodium-Potassium Pump

1. increase
2. decrease
3. true
4. yes

Concept 4: pH in Homeostasis

1. 7.0, 7.4
2. hydrogen, hydroxide

Concept 5: Protein Buffers

1. hydrogen
2. lower, below
3. hydrogen, chemical reactions

Section 7.7 Reinforcement

1. a state of relative stability
2. narrow
3. 7.0, 7.4
4. buffer; a molecule that can accept or donate hydrogen ions
5. B, C
6. entering
7. false

8. high, low, high, low
9. protein
10. false
11. lower
12. homeostasis; a state of relative stability
13. Facilitated diffusion causes sodium ions to enter a cell and potassium ions to leave a cell.
14. homeostasis
15. constant
16. out of, into
17. false
18. too many
19. false
20. protein channels
21. buffers
22. B
23. E
24. A
25. F
26. C
27. D

Comprehensive Review (Chapters 1–7)

28. electron
29. true
30. A, D
31. A
32. abstract
33. 2 cm
34. true

Section 7.8 Protein Synthesis

Concept 1: Types of Proteins

1. structural, functional
2. activities

Concept 2: Chains of Amino Acids

1. protein
2. 20
3. 50, polypeptides

Concept 3: Synthesis

1. Amino acids are placed in the proper sequence to form a specific protein.
2. nucleus, ribosomes
3. nucleus, ribosome

4. ribosome, order

Concept 4: Receiving Amino Acids

1. meat and many types of plants
2. assembled, energy

Concept 5: The Role of DNA

1. no
2. gene

Concept 6: The Role of RNA

1. messenger RNA (mRNA), transfer RNA (tRNA), ribosomal RNA (rRNA)
2. Transfer RNA (tRNA)

Concept 7: Steps in Protein Synthesis

1. transcription, translation
2. Transcription, translation

Concept 8: Transcription

1. sense
2. mRNA, ribosome

Concept 9: Translation

1. template
2. Peptide

Concept 10: Movement Out of the Cell

1. rough
2. transport, Golgi
3. secretory

Section 7.8 Reinforcement

1. nucleus
2. true
3. order
4. transfer RNA (tRNA)
5. structural, functional
6. C
7. false
8. messenger RNA (mRNA), transfer RNA (tRNA), ribosomal RNA (rRNA)
9. amino acids
10. false
11. assembled, broken down
12. transcription; the process of making a copy of the DNA sense strand in the nucleus
13. messenger RNA (mRNA)
14. structural

15. functional proteins
16. synthesis; the assembly of a structure or substance
17. A, C
18. transcription
19. sequence, specific
20. true
21. 20, proteins
22. Proteins that move out of a cell are assembled by ribosomes in the rough endoplasmic reticulum (RER). The proteins leave the RER in transport vesicles, which are received by the Golgi. The Golgi then packages the proteins into secretory vesicles, which travel toward the plasma membrane and release the proteins outside the cell.
23. C
24. E
25. B
26. D
27. A

Comprehensive Review (Chapters 1–7)

28. green
29. 12,000 meters
30. false
31. base
32. false
33. phosphate heads, lipid tails
34. attitude

Section 7.9 Cell Division

Concept 1: Diploid and Haploid Cells

1. pairs
2. Diploid, 46
3. Haploid
4. reproductive cells (eggs in females and sperm in males)

Concept 2: The Beginning of the Human Life Cycle

1. by the fusion of an egg and a sperm
2. daughter
3. mitosis

Concept 3: Replication

1. replication
2. before
3. sister chromatids
4. 92 chromatids

Concept 4: Interphase

1. interphase
2. The cell continues to perform its specific functions and does not divide, though it is preparing for cell division.
3. interphase

Concept 5: Mitosis

1. prophase, metaphase, anaphase, telophase
2. diploid, two
3. prophase
4. anaphase

Concept 6: Meiosis

1. testes, ovaries
2. two
3. In males, meiosis begins at puberty and continues until death. In females, meiosis begins before birth and ends at menopause.

Section 7.9 Reinforcement

1. mitosis, meiosis
2. C
3. B
4. telophase; the final stage of mitosis during which a cell divides down the middle
5. prophase, metaphase, anaphase, telophase
6. interphase
7. true
8. before cell division, during interphase
9. females
10. true
11. mitosis
12. chromatid; one chromosome in a pair of duplicated chromosomes
13. metaphase
14. The cell continues to perform its specific functions and does not divide, though it is preparing for cell division.

15. 46
16. Haploid
17. meiosis
18. false
19. anaphase, metaphase, prophase, telophase
20. identical
21. zygote
22. A, B, F
23. C
24. D
25. B
26. F
27. A
28. E

Comprehensive Review (Chapters 1–7)

29. true
30. Free ribosomes are found in a cell's cytoplasm and make proteins that stay within a cell. Bound ribosomes are attached to the nuclear envelope or RER and make proteins that travel out of a cell.
31. below
32. y-axis
33. law
34. transcription, translation
35. facts

Chapter 7 Review

1. replication
2. Facilitated diffusion does not require energy because atoms are still moving from areas of high concentration to areas of low concentration.
3. C
4. ribosome, messenger
5. around and inside the mitochondria
6. diffusion
7. in the nucleus
8. false
9. In translation, a ribosome assembles amino acids as dictated by mRNA. Translation happens at the ribosome.
10. glucose, phosphate, diphosphate

11. endoplasmic reticulum

12. Downhill reactions do not require energy, whereas uphill reactions do require energy. (Examples will vary but may include:) osmosis, diffusion, or facilitated diffusion (downhill reactions); and the use of pumps, exocytosis, phagocytosis, pinocytosis, or receptor-mediated endocytosis (uphill reactions).

13. high, low

14. homeostasis

15. false

16. The Golgi receives transport vesicles and packages the proteins therein into secretory vesicles.

17. false

18. glycolysis, prep reaction, citric acid cycle, electron transport chain

19. catabolic, releases

20. Osmosis

21. diffusion

22. anabolic

23. Mitosis happens in most cells. One diploid cell divides into two identical diploid daughter cells. Meiosis only happens in the testes and ovaries. One diploid cell divides into haploid cells.

24. false

25. polypeptides

26. To counteract facilitated diffusion, the sodium-potassium pump uses energy to push sodium ions out of the cell and potassium ions into the cell.

27. D

Comprehensive Review (Chapters 1–7)

28. C
29. E
30. I
31. H
32. A
33. D
34. G
35. J
36. F
37. B
38. L
39. K

Chapter 8 Human Body Tissues

Section 8.1 Characteristics of Tissue

Concept 1: What Are Tissues?

1. specialized
2. tissue

Concept 2: Types of Tissue

1. epithelial tissue, connective tissue, muscle tissue, nerve tissue
2. Epithelial
3. structure, protection
4. Muscle, nerve, electrical

Concept 3: Tissues Make Up Organs

1. organ
2. false

Concept 4: Blood Supply for Tissues

1. oxygen
2. blood supply

Concept 5: Vascular Tissue

1. direct
2. muscle tissue, tissue in the lungs

Concept 6: Avascular Tissue

1. diffusion
2. avascular
3. basement
4. epithelial, vascular

Section 8.1 Reinforcement

1. true
2. B
3. A tissue is a group of cells working together to do a job. An organ is different types of tissue working together to do a job.
4. true

5. epithelial tissue, connective tissue, muscle tissue, nerve tissue
6. vascular; having direct access to a blood supply
7. Epithelial
8. true
9. organ
10. blood supply
11. false
12. vascular
13. A
14. diffuse
15. tissue; a group of cells working together to do a job
16. lungs, blood
17. true
18. connective tissue, epithelial tissue, muscle tissue, nerve tissue
19. epithelial tissue

Comprehensive Review (Chapters 1–8)

20. outcome
21. above; beyond
22. 10 millimeters
23. microtubules
24. C
25. false
26. phenomenon
27. muscle tissue, tissue in the lungs

Section 8.2 Epithelial Tissue

Concept 1: Epithelium

1. Epithelial tissue
2. sheets
3. glands

Concept 2: Layers of Epithelial Tissue

1. outermost, innermost
2. connective
3. epithelial tissue

Concept 3: Apical and Basal Surfaces

1. apical
2. basal

Concept 4: Epithelial Cell Shapes

1. squamous
2. Transitional
3. tall
4. cuboidal

Concept 5: Epithelial Cell Arrangements

1. simple, stratified, pseudostratified
2. simple
3. heights
4. stratified

Concept 6: Simple Squamous Epithelium

1. simple squamous epithelium
2. diffuse
3. air sacs, blood

Concept 7: Simple Cuboidal Epithelium

1. one, square
2. cuboidal

Concept 8: Simple Columnar Epithelium

1. the lining of the digestive tract, from the stomach to the intestines; small intestine; fallopian tubes
2. simple columnar

Concept 9: Pseudostratified Columnar Epithelium

1. trachea
2. pseudostratified columnar

Concept 10: Stratified Squamous Epithelium

1. Stratified squamous
2. reproduce

Concept 11: Transitional Epithelium

1. Transitional, transitional
2. expand, recoil

Concept 12: Glands

1. Endocrine
2. Exocrine
3. endocrine gland
4. unicellular, multicellular

Section 8.2 Reinforcement

1. produces, secretes

2. windpipe
3. goblet cell
4. A, D
5. transitional epithelium
6. true
7. pseudostratified, simple, stratified
8. Exocrine glands release products through a duct. Endocrine glands release products into interstitial fluid.
9. false
10. basal, basement
11. stratified
12. true
13. B, C
14. true
15. Columnar epithelial cells are tall.
16. hormones
17. squamous; flat
18. absorption
19. apical
20. A, D
21. mucus
22. squamous—flat; cuboidal—square; columnar—tall; transitional—can change shape
23. basal, shed

Comprehensive Review (Chapters 1–8)

24. scientific method
25. true
26. 48%
27. inside
28. false
29. B
30. solvent concentration
31. 10, 24

Section 8.3 Connective Tissue Proper

Concept 1: Connective Tissue

1. connection, support, protection
2. epithelial
3. connective tissue proper; bone, cartilage, and blood

Concept 2: Extracellular Matrix

1. extracellular

2. liquid, semisolid gel, solid

Concept 3: Extracellular Fibers

1. collagen fibers, reticular fibers
2. Elastic

Concept 4: Fibroblasts

1. collagen, elastin
2. fibroblasts

Concept 5: Adipose Connective Tissue

1. insulates, shock absorber
2. adipocytes
3. energy

Concept 6: Areolar Connective Tissue

1. water, wraps, binds, cushions
2. collagen fibers, elastic fibers, reticular fibers

Concept 7: Reticular Connective Tissue

1. reticular
2. spleen, bone marrow, lymph nodes

Concept 8: Irregular Dense Connective Tissue

1. irregular dense
2. extracellular, fibroblasts

Concept 9: Regular Dense Connective Tissue

1. ligament
2. regular dense

Concept 10: Elastic Connective Tissue

1. elastic
2. heart

Section 8.3 Reinforcement

1. false
2. bone
3. B
4. lower layer of skin
5. fibroblast; a cell that secretes collagen and elastin
6. C
7. false
8. connective
9. areolar connective tissue
10. loose, dense
11. true

12. underlies
13. collagen fibers, elastic fibers, reticular fibers
14. Loose connective tissue is composed of many cells with extracellular fibers winding through them. Dense connective tissue is composed mostly of extracellular fibers with few cells.
15. false
16. extracellular, ground
17. true
18. muscle
19. adipose connective tissue, areolar connective tissue, reticular connective tissue
20. D
21. reticular
22. B
23. A
24. G
25. D
26. C
27. E
28. F

Comprehensive Review (Chapters 1–8)

29. A
30. true
31. D
32. 40 cm
33. histones
34. untested
35. mitosis, meiosis
36. A

Section 8.4 Bone, Cartilage, and Blood

Concept 1: Bone

1. calcium salts, collagen fibers
2. false

Concept 2: Bone Cells

1. lacunae
2. bone cells
3. osteoblast, osteoclast

Concept 3: Types of Bone

1. compact bone, spongy bone
2. compact, spongy

Concept 4: Cartilage

1. extracellular fibers, carbohydrates, water
2. avascular
3. water, collagen

Concept 5: Hyaline Cartilage

1. Hyaline
2. ends, joints

Concept 6: Elastic Cartilage

1. epiglottis
2. Elastic, elastic

Concept 7: Fibrocartilage

1. fibrocartilage
2. vertebrae

Concept 8: Blood

1. plasma, elements
2. plasma
3. nutrients, waste

Section 8.4 Reinforcement

1. A
2. plasma
3. lacunae
4. elastic cartilage, fibrocartilage, hyaline cartilage
5. bones, joints
6. A, C, D
7. false
8. It has an extracellular matrix.
9. platelets, red blood cells, white blood cells
10. true
11. construct
12. true
13. osteoclast; a bone cell that breaks down the bone matrix
14. B
15. A, C
16. fibrocartilage; the strongest type of cartilage; made of thick collagen fibers
17. C
18. calcium, collagen
19. fibrocartilage
20. false
21. A
22. D
23. F
24. B

25. E
26. G
27. C

Comprehensive Review (Chapters 1–8)

28. homeostasis
29. false
30. collagen fibers, elastic fibers, reticular fibers
31. Facts, Sift, Test, Diagnose
32. false
33. four
34. the stomach and intestines
35. smooth endoplasmic reticulum

Section 8.5 Muscle and Nerve Tissue

Concept 1: Excitable Tissue

1. Muscle, nerve
2. action potential
3. true
4. neurotransmitter

Concept 2: Muscle Tissue

1. contract
2. skeletal muscle, smooth muscle, cardiac muscle
3. myocytes, muscle fibers

Concept 3: Skeletal Muscle

1. bone
2. false
3. striations
4. voluntary, conscious

Concept 4: Smooth Muscle

1. Smooth muscle cells do not have striations. They are shaped like spindles and tapered at both ends. Smooth muscles are involuntary muscles.
2. small intestine, blood vessels
3. involuntary, do not
4. true

Concept 5: Cardiac Muscle

1. the heart
2. involuntary, do not
3. intercalated
4. heartbeat

Concept 6: Nerve Tissue

1. cell body, two
2. communicating signals, such as movement and pain, all throughout the body
3. Neuroglia

Section 8.5 Reinforcement

1. B
2. desmosomes
3. false
4. muscle
5. B, C
6. cell body, axon
7. electrical, stimulated
8. voluntary; consciously controlled
9. smooth muscle cell
10. Neuroglia
11. true
12. cardiac muscle, skeletal muscle, smooth muscle
13. cardiac muscle cell
14. true
15. excitable; producing an electrical charge when stimulated
16. true
17. pairs
18. cardiac muscle cell
19. Voluntary muscles are controlled consciously. Involuntary muscles are controlled unconsciously.
20. A, B
21. Excitable
22. B
23. D
24. F
25. C
26. A
27. H
28. E
29. G

Comprehensive Review (Chapters 1–8)

30. B
31. phosphate, sugar, base
32. false
33. true
34. water

35. C
36. calcium salts reinforced with collagen fibers
37. hepat/o; liver

Chapter 8 Review

1. surfaces, tubes, cavities
2. connective tissue
3. basement
4. extracellular
5. apical surface
6. In epithelial tissue, a basement membrane lies beneath the tissue and is in contact with vascular tissue. Nutrients and waste diffuse through the basement membrane between epithelial tissue and the vascular tissue.
7. osteoblasts, osteoclasts
8. simple columnar epithelium
9. true
10. cardiac muscle
11. Dense
12. C
13. stratified squamous
14. transitional; able to change shape and size
15. lacunae
16. action potential
17. false
18. Voluntary muscle is consciously controlled. Involuntary muscle is unconsciously controlled.
19. D
20. elastic
21. false
22. organ
23. regular dense
24. Loose
25. vascular tissue
26. dendrites
27. true
28. one, square
29. calcium, collagen
30. spleen, bone marrow, lymph nodes

Comprehensive Review (Chapters 1–8)

31. B

32. C
33. E
34. G
35. A
36. I
37. H
38. F
39. J
40. D

Chapter 9 Human Body Orientation

Section 9.1 Body Planes and Cavities

Concept 1: Anatomical Position

1. anatomical position
2. forward
3. thumbs

Concept 2: Body Planes

1. midsagittal (median) plane, sagittal plane, frontal (coronal) plane, transverse plane
2. planes
3. anatomical position

Concept 3: Midsagittal and Sagittal Planes

1. midsagittal (median) plane
2. sagittal plane

Concept 4: Frontal Plane

1. frontal
2. true

Concept 5: Transverse Plane

1. top, bottom
2. middle
3. cross-sections

Concept 6: Body Cavities

1. organs
2. bone, connective, epithelial

Concept 7: Dorsal Cavities

1. cranial cavity, spinal cavity
2. cranial cavity

Concept 8: Ventral Cavities

1. thoracic
2. abdominopelvic
3. pelvic

Section 9.1 Reinforcement

1. palms, feet
2. B
3. body cavity
4. true
5. ventral; the front section of the body
6. B, C
7. B
8. cranial, spinal
9. false
10. The midsagittal plane divides the body into equal left and right halves. The sagittal plane divides the body into unequal left and right sections.
11. A, C, D
12. frontal
13. transverse
14. false
15. thoracic cavity
16. false
17. cranial
18. away from the body
19. thoracic; the ventral cavity that houses the heart and lungs
20. B, D
21. transverse plane
22. D
23. C
24. E
25. F
26. B
27. A

Comprehensive Review (Chapters 1–9)

28. midsagittal plane
29. dependent
30. Hydrogen bonds are based on partial charges.
31. facts
32. true
33. E
34. downhill
35. 1
36. skeletal muscle

Section 9.2 Regions of the Body

Concept 1: Axial Versus Appendicular Regions

1. appendicular
2. true
3. axial

Concept 2: Head and Neck

1. cephalic
2. neck
3. (List three:) forehead, scalp, eyes, nose, mouth, cheeks, lips, ears

Concept 3: Trunk

1. pubic region
2. thoracic
3. belly, navel

Concept 4: Abdominopelvic Regions

1. rows, columns
2. the body's, the body's
3. nine

Concept 5: First Row

1. right hypochondriac region, epigastric region, left hypochondriac region
2. epi- + gastr + -ic; pertaining to above the stomach
3. A

Concept 6: Second Row

1. umbilical
2. lumbar, umbilical, lumbar
3. lower back

Concept 7: Third Row

1. stomach
2. ilium
3. right iliac region, hypogastric region, left iliac region

Concept 8: Limbs

1. manus
2. feet
3. The upper limbs are the arms, and the lower limbs are the legs.

Section 9.2 Reinforcement

1. head
2. true
3. groin
4. right lumbar region, umbilical region, left lumbar region
5. B
6. abdominopelvic cavity
7. false
8. B, D
9. right iliac region, hypogastric region, left iliac region
10. false
11. axial region
12. appendicular
13. C
14. hypogastric; below the stomach
15. neck
16. true
17. thoracic region, abdominal region, pelvic region, pubic region
18. appendicular; referring to the appendages (limbs)
19. true
20. B
21. pedal
22. K
23. E
24. M
25. F
26. I
27. J
28. L
29. B
30. D
31. A
32. H
33. G
34. C

Comprehensive Review (Chapters 1–9)

35. middle
36. tested
37. prophase, metaphase, anaphase, telophase
38. fact
39. In anatomical position, a person stands upright with feet apart, arms at the sides, feet and palms facing forward, and

thumbs pointing away from the body.

40. cytosine
41. 0
42. true
43. C, D

Section 9.3 Terms of Location

Concept 1: Describing Location
1. other body parts
2. anatomical position
3. false

Concept 2: Superior and Inferior
1. B
2. inferior
3. D
4. superior

Concept 3: Ventral and Dorsal
1. anterior
2. toes
3. back
4. fingernails
5. front
6. tip of the nose

Concept 4: Medial, Lateral, and Intermediate
1. C
2. midsagittal
3. intermediate
4. D
5. lateral

Concept 5: Proximal and Distal
1. proximal
2. distal
3. distal
4. limbs
5. distal

Concept 6: Superficial and Deep
1. heart
2. closer
3. surface
4. skin
5. farther

Section 9.3 Reinforcement
1. intermediate
2. C

3. superior, inferior
4. B
5. false
6. surface
7. front, back
8. B
9. deep
10. false
11. B
12. midsagittal
13. B
14. anterior
15. false
16. head
17. B
18. true
19. anatomical position
20. stomach
21. lateral
22. posterior
23. C
24. D
25. G
26. H
27. I
28. E
29. F
30. A
31. B
32. J
33. K

Comprehensive Review (Chapters 1–9)
34. ligament
35. one-half
36. 2.376 kg
37. polymer
38. true
39. B, C
40. independent
41. In facilitated diffusion, atoms move into or out of a cell via protein channels.
42. axial region

Section 9.4 Body Organization

Concept 1: Five Levels of Organization
1. organisms, body systems, organs, tissues, cells
2. body systems

Concept 2: Cell Level
1. microvilli
2. parietal cells
3. mucus

Concept 3: Tissue Level
1. two
2. contracts
3. tissue

Concept 4: Organ Level
1. mucosa, serosa
2. lamina propria
3. mucosa

Concept 5: Body System Level
1. organs
2. Digesting
3. 11
4. integumentary system, skeletal system, muscular system, nervous system, endocrine system, respiratory system, cardiovascular system, lymphatic system, digestive system, urinary system, reproductive systems

Concept 6: Organism Level
1. community
2. interdependent

Section 9.4 Reinforcement
1. A
2. true
3. mucosa
4. cells, tissues, organs, body systems, organisms
5. A
6. cell
7. body system
8. false
9. tissue; a group of cells working together to do a job
10. false
11. microvilli

12. tissue
13. body systems, cells, organisms, organs, tissues
14. 11
15. false
16. cardiovascular system, digestive system, endocrine system, integumentary system, lymphatic system, muscular system, nervous system, reproductive systems, respiratory system, skeletal system, urinary system
17. parietal
18. body systems
19. B, D
20. organism
21. body system level
22. D
23. B
24. C
25. A
26. E

Comprehensive Review (Chapters 1–9)

27. between
28. testable, observable
29. facts
30. 3.14
31. shared
32. C
33. false
34. dense connective tissue
35. true

Section 9.5 Homeostasis in the Body

Concept 1: Reviewing Homeostasis

1. homeostasis
2. glucose

Concept 2: Negative Feedback

1. negative feedback
2. stop

Concept 3: Body Temperature

1. homeostasis
2. increasing
3. 37, 98.6

Concept 4: Blood Glucose Concentration

1. 90 mg/100 mL
2. respiration
3. glucose

Concept 5: High Blood Glucose Concentration

1. rise
2. insulin
3. cells, liver

Concept 6: Low Blood Glucose Concentration

1. glucagon
2. glycogen
3. increase

Concept 7: Blood pH

1. raises
2. 7.35, 7.45
3. fall

Section 9.5 Reinforcement

1. glucagon
2. liver
3. fall
4. false
5. kidney
6. insulin
7. true
8. insulin
9. glucagon; a hormone secreted by the alpha cells of the pancreas that signals the liver to break down glycogen into glucose
10. glycogen
11. raise
12. glucagon
13. The body takes action to correct a concentration or factor back to its set value. Once the correction is complete, the cycle stops.
14. false
15. products, actions, stop
16. glucagon
17. evaporates
18. 37°C (98.6°F)
19. homeostasis; a state of relative stability
20. true

21. basic, 7.35, 7.45

Comprehensive Review (Chapters 1–9)

22. 0, 14
23. collagen fibers, elastic fibers, reticular fibers
24. true
25. hypothesis
26. 500
27. microfilaments, intermediate filaments, microtubules
28. pseudo-
29. a molecule containing few atoms
30. body system

Chapter 9 Review

1. midsagittal (median) plane, sagittal plane, frontal (coronal) plane, transverse plane
2. away from
3. true
4. D
5. distal
6. false
7. C
8. inferior
9. frontal
10. false
11. integumentary system, skeletal system, muscular system, nervous system, endocrine system, respiratory system, cardiovascular system, lymphatic system, digestive system, urinary system, reproductive systems
12. C
13. rise
14. true
15. body system
16. spinal
17. insulin
18. ventral
19. false
20. 90 mg/100 mL
21. cells, tissues, organs, body systems, organisms
22. right hypochondriac region, epigastric region, left hypochondriac region

23. true
24. D
25. 37°C (98.6°F)
26. appendicular
27. 7.35, 7.45

Comprehensive Review (Chapters 1–9)

28. F
29. B
30. A
31. M
32. H
33. D
34. L
35. I
36. J
37. E
38. K
39. C
40. N
41. G

Chapter 10 Human Body Systems

Section 10.1 The Integumentary System

Concept 1: Functions of the Integumentary System

1. skin, hair, nails, glands
2. (List three:) protects the body; maintains body temperature; makes vitamin D; removes waste; perceives pressure, touch, pain, and temperature

Concept 2: Skin

1. epidermis
2. true
3. hypodermis

Concept 3: Epidermis

1. keratinocytes
2. true
3. stratified
4. stratum corneum, stratum lucidum, stratum granulosum, stratum spinosum, stratum basale
5. four

Concept 4: Dermis

1. middle
2. sweat glands, sebaceous glands

Concept 5: Hypodermis

1. hypodermis
2. (List two:) connects the skin and muscles, insulates the body, protects deeper tissues

Concept 6: Hair and Nails

1. dead
2. keratin

Section 10.1 Reinforcement

1. epidermis, dermis, hypodermis
2. false
3. B
4. false
5. C, D
6. deepest layer
7. keratin; a tough, water-resistant protein
8. five
9. hypodermis
10. keratin
11. keratin
12. true
13. dermis
14. false
15. touch, pressure, temperature, pain
16. protects the body; maintains body temperature; makes vitamin D; removes waste; perceives pressure, touch, pain, and temperature
17. deep
18. D
19. sweat glands, sebaceous glands
20. true

Comprehensive Review (Chapters 1–10)

21. false
22. observation
23. independent
24. ab-; away from
25. true
26. stratum basale, stratum spinosum, stratum granulosum, stratum lucidum, stratum corneum
27. D
28. transcription, translation
29. collagen
30. transverse plane

Section 10.2 The Skeletal System

Concept 1: Functions of the Skeletal System

1. bone tissue, cartilage
2. (List four:) protects the body by surrounding internal structures; provides support, structure, and shape for the body; produces red blood cells; facilitates body movement; stores calcium
3. joints

Concept 2: Axial Versus Appendicular Skeleton

1. skull, thoracic cage, spine
2. pectoral girdle, pelvic girdle, upper limbs, lower limbs

Concept 3: Skull

1. Cranial, facial
2. mandible (jawbone)

Concept 4: Thoracic Cage

1. true ribs, false ribs, floating ribs
2. thoracic

Concept 5: Spine

1. cervical region, thoracic region, lumbar region, sacral region
2. intervertebral
3. spinal cord

Concept 6: Pectoral Girdle

1. scapula, clavicle
2. pectoral

Concept 7: Pelvic Girdle

1. hip
2. true

Concept 8: Upper Limbs

1. radius, ulna
2. arms, hands

Concept 9: Lower Limbs

1. tibia, fibula
2. legs, feet

Concept 10: Joints

1. connections
2. movement
3. gliding joint, hinge joint, pivot joint, condylar joint, saddle joint, ball-and-socket joint

Section 10.2 Reinforcement

1. pelvic
2. D
3. joints
4. pectoral; relating to the shoulder joints
5. C
6. false
7. cervical region, thoracic region, lumbar region, sacral region
8. sternum
9. C, D
10. mandible (jawbone)
11. C
12. false
13. A
14. appendicular; relating to the limbs
15. axial
16. true
17. bone tissue, cartilage
18. pectoral
19. protects the body by surrounding internal structures; provides support, structure, and shape for the body; produces red blood cells; facilitates body movement; stores calcium
20. true
21. left ilium, left ischium, left pubis, right ilium, right ischium, right pubis

Comprehensive Review (Chapters 1–10)

22. high heat, low pH level
23. no nuclei
24. itself
25. true
26. 200 mm
27. false
28. ad-; toward
29. thoracic region, abdominal region, pelvic region, pubic region
30. contract
31. hypodermis

Section 10.3 The Muscular System

Concept 1: Functions of the Muscular System

1. voluntary
2. (List three:) holds the parts of the body in position, enables the movement of body parts, helps maintain body temperature by producing heat, protects the internal organs

Concept 2: Muscles of the Human Body

1. skeletal muscle, smooth muscle, cardiac muscle
2. triceps brachii, biceps brachii

Concept 3: Muscle Contraction

1. origin
2. insertion
3. (List three:) flexion, extension, abduction, adduction, rotation

Concept 4: Flexion

1. reduces
2. ulna
3. (List two:) tilting your head toward your chest, bending your knee to raise your lower leg, raising your arm forward, bringing your forearm toward your upper arm

Concept 5: Extension

1. flexion
2. false
3. increases

Concept 6: Abduction and Adduction

1. away from
2. toward

Concept 7: Rotation

1. rotation
2. sternocleidomastoid

Section 10.3 Reinforcement

1. pulls
2. skeletal muscle, smooth muscle, cardiac muscle
3. frontal, midsagittal
4. adduct
5. true
6. movable
7. abduction
8. A
9. holds the parts of the body in position, enables the movement of body parts, helps maintain body temperature by producing heat, protects the internal organs
10. false
11. extension; a directional movement that moves a body part along the sagittal plane to decrease the angle between bones or between a limb and the body
12. Flexion
13. A, D
14. true
15. adduction
16. sagittal
17. abduction; a directional movement in which a body part moves along the frontal plane away from the middle (midsagittal plane) of the body
18. immovable
19. true
20. abduction
21. left

Comprehensive Review (Chapters 1–10)

22. false
23. toward
24. catabolic, releases
25. false
26. 0.1
27. natural
28. guanine
29. nucleus
30. D
31. neurons

Section 10.4 The Nervous System

Concept 1: Functions of the Nervous System

1. brain, spinal cord, nerves
2. (List two:) receives external sensory information (for example, sound, smell, sight, and touch); processes and interprets sensory information; responds to sensory information by transmitting impulses to control body parts

Concept 2: CNS and PNS

1. CNS, PNS
2. false

Concept 3: Brain

1. brain
2. cerebellum
3. frontal lobe, parietal lobe, temporal lobe, occipital lobe

Concept 4: Spinal Cord

1. vertebrae
2. nerves

Concept 5: Afferent and Efferent Nerves

1. efferent, motor
2. afferent, sensory

Concept 6: Somatic and Autonomic Nerves

1. efferent
2. voluntary
3. involuntary, organs

Concept 7: Sympathetic and Parasympathetic Nerves

1. Sympathetic
2. Parasympathetic

Section 10.4 Reinforcement

1. receives external sensory information (for example, sound, smell, sight, and touch); processes and interprets sensory information; responds to sensory information by transmitting impulses to control body parts
2. efferent
3. false

4. brain, spinal cord
5. D
6. true
7. cerebrum
8. false
9. brain, spinal cord, nerves
10. A, C
11. cerebellum
12. afferent, sensory
13. true
14. afferent; transmitting toward the CNS
15. spinal cord
16. somatic nerves, autonomic nerves
17. CNS, body
18. false
19. parasympathetic; relating to slowing the body down
20. autonomic nerves
21. Efferent

Comprehensive Review (Chapters 1–10)

22. inside
23. facts, sift, test, diagnose
24. Biology
25. 200 people
26. anabolic
27. endocrine
28. thoracic
29. adduction
30. Structural proteins make up tissues. Functional proteins perform various tasks in the body.
31. ribosomes

Section 10.5 The Endocrine System

Concept 1: Functions of the Endocrine System

1. hormones
2. (List one:) releases hormones to influence the functions of other organs, maintains homeostasis, helps regulate body functions
3. (List three:) hypothalamus, pineal gland, pituitary gland, thyroid gland, thymus gland,

adrenal glands, pancreas, ovary, testis

Concept 2: Hormones

1. hormone
2. endocrine, organ
3. tropic hormones, nontropic hormones

Concept 3: Pituitary Gland

1. base of the brain
2. growth hormone (GH), prolactin, adrenocorticotropic hormone (ACTH), thyroid-stimulating hormone (TSH), follicle-stimulating hormone (FSH), luteinizing hormone (LH)

Concept 4: Thyroid Gland

1. thyrotropin
2. triiodothyronine (T_3), thyroxine (T_4), calcitonin
3. metabolic rate

Concept 5: Calcitonin

1. bones, intestines, kidneys
2. remove

Concept 6: Parathyroid Glands

1. parathyroid
2. raises

Section 10.5 Reinforcement

1. calcitonin, parathyroid hormone (PTH)
2. lower
3. releases hormones to influence the functions of other organs, maintains homeostasis, helps regulate body functions
4. hormone
5. true
6. parathyroid hormone (PTH)
7. A, B, D
8. (List five:) hypothalamus, pineal gland, pituitary gland, thyroid gland, thymus gland, adrenal glands, pancreas, ovary, testis
9. Thyroid-stimulating hormone (TSH)
10. true
11. calcitonin; a hormone released by the thyroid gland that

lowers the level of calcium in the blood

12. false
13. pituitary gland
14. parathyroid; a gland located on the dorsal surface of the thyroid that releases parathyroid hormone (PTH)
15. true
16. A, B, E
17. calcitonin
18. a nonendocrine organ or tissue
19. endocrine; relating to the secretion of products directly into interstitial fluid
20. false
21. pituitary gland

Comprehensive Review (Chapters 1–10)

22. within
23. false
24. protons, neutrons
25. two
26. true
27. cerebrum
28. collagen fiber
29. deep
30. attitude
31. false

Section 10.6 The Respiratory System

Concept 1: Functions of the Respiratory System

1. breathing
2. inhales oxygen-rich air, exchanges respiratory gases to bring oxygen into the body and discard carbon dioxide, exhales carbon dioxide
3. oxygen, carbon dioxide

Concept 2: Volume and Air Pressure

1. fall
2. rise
3. 760
4. high, low

Concept 3: Lungs and Diaphragm

1. larger

2. diaphragm
3. lung

Concept 4: Inspiration

1. decreases
2. inspiration
3. passively

Concept 5: External Respiration

1. air, blood
2. oxygen, carbon dioxide

Concept 6: Internal Respiration

1. all throughout the body
2. oxygen, carbon dioxide

Concept 7: Expiration

1. expiration
2. relax
3. inside, outside

Section 10.6 Reinforcement

1. rise
2. out
3. in the lungs
4. external
5. false
6. expiration; the process of breathing out
7. in
8. expand
9. false
10. 760
11. high, low
12. increase
13. true
14. inspiration; the process of breathing in
15. internal
16. false
17. within
18. fall
19. outside the lungs
20. A, C
21. inside the lungs
22. (List two:) inhales oxygen-rich air, exchanges respiratory gases to bring oxygen into the body and discard carbon dioxide, exhales carbon-dioxide-rich air

Comprehensive Review (Chapters 1–10)

23. A

24. calcitonin
25. true
26. introduction
27. 244 cm
28. polyunsaturated
29. cardi; heart
30. false
31. desmosomes
32. red blood cells, white blood cells, platelets

Section 10.7 The Cardiovascular System

Concept 1: Functions of the Cardiovascular System

1. heart, blood vessels
2. (List two:) transports oxygen-rich blood all throughout the body; circulates nutrients, hormones, and other important substances in the blood; collects and transports waste produced by cells; helps regulate body temperature

Concept 2: Heart

1. heart
2. List right atrium, left atrium, right ventricle, left ventricle
3. Blood flows into the right atrium and then into the right ventricle. From the right ventricle, blood is pumped to the lungs, where it gains oxygen. Then, from the lungs, blood flows into the left atrium. Blood enters the left ventricle, where it is pumped to the rest of the body.

Concept 3: Heart Valves

1. valves
2. AV, SL
3. (See Figure 10.18 in the text.)

Concept 4: Blood Vessels

1. Arteries
2. body, heart
3. Capillaries

Concept 5: Pulmonary Circulation

1. heart, lungs
2. carbon dioxide, oxygen

Concept 6: Systemic Circulation

1. heart and rest of the body
2. oxygen, carbon dioxide

Section 10.7 Reinforcement

1. atria
2. true
3. ventricle
4. air, blood
5. ventricle; a bottom chamber of the heart
6. to keep blood flowing in the right direction
7. lungs
8. B, C
9. closed
10. (List two:) transports oxygen-rich blood all throughout the body; circulates nutrients, hormones, and other important substances in the blood; collects and transports waste produced by cells; helps regulate body temperature
11. ventricles
12. false
13. left
14. left side
15. Capillaries
16. false
17. ventricle
18. true
19. Arteries carry blood from the heart to the body, and veins carry blood from the body to the heart.
20. rest of the body

Comprehensive Review (Chapters 1–10)

21. hydrogen
22. simple, stratified, pseudostratified
23. false
24. pinocytosis
25. -cyte
26. fact
27. ³⁄₁₆ of the circle
28. thoracic region
29. within
30. true

Section 10.8 The Lymphatic System

Concept 1: Functions of the Lymphatic System

1. lymphatic vessels, lymph, lymphatic organs (spleen, thymus, and lymph nodes)
2. returns fluid leaked from capillaries back to the cardiovascular system, defends the body against disease

Concept 2: Lymph

1. lymph
2. capillaries

Concept 3: Lymph Nodes

1. lymph nodes
2. destroy

Concept 4: Spleen and Thymus

1. spleen
2. thymus

Concept 5: Lymphocytes

1. white
2. in bone marrow

Section 10.8 Reinforcement

1. plasma
2. true
3. lymph
4. lymph; the fluid that is circulated through the lymphatic system
5. false
6. returns fluid leaked from capillaries back to the cardiovascular system, defends the body against disease
7. heart
8. spleen
9. lymph
10. thymus; a lymphatic organ located in the chest that houses white blood cells as they mature and signals bone marrow to produce white blood cells
11. lymphocytes
12. true
13. in the abdominal cavity
14. The lymph nodes are working to eliminate infection.

15. true
16. B
17. lymph
18. false

Comprehensive Review (Chapters 1–10)

19. false
20. scientific theories
21. smooth muscle, cardiac muscle
22. view
23. 24%
24. acid
25. absorption
26. false
27. Pulmonary
28. raise

Section 10.9 The Digestive System

Concept 1: Functions of the Digestive System

1. ingestion, digestion, absorption, defecation
2. (List two:) intakes food into the body, breaks down food (mechanically and chemically) into nutrients, absorbs nutrients into the bloodstream, removes solid waste from the body through defecation

Concept 2: Path of Food

1. alimentary
2. mouth, pharynx, esophagus, stomach, small intestine, colon, rectum, anus
3. peristalsis

Concept 3: Ingestion and Digestion

1. in the mouth
2. macromolecules
3. mechanical digestion, chemical digestion

Concept 4: Mechanical Digestion

1. Mechanical
2. teeth
3. in the small intestine

Concept 5: Chemical Digestion

1. Chemical
2. saliva

3. stomach

Concept 6: Absorption

1. digestion
2. Absorption
3. small intestine

Concept 7: Defecation

1. absorbed
2. cellulose

Section 10.9 Reinforcement

1. absorption
2. digestive system
3. false
4. C
5. peristalsis
6. (List three:) intakes food into the body, breaks down food (mechanically and chemically) into nutrients, absorbs nutrients into the bloodstream, removes solid waste from the body through defecation
7. feces
8. alimentary
9. B
10. digestion; breaking down food into macromolecules that can be absorbed by the blood
11. true
12. mechanical digestion
13. false
14. B, D
15. false
16. absorption; the process of taking macromolecules out of food and putting them into the blood
17. chemical digestion
18. true
19. liver

Comprehensive Review (Chapters 1–10)

20. permeable
21. cuboidal
22. true
23. kidney
24. 7
25. capillaries
26. peptide
27. specialized

28. false
29. theory

Section 10.10 The Urinary System

Concept 1: Functions of the Urinary System

1. kidneys, ureters, urinary bladder, urethra
2. (List two:) filters waste products out of blood, stores and removes waste from the body, produces hormones, maintains homeostasis of pH and water levels

Concept 2: Kidneys

1. Blood, blood, urine
2. remain, urine
3. nephron

Concept 3: Nephrons

1. glomerulus
2. renal tubule
3. filtration, reabsorption, secretion

Concept 4: Filtration

1. filtration
2. protein
3. filtrate

Concept 5: Reabsorption and Secretion

1. reabsorption
2. secretion

Concept 6: Urinary Tract

1. ureters, urinary bladder, urethra
2. peristalsis

Section 10.10 Reinforcement

1. pH
2. true
3. afferent, efferent
4. nephron; the basic unit of the kidney
5. filtration, blood
6. false
7. filtrate
8. secretion
9. (List one:) filters waste products out of blood, stores and removes waste from the body,

produces hormones, maintains homeostasis of pH and water levels
10. renal tubule, capillaries
11. urethra
12. filtrate, blood
13. urinary bladder
14. filtrate
15. urine
16. secretion; moving molecules from the blood into filtrate after filtration
17. blood
18. C, D
19. false
20. ureter
21. protein

Comprehensive Review (Chapters 1–10)

22. glucagon
23. outcome
24. false
25. Facts
26. white
27. plasma membrane, nucleus, cytoplasm
28. sperm in males, egg cells in females
29. saturated fat
30. chemical digestion
31. false

Section 10.11 The Reproductive Systems

Concept 1: Functions of the Reproductive Systems

1. life
2. (List three:) produces gametes, facilitates conception, protects and nourishes the developing fetus, expels a baby from the body

Concept 2: Ovaries

1. ovaries
2. menstruation

Concept 3: Fallopian Tubes and Uterus

1. fallopian tube
2. endometrium
3. estrogen, progesterone

Concept 4: Vagina, External Genitalia, and Mammary Glands

1. acidic
2. mammary gland

Concept 5: Testes

1. testes
2. epididymis

Concept 6: Ductus Deferens and Accessory Organs

1. semen
2. urethra
3. the process by which sperm exit the body

Concept 7: Penis

1. penis
2. blood

Section 10.11 Reinforcement

1. the shedding of the innermost layer of the uterus each month
2. alkaline, acidic
3. estrogen, progesterone
4. true
5. ejaculation
6. ovary, uterus
7. to produce milk after childbirth
8. epididymis
9. epididymis; the structure that stores sperm after they have completed their development
10. false
11. scrotum
12. sperm, fluids released from the accessory organs (fructose and alkaline fluids)
13. false
14. ovulation; the release of an egg from an ovary
15. endometrium
16. (List two:) produces gametes, facilitates conception, protects and nourishes the developing fetus, expels a baby from the body
17. vagina
18. ovaries, fallopian tubes, uterus, vagina, external genitalia, mammary glands
19. true
20. testes and scrotum, epididymis, ductus deferens, accessory organs, penis
21. B

Comprehensive Review (Chapters 1–10)

22. vascular tissue
23. anatomical position
24. phenomenon
25. physi + o + -logy; the study of function
26. ureters, urinary bladder, urethra
27. explanation
28. electron
29. true
30. B, C
31. bottom

Chapter 10 Review

1. brain, spinal cord, nerves
2. lymphatic system
3. D
4. sebum
5. sympathetic nerves, parasympathetic nerves
6. bones, intestines, kidneys
7. false
8. mechanical digestion
9. kidney
10. (List one:) releases hormones to influence the functions of other organs, maintains homeostasis, helps regulate body functions
11. spermatogenesis
12. true
13. increases
14. insertion
15. motor nerves
16. filtrate
17. carbon dioxide
18. blood
19. lymphatic vessels, lymph, lymphatic organs
20. false
21. oxygen, carbon dioxide
22. Abduction
23. atria
24. endometrium, vagina
25. B
26. cerebellum
27. Blood flows into the right atrium and then into the right ventricle. From the right ventricle, blood is pumped to the lungs, where it gains oxygen. Then, from the lungs, blood flows into the left atrium. Blood enters the left ventricle, where it is pumped to the rest of the body.
28. true
29. (List four:) hypothalamus, pineal gland, pituitary gland, thyroid gland, thymus gland, adrenal glands, pancreas, ovary, testis
30. epidermis

Comprehensive Review (Chapters 1–10)

31. C
32. B
33. J
34. G
35. I
36. E
37. L
38. A
39. F
40. H
41. K
42. M
43. D